Update in Cosmetic Dermatology

Antonella Tosti • Doris Hexsel
Editors

Update in Cosmetic Dermatology

Springer

Editors
Prof. Antonella Tosti, M.D.
Leonard M. Miller School of Medicine
Department of Dermatology
University of Miami
Miami
Florida
USA

Dr. Doris Hexsel, M.D.
Clinica Hexsel de Dermatologia
Pontifícia Universidade Católica do Rio
Brazilian Center for Studies in Dermatology
Porto Alegre
Rio Grande do Sul
Brazil

ISBN 978-3-642-34028-4 ISBN 978-3-642-34029-1 (eBook)
DOI 10.1007/978-3-642-34029-1
Springer Heidelberg New York Dordrecht London

Library of Congress Control Number: 2013933385

Printed on acid-free paper

Springer is part of Springer Science+Business Media (www.springer.com)

Contents

1 **Skin Evaluation Systems** 1
Débora Zechmeister do Prado, Amanda Stapenhorst, Carolina Siega, and Juliana Schilling de Souza

2 **Cellulite** 21
Doris Hexsel and Rosemarie Mazzuco

3 **Acne** 33
Gabriella Fabbrocini and Maria Pia De Padova

4 **Subcision®** 51
Mariana Soirefmann and Rosemari Mazzuco

5 **Hirsutism** 65
Ticiana C. Rodrigues and Poli Mara Spritzer

6 **Striae Distensae** 75
Taciana Dal'Forno

7 **Cosmeceuticals in Dermatology** 87
Aurora Tedeschi, Lee E. West, Laura Guzzardi, Karishma H. Bhatt, Erika E. Reid, Giovanni Scapagnini, and Giuseppe Micali

8 **Photodynamic Therapy** 115
Mariana Soirefmann, Manoela Porto, and Gislaine Ceccon

9 **Botulinum Toxins** 131
Doris Hexsel and Cristiano Brum

10 **Cryosurgery** 145
Cleide Eiko Ishida

11 **Electrosurgery** 165
Sarita Martins de Carvalho Bezerra and Marcio Martins Lobo Jardim

12 **Injectable Treatments for Fat** 181
Adam M. Rotunda

13 Cosmetic Procedures in Asian Skin 203
Evangeline B. Handog, Ma. Teresita G. Gabriel, and Jonathan A. Dizon

Index 215

Skin Evaluation Systems

1

Débora Zechmeister do Prado, Amanda Stapenhorst, Carolina Siega, and Juliana Schilling de Souza

Core Messages

- Skin evaluation and its correct interpretation are of extreme importance for clinical diagnosis and also in research.
- Skin evaluation must start with a clinical exam and different assessment methods can be chosen according to the conditions or treatment results to be assessed.

1.1 Introduction

Skin evaluation and its correct interpretation are of extreme importance. Skin evaluation requires efficient and well-defined methods to diagnose the skin conditions or diseases and also to follow treatment response. These methods include the use of technological and validated resources, such as devices and scales.

In this chapter, qualitative, semiquantitative, and quantitative skin evaluation methods will be discussed. The qualitative methods are subjective and range from physical examination to the clinical evaluations, including the photographic documentation. The semiquantitative methods include the grade and photographic scales,

D.Z. do Prado (✉)
Independent Clinical Research Consultant,
Porto Alegre, RS, Brazil
e-mail: dezech@terra.com.br

A. Stapenhorst
Department of Biomedicine, Brazilian Center for Studies in Dermatology, Universidade Federal de Ciências da Saúde de Porto Alegre – (UFCSPA), Porto Alegre, RS, Brazil

C. Siega • J.S. de Souza
Department of Research, Brazilian Center for Studies in Dermatology, Sociedade Brasileira de Profissionais em Pesquisa Clínica – SBPPC, Porto Alegre, RS, Brazil

A. Tosti, D. Hexsel (eds.), *Update in Cosmetic Dermatology*,
DOI 10.1007/978-3-642-34029-1_1, © Springer-Verlag Berlin Heidelberg 2013

which were created to facilitate the rating of specific skin conditions. Quantitative methods are based on objective measurements of certain skin features, such as photodamage signs, pigmentation, sebum, and hydration.

1.2 Qualitative Evaluation of Skin

1.2.1 Clinical Exam

The dermatological exam begins with physician's questions to the patients about their skin condition and related symptoms. Demographic data, including age, gender, and race, besides previous conditions, medications, and family medical history are important elements. The skin should be always evaluated in a well-illuminated place, with direct light. The exam is performed from head to toe, including hair, mucosa, nails, and ganglions. It is also recommended using instruments, such as dermatoscope, Wood's lamp, and digital photography, according to each patient's needs.

1.2.1.1 Dermatoscope

The dermatoscope is a magnifier used to diagnose skin pigmentation disorders and to distinguish benign from malignant lesions, including melanomas [32]. Digital dermatoscopes allow keeping and enlarging images and for further analysis (Fig. 1.1).

1.2.1.2 Wood's Lamp

Wood's lamp is an ultraviolet light used to diagnose some hair and skin conditions (Fig. 1.2) such as melasma, vitiligo, and porphyria. When fluorescence is applied onto the skin, the epidermal pigment is highlighted, but the same does not happen to the dermal pigment.

1.2.1.3 Photographic Documentation

Photographic assessment of the skin can be important to record patient's medical history, to follow up patients, and also when a second opinion is sought. Photographic assessment significantly improves patients' understanding on their diagnostic and treatment progression [27].

Before acquiring the images, it is suggested to ask patients to sign an informed consent form for photographs, especially if the patient can be recognized. Define high-quality standards to create and maintain photographic patient records as well as to guarantee and maintain patient anonymity and confidentially [19].

Standard photographic methodology is recommended to collect and store patient's images. The images should be always taken using the same parameters, such as camera settings, patient position, and light. Some pictures require a point-source flash, while others require elimination of shadows caused by using a ring flash [19].

The minimum setup needed to document face and body is composed by digital camera; proper light source; appropriate computer to store, analyze, and display the digital files; and a trained photographer.

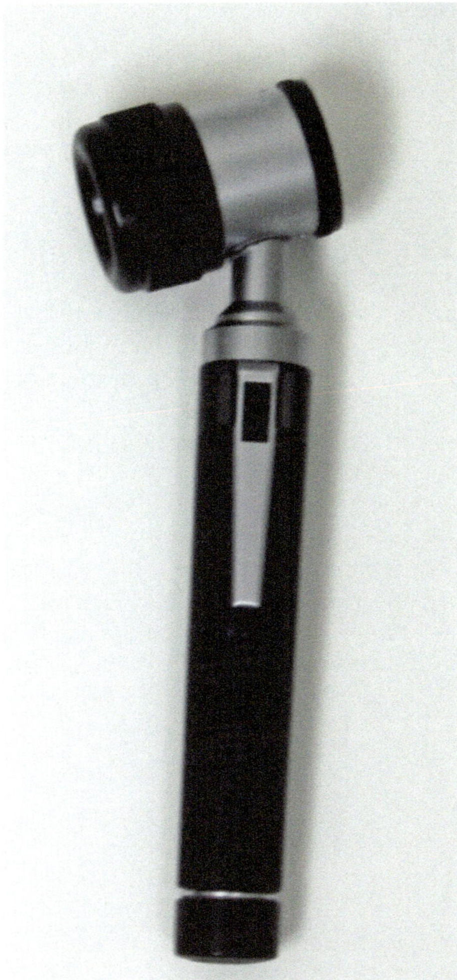

Fig. 1.1 Digital dermatoscope, used to diagnose pigmentation disorders

The photographer is responsible for controlling the standards previously defined when taking the photographs. Moreover, he/she must be patient, especially early on to keep the patient calm to achieve good quality images.

Most of the current digital cameras available in the market offer high resolution. For dermatological use, a resolution of four million pixels is enough [27]. Low-resolution images should be avoided.

Light source positioning is crucial for the photograph quality. Wrong positioning of the lights can create shadows, compromising the skin evaluation. The background must be neutral, monochromatic, and non-reflective, preferably dark. A dark and opaque background provides greater control of the illumination over the subject. The positioning of light source should be the same at all time points for the same subject.

The relatively equal position of the subject to the camera enables the acquisition of the same field size before and after treatment. Makeup, jewelry, and clothing that might interfere the images should be removed. For facial photographs, usual

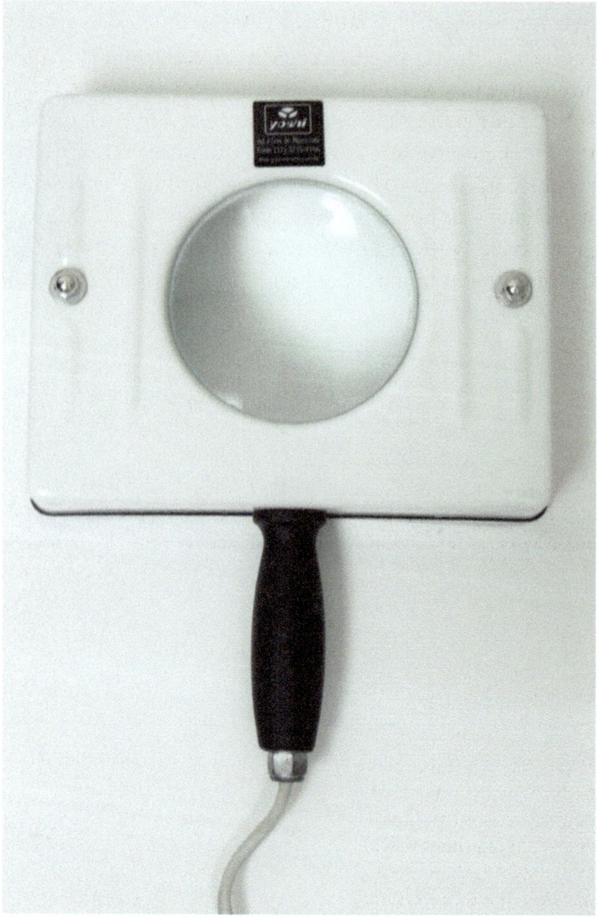

Fig. 1.2 Wood's lamp, an ultraviolet light used to diagnose hair and skin conditions

positions are front, oblique view (45°), and lateral (left and right), and a neutral face expression during the shoot is required (Fig. 1.3).

A standardized setup and imaging procedure is recommended for better correlations between before and after treatment images. Further correlation between the two images could be accomplished using anatomical landmarks. The after treatment image should be compared to the before image immediately after acquisition for consistency and to retake if necessary.

Some objective imaging tools were developed to standardize the photographic position and to assure the photographic quality. Companies like Canfield Scientific™ and FotoFinder Systems™ developed a series of methods and equipments to obtain standardized, reproducible, serial medical photographs and documentation reducing the photographic variables of images.

The OMNIA Imaging System (Canfield Scientific, USA) is a device that standardizes nine photographic angle positions (90°, 67.5°, 45°, 22.5° for left and right

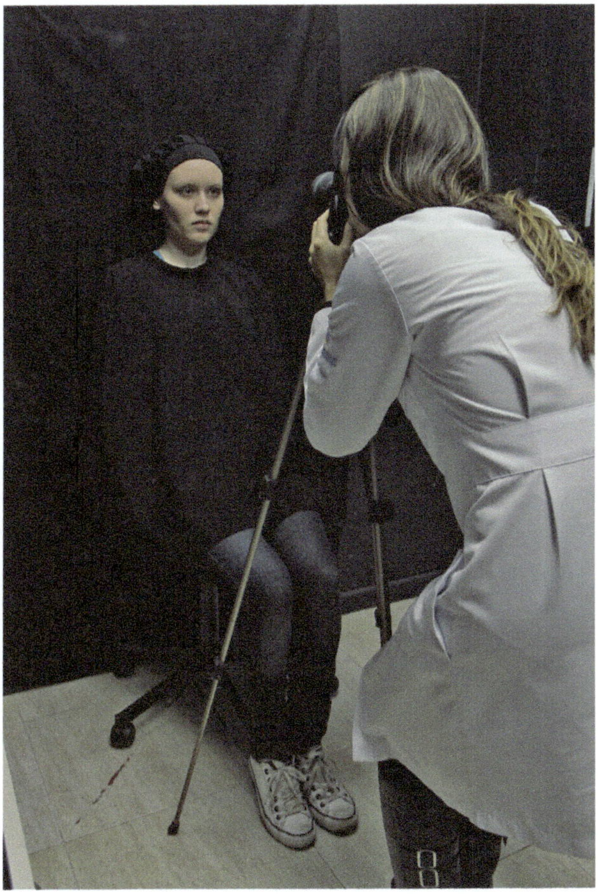

Fig. 1.3 Photographic studio

sides and center 0°) (Fig. 1.4). It can also be coupled with image software such as Mirror™ (Canfield Scientific™, USA), which will be discussed in Sect. 1.4.1.

FotoFinder™ is a photographic system that can be customized for a specific study. All images can be exported and sent to a central server database maintaining their authenticity. Another integrated option is FotoFinder Mediscope Towerstation™, which automatically controls a digital camera permanently connected to the computer.

1.2.2 Qualitative Skin Scales

Qualitative scales permit a more specific evaluation of the skin characteristics, increasing the accuracy of the evaluation. A number of scales have been developed, and the most used for cosmetic purposes are mentioned below.

The Fitzpatrick classification (Table 1.1) known as the Fitzpatrick skin types or Fitzpatrick phototypes depends on the amount of melanin in the skin. It allows evaluating the pigment sensibility to UV light [15].

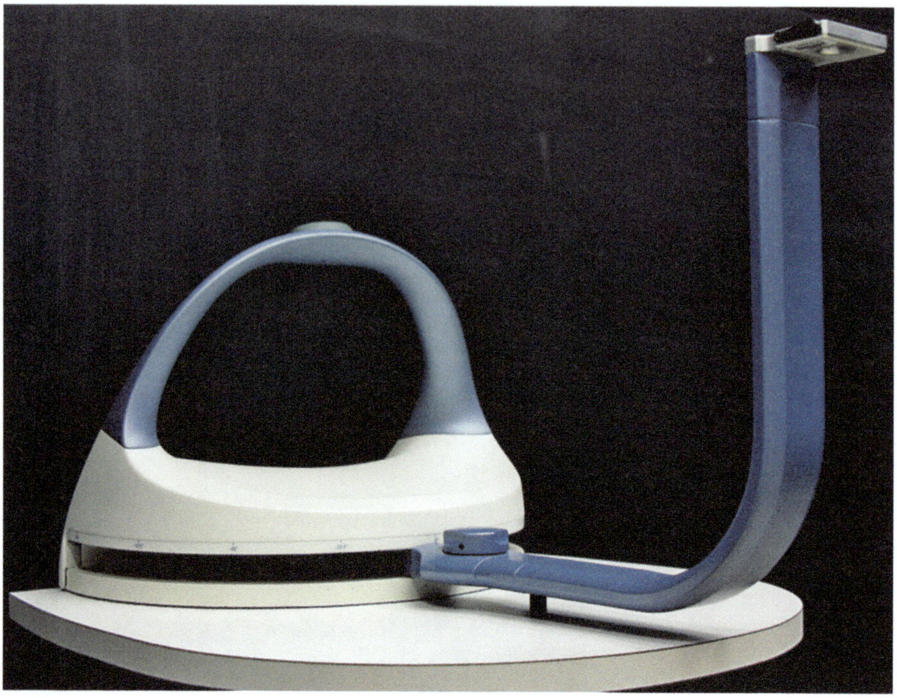

Fig. 1.4 Omnia™ device used to take standard photographs

Table 1.1 Fitzpatrick skin classification

Skin type	Skin color	Tanning ability
I	Pale skin	Always burns, does not tan
II	Fair skin	Burns easily, tans poorly
III	Darker white skin	Tans after initial burn
IV	Light brown skin	Burns minimally, tans easily
V	Brown skin	Rarely burns, tans darkly easily
VI	Dark brown or black skin	Never burns, always tans darkly

Source: Fitzpatrick [15]

The Glogau scale (Table 1.2) is another qualitative skin scale [16]. It is a systematic skin classification of photoaging that permits comparison of therapies and clinical results. Clinical signs of photoaging of the skin include rhytids, lentigines, keratoses, telangiectasia, loss of translucency, loss of elasticity, wrinkles, and sallow color.

The Baumann scale, also called Skin Type Indicator (Table 1.3), identified 16 skin types categorized according to four scales: oily versus dry (O/D), sensitive versus resistant (S/R), pigmented versus nonpigmented (P/N), and tight versus wrinkled (T/W). By answering a 64-question test, the reader is assigned a four-letter type ("OSNW," for example, would mean that a person's skin has been rated as oily, sensitive, and nonpigmented, with a tendency to wrinkle) [5].

Table 1.2 Glogau classification of aging skin

Skin type	Description	Characteristics
Type I	Mild	Early photoaging Early pigmentary changes No keratoses Fine wrinkles Early 20s or 30s
Type II	Moderate	Early to moderate photoaging Early senile lentigines No visible keratoses 30s to 40s
Type III	Advanced	Advanced photoaging Dyschromia and telangiectasia Visible keratoses Wrinkles at rest 50 plus
Type IV	Severe	Severe photoaging Dynamic and gravitational wrinkling Multiple actinic keratoses 60s or 70s

Source: Glogau [16]

Table 1.3 The Baumann Skin Type Indicator

	Oily		Dry		
	Pigmented	Nonpigmented	Pigmented	Nonpigmented	
Wrinkled	OSPW	OSNW	DSPW	DSNW	Sensitive
Tight	OSPT	OSNT	DSPT	DSNT	Resistant
Wrinkled	ORPW	ORNW	DRPW	DRNW	Sensitive
Tight	ORPT	ORNT	DRPT	DRNT	Resistant

Abbreviations: *D* dry, *N* nonpigmented, *O* oily, *P* pigmented, *R* resistant, *S* sensitive, *T* tight, *W* wrinkled

1.3 Semiquantitative Skin Evaluation

Semiquantitative evaluation qualifies the object, turning them into numbers in order to quantify them. However, it is important to differentiate between ordinal scales in which numbers are assigned to range a condition and those in which the ranking generates a sum, as the Likert scale [31].

The Likert scale is a popular method that allows the researcher to quantify opinion-based items. Questions are typically grouped together and rated or responded to base on a five-point scale. This scale typically ranges in order from one extreme to the other, such as (1) very interested, (2) somewhat interested, (3) unsure, (4) not very interested, and (5) not interested at all.

Table 1.4 Ranges of Griffiths scale

Store	Damage
0	No damage
2	Mild damage
4	Moderate damage
6	Moderate/severe damage
8	Severe damage

Source: Griffiths et al. [17]

In general, the semiquantitative scales are developed to evaluate a specific skin condition or a treatment. They can be also photonumeric. On the following examples of semiquantitative methods (scales), some specific cosmetic skin conditions will be better explained.

1.3.1 Skin Aging

Griffiths developed a photonumeric scale to assess the severity of cutaneous photodamage and its response to treatment [17] (Table 1.4).

An analogical visual scale for lip volume evaluation was developed by Rossi and colleagues [36]. This scale is very useful for soft tissue augmentation treatment evaluation. Another validated scale for evaluation of lip fullness was developed and published by Carruthers and colleagues [9].

Shoshani and coauthors validated the Modified Fitzpatrick Wrinkle Scale (MFWS) as a nasolabial wrinkle severity assessment tool. It is a reliable method for the quantitative evaluation of the nasolabial folds [38].

Day and coauthors proposed the Wrinkle Severity Rating Scale to describe the facial folds appearance. It ranges from extreme (score 5) to nonexistent (score 0) [11].

Other semiquantitative dermatological scales include: Fitzpatrick for perioral facial wrinkles [14], Lemperle Wrinkles Scale [30], Facial Attributes Scale [33], among others (Table 1.4).

1.3.2 Pigmentary Disorders

The visual hyperpigmentation scale consists of a series of plastic cards, printed with 10 different skin colors (A–J) and 10 pigment scores for each skin color (1–10), corresponding to 100 possibilities to graduate hyperpigmentation [41].

Melasma Area and Severity Index (MASI) is a score that objectively measures the severity of melasma [28]. It is obtained through the visual inspection of the face, without any risks for the patient. The face is divided in four areas: forehead, right malar region, left malar region, and chin, corresponding to 30, 30, 30, and 10 % of the face, respectively. Before calculating the MASI, it is necessary to graduate the areas of the face according to the following variables: afflicted area, hyperpigmentation, and homogeneity of hyperpigmentation. Pandya and colleagues assessed this tool, and state MASI is a reliable measure of melasma severity [35].

Hyperpigmentation/melasma status [42], color designation of melasma [18], and physician and patient global assessment (PGA) [42] are other commonly utilized tools to evaluate melasma improvement with therapy.

Wood's light is also a useful tool in the assessment of melasma (see Sect. 1.2.1.2). Although it does not measure melasma severity, it can accurately assist in the determination of the presence or absence of pigmentation and its location. It can also distinguish between pigmentary changes and changes due to superficial circulation or scarring.

1.3.3 Botulinum Toxin

Some photonumerical scales were created to evaluate the areas of face treated by botulinum toxin.

The four-point glabellar frown line scale was developed and validated by Hornek and colleagues (The Smile Group). It consists of an atlas with standardized photographs of glabellar frown lines [25]. Years later, the same group led by Hund developed the four-point clinical severity scores for lateral canthal lines (crow's feet) [26].

Other validated grading scales for dynamic wrinkles (those that could be treated with botulinum toxin) were published, such as the validated grading scale for crow's feet [6], validated grading scale for marionette lines [8], and validated grading scale for forehead lines [7].

Minor's test or iodine-starch test evaluates before and after hyperhidrosis treatments by showing residual areas of sweating in the treated areas. The colorful complex formed by Minor's test allows the visualization of the area covered by the effects of botulinum toxin on sweat glands, also known as diffusion or fields of anhydrotic effect. Hexsel and coauthors reinforced a standardized technique to perform Minor's test and created the Sweating Intensity Visual Scale. It is an objective scale to grade the sweat intensity and can be used to categorize degree of hyperhidrosis [22].

1.3.4 Cellulite

While the previous classification of cellulite [34] describes different grades of cellulite, which is very important, there are additional key morphological aspects that affect cellulite severity and, therefore, can be targeted by treatment options. For this reason, Hexsel, Dal'Forno and Hexsel created and validated the cellulite severity scale (CSS) [21] as a new method to objectively measure and grade cellulite severity. The proposed new scale expands the current classification allowing a comprehensive measurement of the intensity of the condition. Four important clinical and morphological aspects and the previous classification are assessed in this scale: A) Number of evident depressions; B) Depth of depressions; C) Morphological appearance of skin surface alterations; D) Grade of laxity, flaccidity, or sagging skin; E) Classification by Nürnberger and Müller. It is an objective method that can facilitate patient follow-up and measure treatment outcomes.

1.3.5 Quality of Life

There are scales developed with the aim of measuring the impact of some diseases or conditions in patient's quality of life. Some of the most used scales include the DLQI for all cutaneous diseases [2], melasma quality of life questionnaire (MelasQol) [4], the Acne Quality of Life Scale [20], Psoriasis Disability Index [13], and Cellulite Quality of Life Scale (Celluqol®) [23].

1.4 Quantitative Skin Evaluation

1.4.1 Imaging Measurement Tools

In vivo imaging of the skin has improved the assessment of initial versus treated skin within cosmetic procedures and research.

Unfortunately, many of these systems use software exclusively for PCs with Windows operating systems. Thus, they cannot take advantage of the graphics presentation possible with the speed of Apple's new Power Mac G5 with its 64-bit processor offering 8 GB of RAM [1].

1.4.1.1 Three-Dimensional Skin Microphotography

Three-dimensional microphotography with equipments like Primos™ measurement device (Canfield Scientific™) has been shown to quantitatively measure skin roughness, wrinkles, and nodule formations and to track changes over time. It can help evaluating the efficacy of non-ablative laser therapy used to minimize acne scarring and facial lines.

The absolute measurement of wrinkle depth by light transmission of a silicone replica (Skin-Visiometer® SV 600) is considered a simple way to diagnose the topography of the skin surface. The device works based upon a parallel light source and a black and white CMOS camera with 640 * 480 pixels that reads the topography of the skin by light transmission of a very thin, especially blue-dyed silicone. The very viscous two-part silicone, mixed under vacuum to avoid bubbles, fills even the smallest skin depths and reproduces them in detail. The replica reproduces the heights and depths of the skin as a negative, that is, wrinkles are higher in the replica as the silicone is thicker in this place. These special parameters have been created to describe the skin topography volume and unfolded surface, which can be displayed quickly in a colored 3D image.

Skin Evidence™ (La Licorne, France) and Visioscope® (Courage-Khazaka, Germany) are also capable of analyzing skin relief (see Sect. 1.4.1.3).

1.4.1.2 Quantitative Reproducible Facial Image Analysis

Visia™ and Visia™ CR (Canfield Scientific™, USA) are imaging booths in a self-contained unit that generates quantitative values for skin features. It provides new detection and analysis of subsurface vascular and melanin conditions. It separates the color signatures of red and brown skin components for analysis of conditions

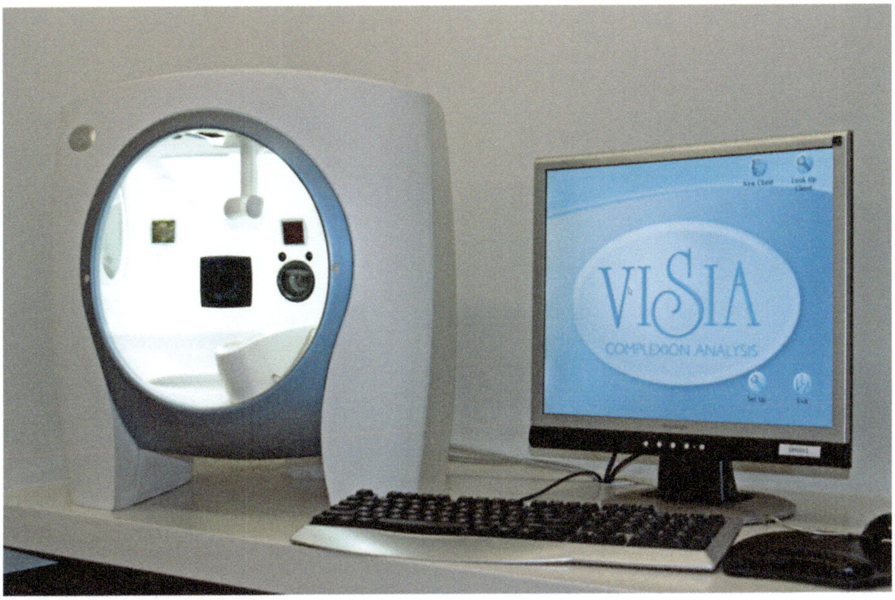

Fig. 1.5 Visia™ imaging booth

such as rosacea, spider veins, melasma, acne, and wrinkles. There is a true UV photo mode that provides the most complete data for sun damage and a UV fluorescence imaging to reveal porphyry (*P. acnes*). It consists of an interactive system through which the dermatologist uses a digital imaging booth with a high-resolution camera to process images with proprietary software (Fig. 1.5). The software is designed to evaluate skin surface imperfections and show the patient the potential results of cosmetic procedures [1]. All the high-resolution images are stored in file, registered under the patient's name, allowing a complete procedure follow-up.

Mirror™ imaging software (Canfield Scientific™, USA) can simulate treatment results and also objectively measure some efficacy parameters expressed in centimeters, such as brown lift (Fig. 1.6) and field effects promoted by botulinum toxin action (Fig. 1.7). Furthermore, this software measures and analyzes facial angles which can be helpful in preoperative analysis and planning the procedure [46]. The ease and speed of image alteration lies at the heart of this sophisticated software, making patient consultations streamline and informative.

The Visioscan® VC 98 (Courage-Khazaka, Germany) is an accurate equipment that provides a high degree of stability visualizing a sharp, non-glossy image of the skin surface shown by a special UV-A light video camera with a high-resolution black and white video sensor and a ring-shaped UV-A light source for uniform illumination of the skin. The device can be used in various fields of application, such as the clinical diagnosis in dermatology, due to its capacity to quantitatively and qualitatively describe clinical parameters of the skin surface: skin smoothness, skin roughness, scaliness, and wrinkles.

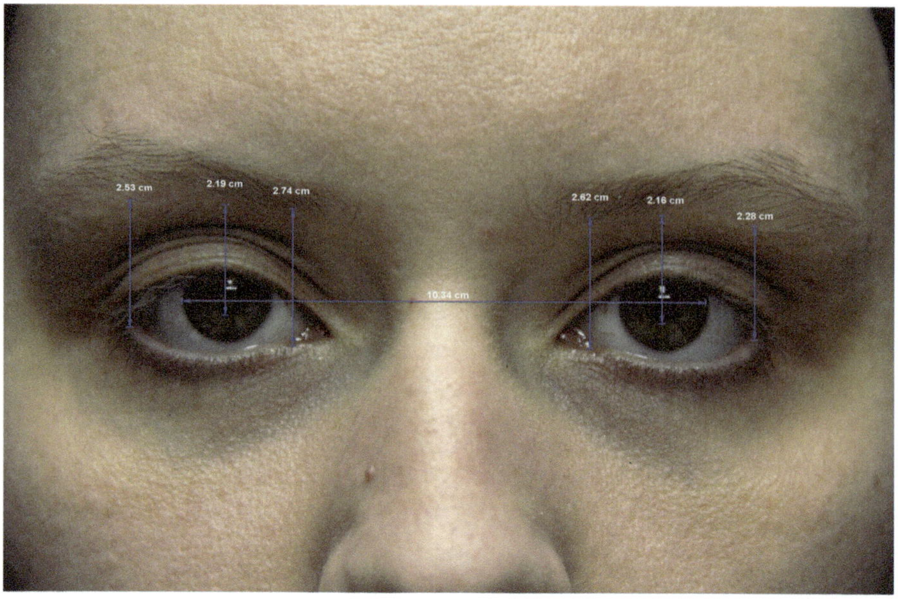

Fig. 1.6 Results of a patient before and after treatment measured by Mirror™ imaging software

1.4.1.3 Biometrical Image Tools

Skin Evidence™ Visio (La Licorne, France) is a biometrical tool designed to facilitate an early and accurate diagnosis and to evaluate objectively the treatment results (Fig. 1.8). It is an imaging device that contains standardized illumination with normal and polarized light together with a quantitative analysis for skin surface (cutaneous microrelief) [3], pigmentation, vascular abnormalities, sebum measurement, hair distribution, and growth (Fig. 1.9). Skin Evidence™ is a system based on four separate parts: a high-performance computer, a video probe, a unified probe, and software. The probes are connected to the computer by a USB cable.

Visioscope® BW 30 (Courage-Khazaka, Germany) is a handheld video camera with a special UV light source designed to visually magnify skin, hair, and scalp on a video screen. The camera shows a skin area of 6×8 mm and monitors the skin texture (smoothness, wrinkles), desquamation (scaliness), skin impurities (reddening, pigmentation spots, acne, comedones, etc.), hair structure, dandruff, and condition of the scalp. There is also a color version (Visioscope® Color 32) that is a handheld video camera connected with a video monitor very similar to Visioscope BW 30, with white light source instead to UV light. It is recommended for use in viewing and diagnosing skin, hair, and scalp conditions. The camera records a color view of 6×8 mm.

Dermascan® (Cortex Technology, Denmark) is a high-resolution ultrasound equipment (Fig. 1.10) that provides a dimensional measurement and diagnoses the structural changes of the skin. It displays the layers of the epidermis, dermis, and subcutaneous tissues in a color LCD panel, in 2D or 3D resolution. The exam is

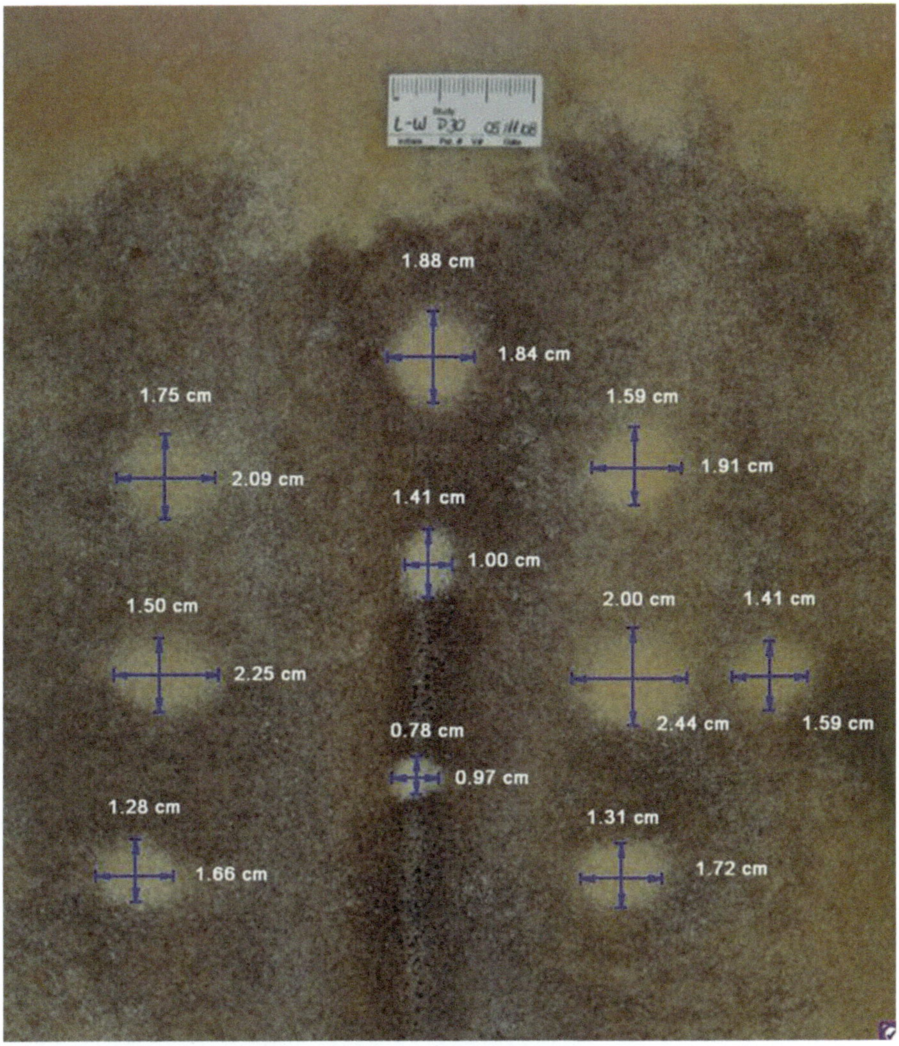

Fig. 1.7 Measurement of botulinum toxin action halos by Mirror™ imaging software

quick and does not cause any harm to the patient, being a positive way to keep the progress of the treatment, tracking before and after of the same skin site enabling a comparison of trends in skin condition. It has been mainly used for the assessment of photoaging and cellulite.

Reflectance confocal microscopy technology is a technique that allows physicians to obtain high-resolution optical images that are acquired point-by-point and reconstructed with a computer, allowing three-dimensional reconstructions of topologically complex objects. It provides direct, noninvasive, serial optical sectioning of intact, thick, living specimens with a minimum sample preparation as well as a

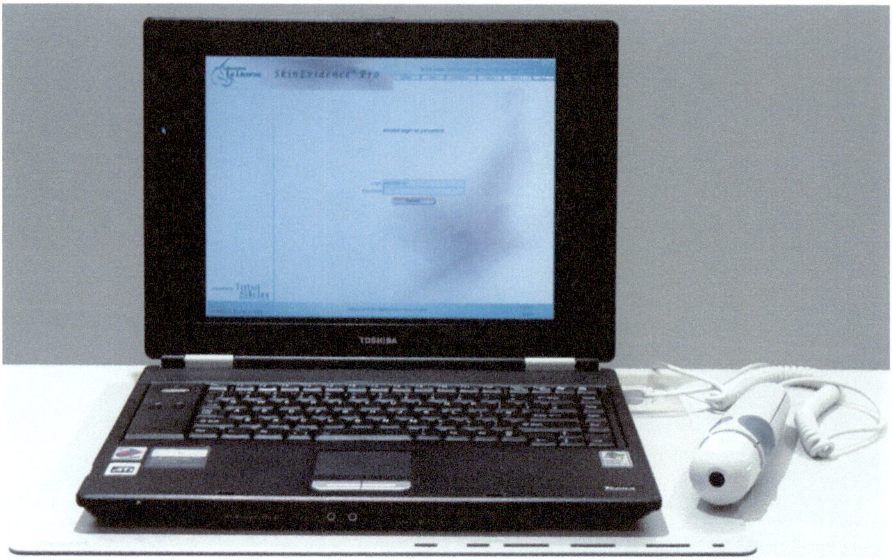

Fig. 1.8 Skin Evidence™ device

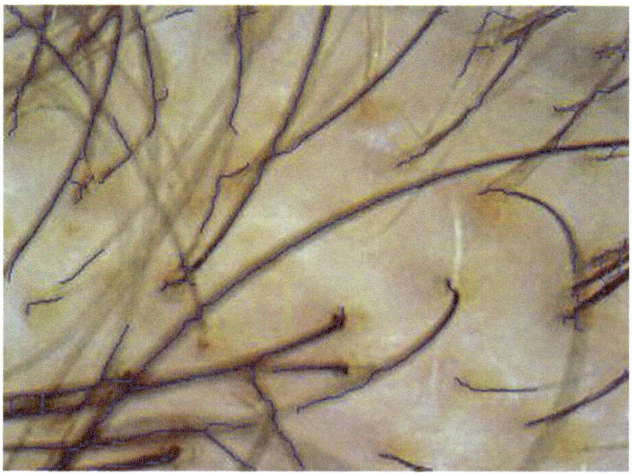

Fig. 1.9 Hair evaluation by the Skin Evidence™ device

marginal improvement in lateral resolution. With this technology it is possible to examine cellular and structural details, including the nucleus, blood circulation, and microvascularization, without the necessity to process the tissue as in the histology. The first works in the area characterized the morphology of the normal skin, whereas the following publications elucidated the biggest histological parameters of a series of inflammatory and proliferated injuries of skin's conditions as skin cancer. The VivaScope® (Lucid Inc, USA) is the pioneer in the development of the reflectance confocal microscopy technology.

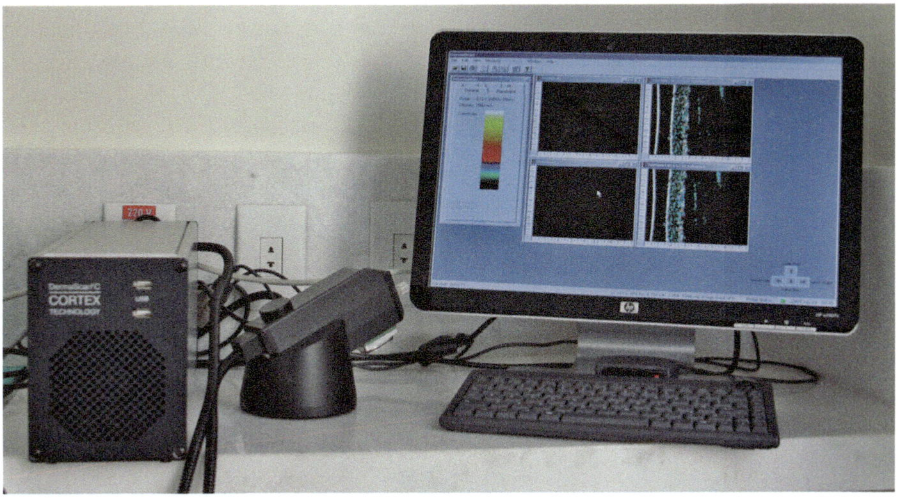

Fig. 1.10 Dermascan® device

Confocal Raman spectroscopy is a spectroscopic technique used to study vibrational, rotational, and other low-frequency modes in a system. It is a noninvasive optical technique that can probe the molecular structure and conformation of biochemical constituents. This technology can monitor the amount of chemical compounds, in vivo. Confocal Raman microspectroscopy is able to determine depth profiles of water concentration in the skin [44]. Advances in Raman hardware and probe design have reduced spectral acquisition times, paving the way for clinical applications. In vivo real-time Raman can be a very promising research and practical technique for skin evaluation [45].

Magnetic resonance imaging (MRI) is a medical imaging technique most commonly used in radiology to visualize the internal structure and function of the body. MRI provides much greater definition between the different soft tissues of the body than computed tomography (CT), making it especially useful in neurological, musculoskeletal, cardiovascular, and other areas, such as dermatological imaging. Hexsel and coauthors evaluated 30 female patients and compared subcutaneous tissue in areas with and without cellulite on the buttocks of the same subjects using MRI, a noninvasive technique. Results of the MRI analysis showed that cellulite depressions on the buttocks were significantly associated with the presence of underlying fibrous septa [24].

1.4.2 Skin Features Measure Tools

1.4.2.1 Skin Reflectance Instruments

This kind of instruments quantify pigmentation based upon reflectance spectroscopy, that is, by measuring the intensity of light reflected from the skin. There are two types of instruments: narrowband reflectance spectrophotometers and tristimulus reflectance colorimeters.

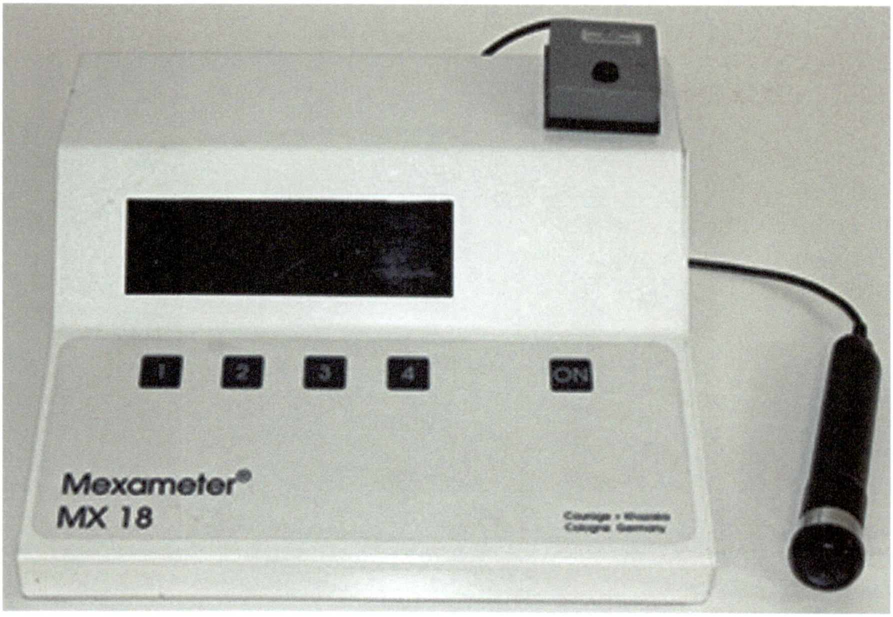

Fig. 1.11 Mexameter®

The two commercially available narrowband reflectance spectrophotometers most used are Mexameter® MX (Courage-Khazaka, Germany) and DermaSpectrometer (Cortex Technology, Denmark). Mexameter® MX (Courage-Khazaka, Germany) contains diodes emitting light at three wavelengths 568 nm (green), 669 nm (red), and 880 (infrared) (Fig. 1.11) [10]. It measures the major components of the color of the skin: melanin and hemoglobin (erythema). The probe is placed on the skin, and the reading of reflected light is showed on the screen. Hemoglobin, the chromophore primarily responsible for the skin's erythema, absorbs primarily in the green wavelengths (568 nm), and melanin, responsible for pigmentation, absorbs in all wavelengths but especially in the red spectrum (669 nm). The melanin index is calculated from the intensity of the absorbed and reflected light at wavelengths 660 and 880 nm. Therefore, the degree of pigmentation in a patient with melasma may be quantified for melanin ranging from white (1) to black (1,000). The erythema index is computed from the absorption and reflection of light at 565 and 660 nm. Similarly, the DermaSpectrometer's diodes emit light at wavelengths 568 nm (green) and 655 nm (red), and based upon absorption and reflectance determine erythema and melanin indexes.

The tristimulus colorimeters commonly used are the Chromameter CR200 and CR300 (Konica Minolta Holdings, Inc., Japan) and the Photovolt ColorWalk colorimeter (Protovolt Instruments Inc, USA). The tristimulus colorimeters are capable of measuring all colors in contrast to the narrowband, simple reflectance meters that measure only the intensity of erythema and melanin. With the tristimulus reflectance colorimeters, a pulsed xenon arc lamp is utilized as the light

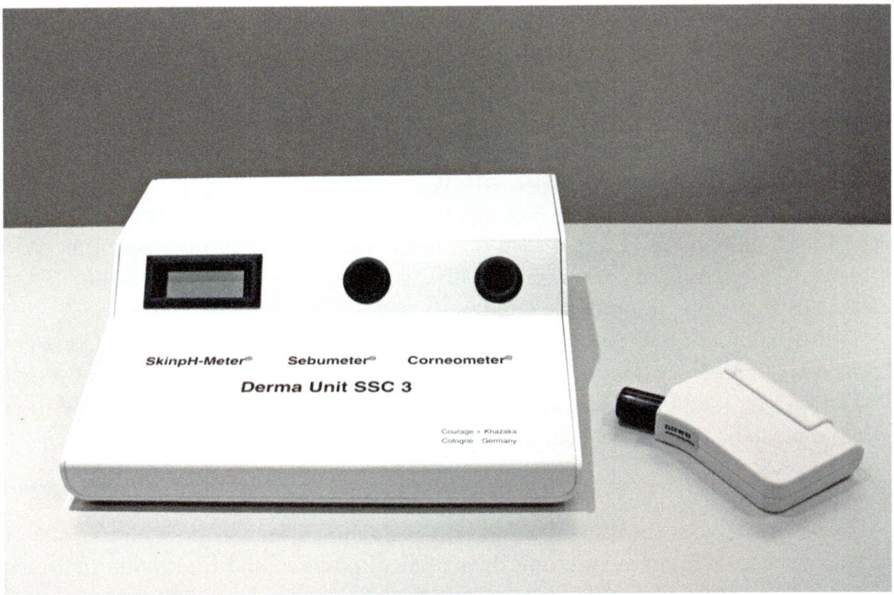

Fig. 1.12 Corneometer- pH-Meter-Sebumeter®

source, and light reflected from the skin is analyzed at three wavelengths 450, 560, and 600 nm.

Clarys and coauthors compared two types of skin reflectance instruments: Minolta Chromameter CR200 and Mexameter® MX16. Color measurements were compared in vitro on standardized color charts and subsequently in vivo on different skin areas. The in vitro and in vivo repeatability as well as the sensitivity of the three instruments was rather good. The Chromameter and the two narrowband reflectance instruments were able to characterize skin color and small skin color changes [10]. Other study from Shriver and coauthors [39] also compared these two types of reflectometers. They conclude that the narrowband reflectance spectroscope is the preferred instrument as the melanin index and it is less likely to be influenced by the levels of hemoglobin in the skin [10].

1.4.2.2 Skin Barrier and Skin Surface Parameters

Courage-Khazaka (Germany) produces a three in one device which measures different skin characteristics, called Corneometer-pH-Meter-Sebumeter® (Fig. 1.12). The Corneometer® measures the stratum corneum's hydration levels, which is essential for a well-functioning skin barrier [29]. The measurement is based on the amount of the dielectric constant of the water in the superficial layer of the stratum corneum, ensuring that the measurement is not influenced by the capillary blood vessels. The pH Meter® measures the pH level on the skin surface. The skin pH is an important parameter [12] to assess the quality of the hydrolipidic film. These measures are mainly used to test the effects of soaps, cleansers, or detergents. The measurement is made through a probe, connected to an electronic meter that displays the pH reading. The Sebumeter® is responsible for measuring the amount of sebum on the skin [43]. The measurement is based on the principle of grease-spot photometry, when the measuring head of the cassette is placed on the skin (Fig. 1.12) [40].

1.4.2.3 Skin Elasticity Measurement

Cutometer® (Courage-Khazaka, Germany) is a device used to measure skin elasticity [37]. A probe is used to perform the measurements. When pressed on the skin, the result is a temporary vacuum that lifts, stretches, and releases the skin. These deflections are optically recorded and evaluated.

The elasticity measurement by Elastomer® EM 25 (Courage-Khazaka, Germany) indicates the biological skin age and is performed very quickly by the well-established suction method. The result is shown in percentage in the display. The interpretation can be done with a chart according to the age.

Conclusion

In recent years, several advances in skin evaluation systems allow state-of-the-art patient care while streamlining their clinical practice and improving their academic and research skills.

These technologies offer both enhanced clinical examination and improved methods of analyzing, grading, and standardizing results of daily practice and clinical research.

References

1. Abramovits W, Stevenson LC (2003) Changing paradigms in dermatology: new ways to examine the skin using noninvasive imaging methods. Clin Dermatol 21:353–358
2. Anderson RT et al (1997) Development and validation of a quality of life instrument for cutaneous diseases. J Am Acad Dermatol 37:41–50
3. Atrux-Tallau N et al (2008) Effects of physical and chemical treatments upon biophysical properties and micro-relief of human skin. Arch Dermatol Res 300(5):243–251
4. Balkrishnan R et al (2003) Development and validation of a health-related quality of life instrument for women with melasma. Br J Dermatol 149(3):572–577
5. Baumann L (2008) Understanding and treating various skin types: the Baumann skin type indicator. Dermatol Clin 26:359–373
6. Carruthers A, Carruthers J, Hardas B et al (2008) A validated grading scale for Crow's feet. Dermatol Surg 34(Special Issue 2):167–172
7. Carruthers A, Carruthers J, Hardas B et al (2008) A validated grading scale for forehead lines. Dermatol Surg 34(Special Issue 2):155–160
8. Carruthers A, Carruthers J, Hardas B et al (2008) A validated grading scale for marionette lines. Dermatol Surg 34(Special Issue 2):173–178
9. Carruthers A, Carruthers J, Hardas B et al (2008) A validated lip fullness grading scale. Dermatol Surg 34(Suppl 2):S161–S166
10. Clarys P, Alewaeters K, Lambrecht R, Barel AO (2000) Skin color measurements: comparison between three instruments: the Chromameter®, the DermaSpectrometer® and the Mexameter®. Skin Res Technol 6(4):230–238
11. Day DJ et al (2004) Wrinkle severity rating scale. Am J Clin Dermatol 5(1):49–52

12. Ehlers C, Ivens UI, Møller ML et al (2001) Females have lower skin surface pH than men. A study on the surface of gender, forearm site variation, right/left difference and time of the day on the skin surface pH. Skin Res Technol 7(2):90–94
13. Finlay AY et al (1987) Psoriasis: an index of disability. Clin Exp Dermatol 12:8–11, In: Dermatology: a practical guide
14. Fitzpatrick RE, Goldman MP, Satur NM (1996) Pulsed carbon dioxide laser resurfacing of photo-aged facial skin. Arch Dermatol 132:395
15. Fitzpatrick TB (1988) Fitzpatrick phototypes. Arch Dermatol 124(6):869–871
16. Glogau RG (1996) Aesthetic and anatomic analysis of the aging skin. Semin Cutan Med Surg 3:134–138
17. Griffiths CEM et al (1992) Photonumeric scale for the assessment of cutaneous photodamage. Arch Dermatol 128:347–351
18. Griffiths CEM, Finkel LJ, Ditre CM, Hamilton TA, Ellis CN, Voorhees JJ (1993) Topical tretinoin (retinoic acid) improves melasma. A vehicle-controlled, clinical trial. Br J Dermatol 129:415–421
19. Grimes PE (2008) Photography in cosmetic surgery. In: Grimes PE (ed) Aesthetics and cosmetic surgery for darker skin types. Lippincott Williams & Wilkins, Philadelphia, pp 62–70
20. Gupta MA et al (1998) The development of an acne quality of life scale: reliability, validity, and relation to subjective acne severity in mild to moderate acne vulgaris. Acta Derm Venereol 78(6):451–456
21. Hexsel D, Dal Forno T, Hexsel CL (2009) Severity scale of cellulite. J Eur Acad Dermatol Venereol 23(5):523–528
22. Hexsel D, Rodrigues TC, Soirefmann M, Zechmeister-Prado D (2010) Recommendations for performing and evaluating the results of Minor's test according to a sweating intensity visual scale. Dermatol Surg 36(1):120–122
23. Hexsel D, Weber MB, Taborda ML et al (2011) CELLUQOL® – a quality of life measurement for patients with cellulite. Surg Cosmet Dermatol 3(2):96–101
24. Hexsel DM, Abreu M, Rodrigues TC et al (2009) Side-by-side comparison of areas with and without cellulite depressions using magnetic resonance imaging. Dermatol Surg 35(10):1471–1477
25. Honeck P, Weiss C, Sterry W, Rzany B, Gladys Study Group (2003) Reproducibility of a four-point clinical severity score for glabellar frown lines. Br J Dermatol 149(2):306–310
26. Hund T, Ascher B, Rzany B (2006) Reproducibility of two four-point clinical severity scores for lateral canthal lines (crow's feet). Dermatol Surg 32(10):1256–1260
27. Kaliyadan F (2008) Digital photography for patient counseling in dermatology – a study. J Eur Acad Dermatol Venereol 22(11):1356–1358
28. Kimbrough-Green CK, Griffiths CE, Finkel LJ et al (1994) Melasma area and severity Index (MASI). Arch Dermatol 130:727–733
29. Leite e Silva VR, Schulman MA, Ferelli C et al (2009) Hydrating effects of moisturizer active compounds incorporated into hydrogels: in vivo assessment and comparison between devices. J Cosmet Dermatol 8(1):32–39
30. Lemperle G et al (2001) A classification of facial wrinkles. Plast Reconstr Surg 108(6):1735–1750
31. Likert R (1932) A technique for the measurement of attitudes. Arch Psychol 140:1–55
32. Magalhães L, Hofmester H (2003) Técnicas Semióticas para Determinação e Avaliação dos Diferentes Tipos de Pele. In: Kede MPV, Sabatovich O (eds) Dermatologia Estética. Atheneu, São Paulo, pp. 25
33. Nkengne A, Bertin C, Stamatas GN et al (2008) Influence of facial skin attributes on the perceived age of Caucasian women. J Eur Acad Dermatol Venereol 22(8):982–991
34. Nürnberger F, Müller G (1978) J Dermatol Surg Oncol 4(3):221–229
35. Pandya AG, Hynan LS, Bhore R et al (2011) Reliability assessment and validation of the Melasma Area and Severity Index (MASI) and a new modified MASI scoring method. J Am Acad Dermatol 64(1):78–83, 83.e1–2
36. Rossi AB, Stamatas G, Ruvolo E, Nkengne A (2008) The validation of a grading scale for lip volume. In: Poster – 66th annual meeting – American Academy of Dermatology, San Antonio, 1–5 Feb 2008

37. Naouri M, Atlan M, Perrodeau E et al (2012) Skin tightening induced by fractional CO(2) laser treatment: quantified assessment of variations in mechanical properties of the skin. J Cosmet Dermatol 11(3):201–6
38. Shoshani D et al (2008) Modified Fitzpatrick wrinkle scale. Dermatol Surg 34(Suppl 1): S85–S91
39. Shriver MD, Parra EJ (2000) Comparison of narrow-band reflectance spectroscopy and tristimulus colorimetry for measurements of skin and hair color in persons of different biological ancestry. Am J Phys Anthropol 112:17–27
40. Pande SY, Misri R (2005) Sebumeter. Indian J Dematol Venerol Leprol 7:444–446
41. Taylor S et al (2006) Visual hyperpigmentation scale. J Am Acad Dermatol 54(5 Suppl 2):S282–S290
42. Taylor SC, Torok H, Jones T, Lowe N, Rich P et al (2003) Efficacy and safety of a new triple-combination agent for the treatment of facial melasma. Cutis 72:67–72
43. Youn SW, Park ES, Lee DH et al (2005) Does facial sebum excretion really affect the development of acne? Br J Dermatol 153(5):919–924
44. Zhang Q, Chan KL, Zhang G, Gillece T, Senak L et al (2011) Raman microspectroscopic and dynamic vapor sorption characterization of hydration in collagen and dermal tissue. Biopolymers 95(9):607–615. doi:10.1002/bip. 21618
45. Zhao J, Lui H, McLean DI, Zeng H (2008) Integrated real-time Raman system for clinical in vivo skin analysis. Skin Res Technol 14(4):484–492
46. Zimbler MC, Ham J (2005) Aesthetic facial analysis. In: Cummings CW, Schuller DE, Thomas JR, Robbins KT, Harker LA (eds) Cummings otolaryngology: head and neck surgery, 4th edn. Mosby Inc., Philadelphia

Cellulite

2

Doris Hexsel and Rosemarie Mazzuco

Core Messages

- Elements that seem to be involved in cellulite's appearance are: adipocyte hypertrophy, connective tissue abnormalities, fibrous septa, and hormonal influences.
- A new cellulite severity scale (CSS) and classification was recently developed. The CSS considers relevant morphological aspects, such as the number of evident depressions, depth of depressions, aspect of raised areas, grade of laxity, flaccidity or sagging skin, and the previous cellulite scale.
- Diagnosis is mainly clinical although magnetic resonance imaging, laser Doppler flowmetry, thermography, and ultrasound can be used for research purposes.
- A series of treatments can treat or improve the appearance of cellulite, such as topical products, oral supplements, devices (mechanical massage, lasers, light sources, radiofrequency, and other technologies), and surgical procedures (Subcision® and liposuction).

D. Hexsel, M.D. (✉)
Department of Dermatology, Pontificia Universidade Catolica do Rio Grande do Sul (PUC-RS), Brazilian Center for Studies in Dermatology, Porto Alegre, RS, Brazil

Brazilian Center for Studies in Dermatology, Porto Alegre, RS, Brazil

782 Dr. Timoteo, St., 90570-040 Porto Alegre, RS, Brazil
e-mail: doris@hexsel.com.br

R. Mazzuco, M.D.
Brazilian Society of Dermatology and Brazilian Society of Dermatologic Surgery, São Paulo, SP, Brazil
e-mail: rosemazzuco@hotmail.com.br

A. Tosti, D. Hexsel (eds.), *Update in Cosmetic Dermatology*,
DOI 10.1007/978-3-642-34029-1_2,

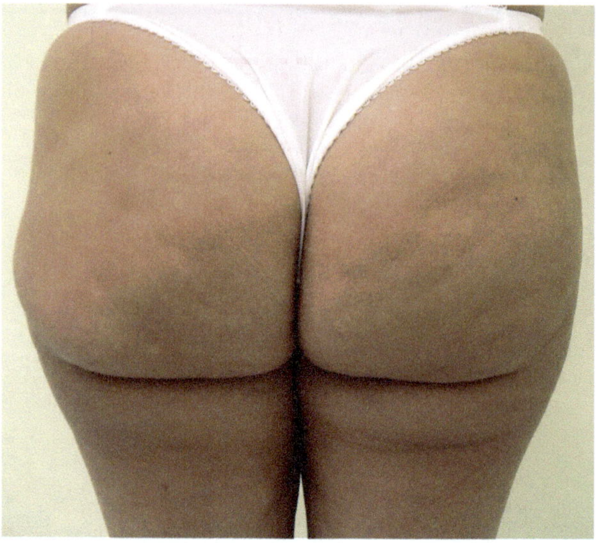

Fig. 2.1 Common aspect of cellulite depressed lesions on the buttocks

2.1 Introduction

Cellulite, also called as edematous fibrosclerotic panniculopathy and local or gynoid lipodystrophy [6], is characterized by irregular relief alterations to the skin surface of the affected areas, giving orange peel, cottage cheese [31], or mattress aspect (Fig. 2.1). It is frequently found on the thighs and buttocks of women. Although cellulite is not a disease, it is considered a noninflammatory phenomenon with alterations in the subcutis.

It is a common clinical condition that usually affects women. It begins in puberty and progresses during the life. Nowadays, some factors involved in the genesis of this condition are better understood [18]. However, there are many other controversial theories that attempt to explain the pathophysiology of cellulite [30].

2.2 Prevalence

Approximately 85–90 % of women over 20 years are believed to have some degree of cellulite [31]. It has been described by Goldman [8] as a normal physiological state in postadolescent women, in which the fat storage in the adipose tissue is maximized ensuring adequate caloric availability for pregnancy and lactation [8]. It is highly prevalent in women of all races but seems to be more common in Caucasian females than in Asian females [1]. Ortonne and colleagues distinguished two subpopulations among women with cellulite by characterizing the "orange peel appearance" and the "shadowed surfaces": those of 21–30 years old, presented large but less numerous dimpled surfaces, and those of more than 30 with smaller and more numerous dimpled surface [25].

It is rarely seen in males, except those with androgen deficiency, such as Klinefelter's syndrome, hypogonadism, and post-castration, and in those patients receiving estrogen therapy for prostate cancer [1].

2.3 Etiology and Pathophysiology

Cellulite was first described by Alquier and Paviot (1920) as a noninflammatory complex cellular dystrophy of the mesenchymal tissue caused by a disorder of water metabolism. Interstitial liquids would produce a saturation of adjacent tissues in this condition [32].

In 1978, Nürnberger and Müller attributed the appearance of cellulite to two factors: the volume of fat cells and the differences of subcutaneous tissue architecture between men and women [24]. In women, fibrous branches perpendicular to the skin's surface separate voluminous lobules in rectangular sections [34] resulting in the dimpled surface characteristic of cellulite.

Considering theories that have emerged on the etiopathogenesis of cellulite, Terranova et al. [34] identifies the following related causes to cellulite: edema resulting from excessive hydrophilia of the intracellular matrix, microcirculatory alteration, and different anatomical conformation of the subcutaneous tissue in women compared to men [34]. Ortonne and colleagues also propose adipocyte hypertrophy, microcirculation disorders, and venous stasis as important elements linked to the cellulite condition. Besides, they refer connective tissue abnormalities and fibrosis as others important elements [25].

Collagen type I was reported as a major target in cellulite [28]. One of the theories on the etiology of cellulite is based on the collagen breakdown in the dermis [7]. Rossi and Vergnanini [32] relate that estrogen provokes alterations in collagen. In fact, cellulite worsens with pregnancy, menstrual cycle, use of contraceptives, and hormonal replacement. Another estrogen's influence related by those authors is the stimulation of lipoprotein lipase, an enzyme responsible for lipogenesis, process which leads to the fat accumulation [32]. Fat accumulation in the buttocks and thighs is also related to the characteristics of the adipocytes in these areas. They have a great number of α-adrenergic receptors which are anti-lipolytic and thus responsible for the resistance of adipose tissue mobilization [28], in contrast to visceral and abdominal fat where there is less α-adrenergic receptors and, for this reason, a better response to lipolysis induced by catecholamines [18]. Skin laxity has also been considered to play an important role in cellulite appearance or worsening [14]. The results of a recent study may corroborate this hypothesis as they suggest the cellulite severity increases with age [16].

2.4 Anatomical Considerations

Cellulite is viewed as the result of a combination of the gender-related dimorphism of the hypodermal tissue and mechanobiological effects of tissue tensions inside this tissue, being thus much more prevalent in women than in men [26].

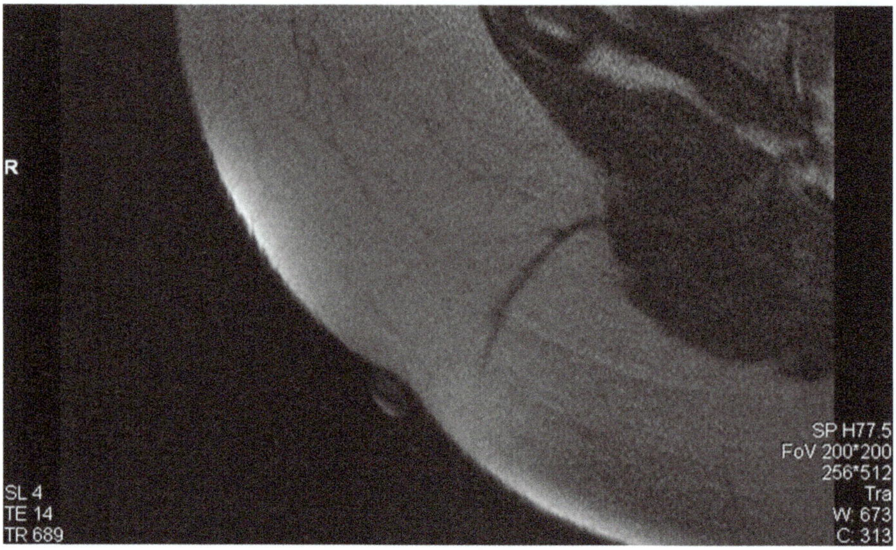

Fig. 2.2 MRI of the subcutaneous septa in cellulite depressed lesion

According to Querleux and colleagues, the results obtained with high-frequency ultrasound confirm an increase in skin thickness in women with cellulite, as well as the presence of deep indentations of adipose tissue into the skin [29]. The standing lobules, called papillae adipose, rise into pits and dells at the surface of the dermis [26].

The bumpy appearance of the skin surface results from the alteration of the network of connective tissue strands normally tethering the dermis to the deeper layers. Some strands are enlarged and fibrosclerotic, whereas other strands become loose. At the latter sites, edema and deposits of proteoglycans may be present in association with alterations in the shape and pattern of distribution of the elastic fibers [26].

The cutaneous alterations found in cellulite are largely due to the subcutaneous fibrous septa present in the dermis and/or in the subcutaneous tissue [14]. In women with cellulite, there are higher percentages of perpendicular fibers in comparison with women (and men) that do not have cellulite [24]. As for the fibers in other directions, women with cellulite have a lower percentage of parallel septa to the skin and higher percentage of angled septa [27]. Corroborating this information, Hexsel and colleagues compared areas of subcutaneous tissue with and without cellulite and have described the presence and characteristics of fibrous septa in the depressed lesions of cellulite (Fig. 2.2). The fibrous septa analyzed were all perpendicular to the skin surface. Furthermore, they were present in 96.7 % of the areas with cellulite depressions, while the percentage to those areas without cellulite was 16.7 % [12]. Under the influence of estrogen, fat is stored in women's buttocks and thighs. The more the fat is stored in predisposed areas, the more apparent is cellulite.

Table 2.1 Cellulite classification according to Nürnberger and Müller

0	No alteration to the skin surface
I	The skin of the affected area is smooth while the subject is standing or lying, but the alterations to the skin surface can be seen by pinching the skin or with muscle contraction
II	The orange skin or mattress appearance is evident when standing, without the use of manipulation (skin pinching or muscle contraction)
III	The alterations described in degree or stage II are present together with raised areas and nodules

2.5 Classification

The evaluation of the patient's degree of cellulite should be done before starting any treatment. This may interfere in the right choice of the procedure and is useful for follow-up of the results. A previous cellulite classification describes different grades from 0 to 3 and is based on the clinical alterations observed in three situations: with the patient at rest, after the application of the pinch test, or muscular contraction (Table 2.1) [24].

A new cellulite severity scale (CSS) and classification for cellulite was developed by Hexsel and colleagues [13]. This new scale has the purpose of creating an objective method to measure cellulite severity and the effects of different modalities. Five key clinical features of cellulite are evaluated:

A. The number of evident depressions
B. Depth of depressions
C. Morphological appearance of the skin surface alterations
D. Grade of laxity, flaccidity, or sagging skin
E. The classification scale originally described by Nürnberger and Müller

The severity of each item is graded from 0 to 3, allowing a final sum of scores that range numerically from 1 to 15. Based on the final numeric score, cellulite is classified as mild, moderate, or severe [13].

Cellulite can be either classified in primary or secondary cellulite. In the primary cellulite there are no causal factors involved, such as previous trauma. In the secondary cellulite, the alterations are due to other factors, such as surgical trauma, mainly from liposuction, injections that cause lipoatrophy, or subcutaneous fibrosis from previous inflammatory or infectious process [14].

2.6 Diagnosis

It is important to ask the patient about medical history and regarding the age at which cellulite appeared, as well as prior occurrence of trauma, liposuction or injections on the affected area, presence of chronic vascular or associated hormonal disorders, and use of any medication that may contribute to the increase in the deposit of fat in the affected area. Diagnosis of the cellulite is done mainly on clinical basis during the physical examination with the patient in the standing position.

Cellulite normally occurs in areas with fat accumulation, such as buttocks, thighs, flanks, abdomen, and upper legs [14, 30]. The characteristic appearance of cellulite is the presence of depressions on the cutaneous surface, surrounded or not by elevations. The depressions can be deep or superficial, single or multiple. The lesions are essentially asymptomatic; nevertheless, sensation of heaviness and pain may occur in the affected areas in advanced degrees of cellulite, probably as a result of nervous terminal compression or inflammatory reactions [14].

For the initial evaluation, it is also important to make an anthropometrical examination, which consists of measuring weight, height, and calculating the body mass index. It is a good method also to evaluate obesity [32], a condition that is associated with the worst degree of cellulite.

Digital photographs should be taken at the initial evaluation and after treatment and should follow the same standardized light patterns, position, and camera settings [17].

Rarely, complementary exams may be indicated for some cases or for research purposes. Ultrasound can be used to study the thickness and the quality of the connective tissue and the edematous component of cellulite [2]. Ultrasound imaging of the skin affected by cellulite at this stage reveals thinning of the dermis with subcutaneous fat pushing upward, which translates into the rumpled skin known as cellulite [7].

Laser Doppler flowmetry (LDF) is an optical technique used to evaluate skin microcirculation which provides information on blood flow and erythema. The radiation is reflected by the skin and converted to electrical signal, which is proportional to the flux of erythrocytes of the blood flow. Hence, it consists in a reliable method to estimate cutaneous microcirculation [2].

Thermography is an effective technique to evaluate the local skin temperature. It is based on the detection of infrared radiation emitted by skin. Areas affected by cellulite present less local skin blood flow, presenting thus lower temperature [2].

Magnetic resonance imaging (MRI) allows to visualize changes in skin architecture caused by cellulite – pointing out clearly in the images the skin fat layers beneath the dermis and down to the level of muscles – as well as to quantify herniations of adipose tissue into the dermis. It is a good method to evaluate cellulite in clinical trials [2] and also to determine anatomical features of cellulite [12].

2.7 Treatments

Many different treatments have been proposed to treat the cellulite. Weight loss is frequently employed as well as skin massage and a variety of topical agents. Mechanical devices, surgical procedures, and oral supplements can also be recommended [31]. Aerobic exercise is capable to burn fat deposits and to improve the body contour.

2.7.1 Manual Lymphatic Drainage

It is performed through compressions over specific lymphatic system sites intending to improve lymphatic flow by removing lymph from tissues. There are four different techniques for manual lymphatic drainage [22]: stationary circles technique, pump technique, scoop technique, and rotary technique.

2.7.2 Topical Treatment

Topical agents are often used by women to treat cellulite. Normally, they are recommended to treat mild-to-moderate cellulite and as an adjuvant treatment for severe cellulite.

Topical anticellulite preparations may be divided in four major groups according to the mechanism of action of its compounds. Active substances used in topical treatments for cellulite act by increasing the microcirculation flow, reducing lipogenesis and promoting lipolysis, restoring the normal structure of dermis and subcutaneous tissue, and preventing free radical formation or scavenge free radicals. Such products normally come in the form of creams, lotions, and gels. These products, which act in both the health and beauty of the skin, have been recently defined as cosmeceuticals and comprise a category placed between cosmetics and pharmaceuticals [11].

The methylxanthines are commonly added in cellulite products. The most used are caffeine, aminophylline, and theophylline, and they are used because of their proposed effect on adipocyte lipolysis via inhibition of phosphodiesterase and increasing cyclic adenosine monophosphate (AMP) [11, 31].

Many herbal extracts are used in slimming products such as verbena, green tea, lemon, and kola nut. The results would be an improvement of the peripheral microcirculation and to facilitate lymphatic drainage [11, 31]. The use of retinoids is shown to be efficient. It increases the dermal content and architecture of collagen and dermoepidermal proteins together with anchoring and elastic fibrils [11, 31].

The clinical efficacy of many active ingredients is limited owing to their inability to penetrate the corneal stratum barrier. For this reason, some topical formulations include skin enhancers, which are substances capable of augmenting cutaneous penetration of the active ingredients [15]. Vitamins, such as ascorbic acid and vitamin E, may work as antioxidants, protecting dermal and subcutaneous cell membranes from free radical toxicity [11].

2.7.3 Oral Treatment

Formulations taken orally also have to reach and act in the target site. Distante and colleagues have proved that plant extracts such as grape (*Vitis vinifera*), *Ginkgo biloba*, Asiatic centella, melilotus (*Melilotus officinalis*), and fucus (*Fucus vesiculosus*) contained in orally administered medication show good bioavailability and are effective in improving all clinical signs and symptoms associated to cellulite [6]. The extract of fucus has an important effect on peripheral fat tissue. Results of a study testing the effect in vitro of wild yam root (*Dioscorea opposita*), cocoa bean (*Theobroma cacao*), horse chestnut tree seed (*Aesculus hippocastanum*), horse chestnut tree bark (*A. hippocastanum*), and tomato (*Solanum ycopersicum*) in adipocytes suggest that those plant extracts have the potential to modulate glycerol release from the adipocytes, stimulating the reduction of fat content in adipose tissue [4].

2.7.4 Endermologie®

It is a French-designed method of deep massage approved also by the United States Food and Drug Administration (FDA) to diminish the appearance of cellulite. During the massage, suction is used to pull the skin into a handheld machine where the skin is compressed and rolled to increase blood and lymphatic flow and to modify the underlying connective tissue [30].

One side effect related to this type of treatment is the possible increase of cutaneous laxity. Besides that, it is not recommended to pregnant women and to people that present with hypertension, diabetes, circulatory disabilities, or excessive skin flaccidity conditions.

2.7.5 Radiofrequency

Radiofrequency (RF) efficiency for different aesthetic and dermatological applications is due to the use of thermal energy, which contracts loose, lax skin through collagen denaturalization. When the collagen is heated, the bonds that are sensitive to heat begin to break and originate a disorganized gel rather than the previous organized crystalline structure. Collagen contraction occurs when the tension of residual crossed intermolecular unions stabilizes to heat. The amount of the tissue contraction depends on various factors, including the highest reached temperature, the RF exposure time, and the mechanical stress applied to the tissue during the heating process [27]. Pino and colleagues [27] have demonstrated that the effect of RF over the connective tissue was evident in the ultrasound images where a visible compression of the entire thickness of the dermis to the muscle could be appreciated but with better results on the thigh. Radiofrequency is indicated for treating cellulite mainly caused or influenced by skin laxity.

2.7.6 Lasers and Lights and Combinations

TriActive™ (Cynosure, Westford, MA, USA) is an FDA-approved device which combines a localized cooling, six diode lasers, and mechanical massage [1]. The low temperature reduces edema, the laser favors blood and lymphatic flow, and the mechanical massage increases local drainage.

VelaShape™ (Syneron Medical Ltd., Yokneam Illit, Israel) is a system based on the application of an infrared light to the skin combined to RF energies and vacuum suction pulses [35]. The IR and RF act synergically, promoting heating in the target tissue, collagen remodeling, and improvement of the adipose tissue metabolic rate. The negative pressure vacuum massage improves circulation and also allows the treatment of both the superficial and deep dermal layers [3]. A recent study has showed the effects of this device on the reduction of cellulite severity and body circumference measures in the buttocks [17].

SmoothShapes™ (Cynosure, Westford, MA, USA) is also approved by FDA and combines 915-nm laser and 615-nm light to mechanical massage. It stimulates metabolism, reducing edema and thus improving the skin appearance. Another relevant effect is over collagen, remodeling the fiber and consequently improving skin appearance. Studies [19, 20] have demonstrated both the safety and efficacy of this device in subjects treated over a 4–6-week period.

2.7.7 Liposuction

Liposuction involves the removal of local adipose tissue deposits to achieve a grater aesthetic body contour. It requires general or local tumescent anesthesia and the use of a small tip suction cannula to remove fat from the selected areas, without altering other skin tissues. Liposuction may decrease the appearance of cellulite because it reduces the local fat volume, and it may also disrupt the fibrous bands that cause the dimpling appearance of the skin surface [30]. Despite that, alterations of the cutaneous surface may result from liposuction being caused by subcutaneous fibrosis. They usually appear late, from 3 months to 1 year after surgery, and may be slight, moderate, or severe [14].

2.7.8 Mesotherapy

Mesotherapy was developed in France, where it is well known and frequently used. It comprises injections of very small doses of solutions – composed by some active substances – into the skin at 2–6 mm depths. Its objective is to inject the medication directly on the affected site. These substances present vascular and lipolytic action [5, 23]. Although the design of injectables is more detailed, among other cautions, extreme care should be taken to ensure the sterility of the formulation.

2.7.9 Subcision®

Subcision® was developed as a treatment for cellulite by Dr. Hexsel and Dr. Mazzuco [9]. It is a surgical technique that does not require incisions and leave no scars. A needle is introduced into the skin, and it is used to cut the fibrous septa responsible for the depressed lesions of cellulite [10].

In this book you will find a specific chapter about Subcision®, in which further information and explanation will be provided.

2.7.10 Carboxytherapy

Carboxytherapy is the therapeutic use of carbon dioxide (CO_2) in its gaseous state, either by transcutaneous or subcutaneous injections. It seems to increase vascular tone and produces active microcirculatory vasodilatation due to the action of CO_2 on arteriole smooth muscle cells. By improving capillary blood flow, it reduces stasis and contributes to the restoration of microvascular tissue unit exchanges [21].

2.8 Prognosis

Cellulite is worsened by age, skin laxity, and weight gain. One of the causes that exacerbate cellulite seems to be the repeated cyclical collagenase production during women's life, in which more and more dermal collagen is destroyed. If the amount of collagen destroyed is enough to weaken the reticular and papillary dermis, it will allow subcutaneous dermis to herniate among the structural fibrous septa found in female fat. If higher amount of subcutaneous fat is present, there will be a more pronounced herniation [12].

The skin laxity, a condition which is also related to the aging process, worsens the cellulite.

Weight gain may also worsen this condition. Weight loss has been suggested as a strategy to reduce cellulite by decreasing the dermal papillae adipose herniation, but it may not affect the underlying connective tissue network [33].

Conclusion

Cellulite is a very common condition which has been more studied in past few decades. Many morphological and physiological aspects have been described, but the precise cellulite's etiology has not been established yet. Many factors are involved in cellulite, such as adipocyte hypertrophy, microcirculation disorders and venous stasis, and connective tissue abnormalities and fibrosis. Recently, hormonal influences in collagen are being mentioned as a relevant cause for cellulite. Skin laxity has also been regarded as another relevant contributor to worsen cellulite, especially in older women. Besides the far known treatments such as diet, exercises, and lymphatic drainage, several other treatments have been developed lately presenting successful results. Devices, such as laser, lights and radiofrequency, are being used to treat this condition as well.

References

1. Avram MM (2004) Cellulite: a review of its physiology and treatment. J Cosmet Laser Ther 6(4):181–185
2. Biefeldt S, Buttgereit P, Brandt M et al (2008) Non-invasive evaluation techniques to quantify the efficacy of cosmetic anti-cellulite products. Skin Res Technol 14(3):336–346

3. Brightman L, Weiss E, Chapas AM et al (2009) Improvement in arm and postpartum abdominal and flank subcutaneous fat deposits and skin laxity using a bipolar radiofrequency, infrared, vacuum and mechanical massage device. Lasers Surg Med 41(10):791–798
4. Cals-Grierson MM (2007) Modulation of activity of the adipocyte aquaglyceroporin channel by plant extracts. Int J Cosmet Sci 29(1):7–14
5. Caruso MK, Roberts AT, Bissoon L et al (2008) An evaluation of mesotherapy solutions for inducing lipolysis and treating cellulite. J Plast Reconstr Aesthet Surg 61:1321–1324
6. Distante F, Bacci PA, Carrera M (2006) Efficacy of a multifunctional plant complex in the treatment of the so called 'cellulite': clinical and instrumental evaluation. Int J Cosmet Sci 28:191–206
7. Draelos ZD (2005) The disease of cellulite. J Cosmet Dermatol 4:221–222
8. Goldman MP (2002) Cellulite: a review of current treatments. Cosmet Dermatol 15(2):17–20
9. Hexsel DM, Mazzuco R (2000) Subcision: a treatment for cellulite. Int J Dermatol 39(7): 539–544
10. Hexsel D, Mazzuco R (2006) Subcision®. In: Goldman MP, Bacci PA, Leibaschoff G, Hexsel D, Angelini F (eds) Cellulite: pathophysiology and treatment. Taylor & Francis, New York, pp 251–262
11. Hexsel D, Soirefmann M (2011) Cosmeceuticals for cellulite. Semin Cutan Med Surg 30(3):167–170
12. Hexsel DM, Abreu M, Rodrigues TC et al (2009) Side-by-side comparison of areas with and without cellulite depressions using magnetic resonance imaging. Dermatol Surg 35(10): 1471–1477
13. Hexsel DM, Dal'forno T, Hexsel CL (2009) A validated photonumeric cellulite severity scale. J Eur Acad Dermatol Venereol 23(5):523–528
14. Hexsel D, Dal'Forno T, Mazzuco R (2010) Definition, clinical aspects, classifications, and diagnostic technique. In: Goldman MP, Hexsel D (eds) Cellulite: pathophysiology and treatment, 2nd edn. Taylor & Francis, New York, pp 13–23
15. Hexsel D, Orlandi C, Zechmeister do Prado D (2005) Botanical extracts used in the treatment of cellulite. Dermatol Surg 31(7 Pt 2):866–872
16. Hexsel DM, Porto MD, Siega C et al Comparative study on the anatomy of adipose tissue in areas with and without raised lesions of cellulite using magnetic resonance imaging. Under submission to Dermatol Surg
17. Hexsel DM, Siega C, Schilling-Souza J et al (2011) A bipolar radiofrequency, infrared, vacuum and mechanical massage device for treatment of cellulite: a pilot study. J Cosmet Laser Ther 13(6):297–302
18. Khan MH, Victor F, Rao B, Sadick NS (2010) Treatment of cellulite: part I. Pathophysiology. J Am Acad Dermatol 62(3):361–370; quiz 371–372
19. Kulick MI (2010) Evaluation of a noninvasive, dual-wavelength laser-suction and massage device for the regional treatment of cellulite. Plast Reconstr Surg 125(6):1788–1796
20. Lach E (2008) Reduction of subcutaneous fat and improvement in cellulite appearance by dual-wavelength, low-level laser energy combined with vacuum and massage. J Cosmet Laser Ther 10(4):202–209
21. Leibaschoff G (2006) Carboxitherapy. In: Goldman MP, Bacci PA, Leibaschoff G, Hexsel D, Angelini F (eds) Cellulite: pathophysiology and treatment. Taylor & Francis, New York, pp 197–210
22. Leibaschoff G (2006) Manual lymphatic drainage. In: Goldman MP, Bacci PA, Leibaschoff G, Hexsel D, Angelini F (eds) Cellulite: pathophysiology and treatment. Taylor & Francis, New York, pp 287–290
23. Leibaschoff G, Steiner D (2006) Mesotherapy. In: Goldman MP, Bacci PA, Leibaschoff G, Hexsel D, Angelini F (eds) Cellulite: pathophysiology and treatment. Taylor & Francis, New York, pp 263–286
24. Nürnberger F, Müller G (1978) So-called cellulite: an invented disease. J Dermatol Surg Oncol 4(3):221–229
25. Ortonne JP, Zartarian M, Verschoore M et al (2008) Cellulite and skin ageing: is there any interaction? J Eur Acad Dermatol Venereol 22(7):827–834

26. Piérard GE (2005) Commentary on cellulite: skin mechanobiology and the waist-to-hip. J Cosmet Dermatol 4(3):151–152
27. Pino ME, Rosado RH, Azuela A et al (2006) Effect of controlled volumetric tissue heating with radiofrequency on cellulite and the subcutaneous tissue of the buttocks and thighs. J Drugs Dermatol 5(8):714–722
28. Pugliese PT (2007) The pathogenesis of cellulite: a new concept. J Cosmet Dermatol 6:140–142
29. Querleux B, Cornillon C, Jolivet Q, Bittoun J (2002) Anatomy and physiology of subcutaneous adipose tissue by in vivo magnetic resonance imaging and spectroscopy: relationships with sex and presence of cellulite. Skin Res Technol 8(2):118–124
30. Rao J, Gold MH, Goldman MP (2005) A two-center, double-blinded, randomized trial testing the tolerability and efficacy of a novel therapeutic agent for cellulite reduction. J Cosmet Dermatol 4(2):93–102
31. Rawlings AV (2006) Cellulite and its treatments. Int J Cosmet Sci 28:175–190
32. Rossi ABR, Vergnanini AL (2000) Cellulite: a review. J Eur Acad Dermatol Venereol 14:251–262
33. Smalls LK, Lee CY, Ehitestone J et al (2005) Quantitative model of cellulite: three dimensional skin surface topography, biophysical characterization and relationship to human perception. Int J Cosmet Sci 27:295–297
34. Terranova F, Berardesca E, Maibach H (2006) Cellulite: nature and aetiopathogenesis. Int J Cosmet Sci 28:157–167
35. Wanitphakdeedecha R, Manuskiatti W (2006) Treatment of cellulite with a bipolar radiofrequency, infrared heat, and pulsatile suction device: a pilot study. J Cosmet Dermatol 5(4): 284–288

Acne

3

Gabriella Fabbrocini and Maria Pia De Padova

Core Messages

- Acne is a chronic inflammatory, exclusively human disease of the pilosebaceous unit, mostly affecting the sebaceous gland follicles – usually referred to as sebaceous follicles – located on the face, chest, shoulders, and back, where they are most common.
- Acne is the most common disease affecting all ages and ethnic groups and is the leading dermatologic diagnosis with 10.2 million diagnoses. Acne is considered a problem that occurs in adolescence, but the prevalence of adult acne is 3 % in men and between 11 and 12 % in women.
- We can distinguish different types of acne: acne neonatorum and infantile, acne vulgaris (teenage acne), adult acne, acne conglobata, acne inversa, and acne fulminans.
- Diet, weight loss, sunlight, and cosmetics/drugs are differently related to acne symptoms.
- The treatment of acne is based on different approaches such as cosmetological and cleansing agents, moisturizing agents, sebum regulators, keratolytics, and photoprotection to support medical treatment based on topical (retinoids, antibiotics, alpha hydroxy acids, and chemical peels) and systemic medical treatment (oral antibiotics, oral isotretinoin, hormonal therapy).

G. Fabbrocini (✉)
Department of Dermatology, University of Naples Federico II,
Via Sergio Pansini, 5 – 80132 Naples, Italy
e-mail: gafabbro@unina.it

M.P. De Padova
Department of Dermatology, "Nigrisoli" Hospital – Bologna,
Viale Ercolani, 9 – 40138 Bologna, Italy
e-mail: depadova.mariapia@libero.it

A. Tosti, D. Hexsel (eds.), *Update in Cosmetic Dermatology*,
DOI 10.1007/978-3-642-34029-1_3, © Springer-Verlag Berlin Heidelberg 2013

3.1 Introduction

Acne is a chronic inflammatory, exclusively human disease of the pilosebaceous unit, mostly affecting the sebaceous gland follicles – usually referred to as sebaceous follicles – located on the face, chest, shoulders, and back, where they are most common. Acne is a problem which has been argued for hundreds of years without any completely satisfactory conclusion being reached. The ancient Greek physicians certainly recognized a condition which Aristotle [1] describes in sufficient detail for there to be little doubt of the identification. Hippocrates [2] also uses the term, but does not state what he means by it, although his wording suggests that it was a well-known and recognized disease. The early Roman physicians, on the other hand, used the word "varus" which is mentioned by Pliny [3] and discussed briefly by Celsus [4]. Acne cannot be regarded as a serious disease or measured in terms of life and death, but it has a nuisance value out of all proportion to its seriousness, affecting, as it does, young people at an age when they are most sensitive to any disfigurement. In fact, acne is considered a common and difficult condition that can affect many aspects of an individual's health-related quality of life. The psychosocial effects of acne can produce anxiety, depression, and other psychological problems [5].

3.2 Incidence

Acne is the most common disease affecting all ages and ethnic groups and is the leading dermatologic diagnosis with 10.2 million diagnoses (25.4 % of the ten most common dermatologic diagnoses) according to a National Ambulatory Medical Care Survey conducted in 1995 in the USA. Although acne is commonly considered a problem that occurs in adolescence (acne affects about 85 % of all adolescents), an increasing number of patients over 25 years of age are consulting for this condition, and most of these are women. The prevalence of adult acne is 3 % in men and between 11 and 12 % in women [6] with a significant decline from 45 years of age [7].

3.3 Classification

3.3.1 Acne Neonatorum

Acne neonatorum occurs in up to 20 % of newborns [8]; it is quite common and is not associated with a later development of acne vulgaris. It typically consists of closed comedones on the forehead, nose, and cheeks, although other locations are possible. Open comedones, inflammatory papules, and pustules can also develop. Neonatal acne is thought to result from stimulation of sebaceous glands by maternal or infant androgens. Parents should be counseled that lesions usually resolve spontaneously within 4 months without scarring. Treatment generally is not indicated, but infants can be treated with a 2.5 % benzoyl peroxide lotion if lesions are extensive and persist for several months [9]. Parents should apply a small amount of benzoyl peroxide to the antecubital fossa to test for local reaction before widespread or facial application. Severe, unrelenting neonatal acne accompanied by other signs of hyperandrogenism should prompt an investigation for adrenal cortical hyperplasia, virilizing tumors, or underlying endocrinopathies.

3.3.2 Infantile Acne

Infantile acne is a rare occurrence and has its onset at 3–6 months and is less common than neonatal acne. It is more common in boys and predominately occurs on the cheeks. Clinically, the lesions range from comedones to inflammatory papulopustules to cysts. Successful therapies include topical tretinoin, benzoyl peroxide, and topical and oral erythromycin. For more serious cases, oral isotretinoin has been reported to successfully treat recalcitrant infantile cystic acne [10, 11]. It is probably associated with a premature secretion of gonad androgens. These patients may develop severe acne as teenagers.

3.3.3 Acne Vulgaris (Teenage Years)

Acne vulgaris is the most frequent form of acne and resolves slowly after the teenage years. Before and during puberty acne vulgaris may arise as result of hormonal changes. Adrenal maturation and gonadal development cause androgen production and subsequent sebaceous gland enlargement. It usually starts at puberty, progresses until the age of 17 or 18, and regresses in the 30s, often leaving indelible scars for the rest of the patient's life. It may involve the chest, the back, and particularly the face (Fig. 3.1). Acne vulgaris is more frequent, but less severe in women than men, and it involves more frequently face in women, but chest in men. Its evolution is unpredictable with the tendency to complete or incomplete remissions particularly in summertime and subintrant exacerbations at the time of the menses, with overwork, etc.

Lesions of all the various stages can be seen at the same time.

3.3.4 Adult Acne

Adult acne can be a continuation of teenage acne or appear de novo. There are no known reasons for why acne persists into adulthood. Women with persistent acne do have greater sebum secretion than those without, and tobacco appears to be a predisposing factor for the condition. Noninflammatory acne (with micro- and macrocomedones) was reported to be more common in women smokers than nonsmokers in the 25–50-year-old age bracket (41.5–9.7 %) [12], a fact confirmed by a subsequent study of male and female patients aged 1–87 years where a greater prevalence was observed among smokers (40.8 %) than nonsmokers (25.5 %) [13]. Tobacco therefore appears to be an aggravating factor for preexisting acne, or a factor for triggering acne in those with a predisposition, rather than a primary cause of the condition. Adult acne may differ clinically showing fewer comedones and more

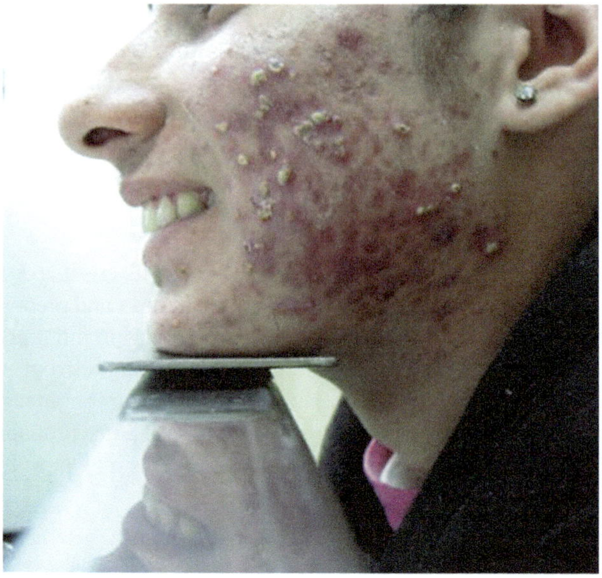

Fig. 3.1 Acne vulgaris

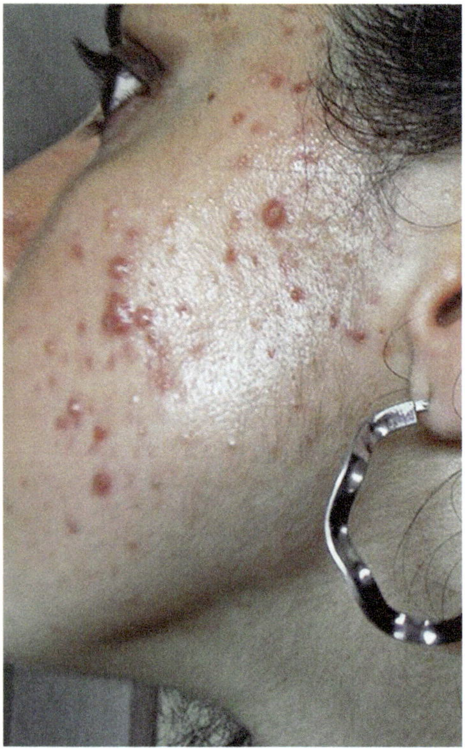

Fig. 3.2 Adult acne

inflammation, affecting most commonly the perioral, chin, and jawline regions (Fig. 3.2). Gary et al. [14] evaluated the incidence of mature acne, and they found that the majority (76 %) of patients with postadolescent acne are women. Of these women, 37 % had features of hyperandrogenicity. External factors including cosmetics, drugs, and occupation have no significant etiological role.

3.3.5 Acne Conglobata

Acne conglobata is a disease characterized by the presence of cystic abscesses, confluent follicular and perifollicular inflammations, and intercommunicating cysts. These lesions affect primarily the face, neck, chest, and shoulders and are the cause of serious and disfiguring scars. This disorder typically begins in adulthood and presents as numerous comedones, papules, pustules, nodules, abscesses, and draining sinus tracts involving the chest, back, and buttocks. These lesions frequently become secondarily infected with gram-positive bacteria and often heal with scarring. Pathology usually reveals inflammatory infiltrate around follicles, which can often disrupt the normal dermal architecture. Acne conglobata is particularly disfiguring and socially detrimental to patients because of its chronicity, severity, and treatment challenge. Patients with this disease are usually from 15 to 25 years of age and have an antecedent history in most cases of acne vulgaris of varying degrees of severity. Acne conglobata may have a fulminating onset and course. Conventional therapy, consisting of antibiotics and local measures, is frequently disappointing. For this reason, systemic agents are indispensable. The choices include oral antibiotics, isotretinoin, and hormonal treatment.

3.3.6 Acne Inversa

Acne inversa (also known as hidradenitis suppurativa) is a chronically relapsing inflammatory disease that is characterized by recurrent draining sinuses and abscesses occurring predominantly in skin folds that carry terminal hairs and apocrine glands. Healing occurs with substantial scarring. Acne inversa has to be differentiated from furuncles, vegetating pyoderma, cutaneous tuberculosis, actinomycosis, lymphogranuloma inguinale, and Crohn's disease [15]. Treatment options include antiseptics, corticosteroids, and antibiotics, such as tetracycline, clindamycin, or rifampicin. Unfortunately, they have all been tried with limited success, and recurrence after stopping the therapy is very common, making the disease a source of frustration for dermatologist and patient alike. Surgical excision and drainage or exteriorization of individual lesions may be useful in the large nodular lesions. Carbon dioxide laser excision is another treatment option. In the last years, several studies have showed the effectiveness of etanercept in the treatment of acne inverse. Etanercept would be a safe and effective therapy for hidradenitis suppurativa and decrease the extent of the disease and improve the quality of life. Future studies are indicated to elucidate fully the role of etanercept in the treatment of hidradenitis suppurativa.

Table 3.1 Drugs that can cause or exacerbate acne

Drug or type l	Examples
Corticosteroids	
Topical	Betamethasone
Oral	Prednisolone
Inhaled	Budesonide
Anabolic steroids/synthetic	Danazol, nandrolone, androgens, stanozolol
Antiepileptics	Carbamazepine, phenytoin, gabapentin, topiramate
Antidepressants	Lithium, sertraline
Antipsychotics	Pimozide, risperidone
Antituberculous	Isoniazid, pyrazinamide
Antineoplastics	Dactinomycin, pentostatin
Antivirals	Ritonavir, ganciclovir
Calcium antagonists	Nilvadipine, nimodipine
Vitamins	Vitamin B12 and other B group vitamins
Miscellaneous	Buserelin Cabergoline Clofazimine Cyclosporin Dantrolene Famotidine Follitropin alpha Isosorbide mononitrate Medroxyprogesterone Mesalazine Ramipril

3.3.7 Acne Fulminans

Acne fulminans is a severe form of cystic acne primarily affecting Caucasian adolescent males. The systemic clinical manifestations of the disease make it likely that the patient will present to his or her primary care provider rather than to a dermatologist. Musculoskeletal symptoms and hematologic manifestations frequently accompany this disorder. It is a rare form of acne characterized by ulcerative nodules and associated with systemic complications. The cause of acne fulminans is not known. The pathogens grown from skin lesions do not differ from those cultured from the skin in acne vulgaris. An associated arthralgia or arthritis frequently occurs. Isotretinoin, prednisone, and minocycline are some of the treatments proposed. However, response to traditional acne therapies is poor.

3.3.8 Acne Cosmetica and Iatrogenic Acne

Acne cosmetic results from the use of cosmetic containing comedogenic substances (such as lanolin, certain vegetable oils, butyl stearate, lauryl alcohol, and oleic acid) and resolves with the cessation of the use of the causative agent. Moreover, there are several drugs that can cause or exacerbate acne (Table 3.1). For these reasons, any medical history must fully investigate family history and exclude the precipitating factors indicated above: medications and comedogenic cosmetics.

3.3.9 Acne Excoriée

Acne induces stress and picking of the spots will aggravate the appearance of the acne patient. This is particularly obvious in acne excoriée, which occurs predominantly in females and often results from personality or psychological problems.

3.4 Etiology

3.4.1 Classical Aspects of Acne Etiology

The etiology of acne is not yet fully clarified, but it is widely accepted that it is multifactorial, with abnormal follicular differentiation and increased cornification, enhanced sebaceous gland activity and hyperseborrhea, bacterial hypercolonization, as well as inflammation and immunological host reaction being the major contributors (see pathogenesis for more details). However, a lot of different factors, such as diet, weight loss, sunlight, and cosmetic, seem to have a controversial role in acne etiology.

3.4.2 Diet and Weight Loss

No direct link has been found between acne and diet [16, 17]. In particular, no effect has been established between chocolate, dairy products, shellfish, or fatty foods [20]. There are some dissenting studies [18] with criticism of studies looking at diet and acne, and some showing exogenous fatty acids can end up in sebaceous gland output. Weight loss and the use of metformin are both associated with lower plasma insulin levels and decreased androgen levels. Insulin-like growth factor levels are reported to be elevated in acne [19, 20]. Hyperinsulinemia can be triggered by some dietary habits such as milk protein consumption [21]. With hyperinsulinemia, there may be an increase in androgen production, resulting in a stimulation of sebaceous glands. It may be that in a small subset of obese acne patients, hyperinsulinemia may stimulate endogenous androgen production resulting in development or worsening of acne. For this cohort of acne patients, a weight loss diet may be indicated [22].

3.4.3 Sunlight and Cosmetics

Although there has been little evidence that sunlight has any reliable beneficial effect on acne [23] and even less so for the role of solariums, there has been a resurgence of interest in this area. Rarely, acne may worsen with sunlight [24]. However, visible light may be relatively benign and useful in treatment by stimulating the natural porphyrins produced by *P. acnes*. Blue and other longer wavelengths may induce a toxic effect on the bacteria inducing their destruction and lessening the clinical disease [25, 26]. This may be augmented by the use of exogenous porphyrins utilizing photodynamic therapy [27, 28]. Some years ago many cosmetics contained comedogenic agents that blocked follicular structures and induced comedonal disease on the cheeks of females. There are still preparations that contain comedogenic substances such as isopropyl myristate. However, as most manufacturers now produce reasonably noncomedogenic products, cosmetics are now an uncommon cause for acneiform conditions [29–31].

3.5 Pathophysiology

Hyperproliferation of the follicular epithelium leads to formation of microcomedones, which are the first acne lesions and can be found in normal-looking skin [32]. The very early stage of acne lesion development, namely, the beginning of microcomedones, is associated with vascular endothelial cell activation and involvement of inflammatory events [33], which corroborates the suggestion that acne may represent a genuine inflammatory disorder without involvement of bacteria in its initiation [34]. Active sebaceous glands are needed for the development of acne. A microscopic plug forms owing to an excess of sebum production and an abnormal keratinization of the follicular lining. Accumulation of this material causes distention. In addition, the enlarged pilosebaceous structure allows the normal follicular bacterium *Propionibacterium acnes* to proliferate, releasing free fatty acids, which are inflammatory. The distended follicular may rupture, causing further inflammatory reaction, leading to the formation of papules, pustules, cystis, and nodules. However, ongoing research is modifying the classical view of acne pathogenesis through identification of upstream mechanisms.

Androgens, skin lipids, inflammatory signaling, and regulatory neuropeptides seem to be mainly involved in this multifactorial process. Moreover, susceptibility is influenced by genetic factors: identical twins, but not nonidentical twins, had identical rates of sebum excretion but different acne severities. This indicates a genetic control of sebum excretion with modification of the development of clinical lesions by environmental factors [35]. Interestingly, evidence of direct genetic association of acne with androgen and lipid abnormalities has been observed: neonatal acne was found to be associated with familial hyperandrogenism [36], inadequate activity of steroid 21-hydroxylase as well as CYP21 gene mutations has been reported to be involved in the pathogenesis of acne [37], and identical sebum excretion rates were described in homozygotic but not in heterozygotic twins. Several clinical observations point to a major role of androgens in the pathogenesis of acne. Androgens play an essential role in increasing the size of sebaceous glands and stimulating sebum production [38] as well as in stimulating keratinocyte proliferation in the ductus seboglandularis and the acroinfundibulum [39, 40]. There is current evidence that regulatory neuropeptides with hormonal and nonhormonal activity may control the development of clinical inflammation in acne. Numerous substance P-immunoreactive nerve fibers were detected in close opposition to the sebaceous glands, and expression of the substance P-inactivating enzyme neutral endopeptidase was observed within sebaceous germinative cells of acne patients [41]. Acne vulgaris is likely to be a genuine inflammatory disease with androgens, regulatory neuropeptides, and environmental factors being agents able to interrupt the natural cycling of the sebaceous follicles and lead microcomedones to form comedones and inflammatory lesion.

3.6 Diagnosis

Acne diagnosis is generally trouble-free, supported by clinical anamnestic information that can help dermatologist to evaluate a potential not common etiology (acneiform drug reaction, halogen acne caused by iodides and bromides). The sprouting of typical acne lesions (comedones, papules, pustules, and nodules) on the face, on the chest, and on the neck is pathognomonic. At times, acne could result in differential diagnosis with a lot of dermatologic disease: in occupational acne, skin lesions are localized in unusual sites as legs and there are no nodules. Acne inverse (hidradenitis suppurativa) affects parts of the body such as the groin and armpits, the breasts, and the hair follicles. Rosacea is characterized by persistent erythema and telangiectasia predominantly of the cheeks frequently followed by papules and pustules but not comedones, the elementary lesion of acne. Perioral dermatitis (probably a rosacea-like disease) affects mostly perioral area and seldom periorbital area. Lupus miliaris disseminatus (granulomatous rosacea) is an uncommon, chronic, inflammatory dermatosis characterized by red-to-yellow or yellow-brown papules of the central face, particularly on and around the eyelids. Pseudofolliculitis of the beard (razor bumps) can make the skin look itchy and red, and in some cases, it can even look like pimples. These inflamed papules or pustules can form especially if the area becomes infected. The extrafollicular hair is a hair that has exited the follicle and reentered the skin. The transfollicular hair never exits the follicle, but because of its naturally curly nature, it curls back into the follicle causing fluid buildup and irritation. The red papules and papular nodules lesions affect the submandibular area. Sometimes, syphilide's follicular lesions could be similar to acne papules.

3.7 Histology

Acne is associated to many histological features. Follicular close-up is a mass of corneocytes strictly collected all around a nonpigmented hair (vellus hair). Microcomedones are visible as sebaceous follicles with a hyperplastic follicular epithelium and a huge lumen colonized by desquamation materials and many bacteria. Slowly the microcomedo could become a closed comedo or an open comedo. Closed comedo (whitehead) is cystic formation of variable dimensions (0.5–2 mm). The entire pilosebaceous unit is distended with inspissated materials (sebum and corneous laminar layers). Follicular epithelium is reduced with atrophy of the sebaceous grapes. All around the microcomedo, we can find atypical ductal structures. Blackheads, also known as open comedo, are follicles that have a wider than normal opening. They are filled with plugs of sebum and sloughed-off cells and have undergone a chemical reaction resulting in the oxidation of melanin. This gives the material in the follicle the typical black color. Papules and pustules can be the evolution of a microcomedo or represent the inflammatory evolution of an open or a closed comedo: we find a huge phlogistic process, spongiosis, and lymphoid cells. Papules and pustules histologically represent suppurative folliculitis with epidermal or dermal perifolliculitis. Sebaceous follicle is expanded with inclusions of leukocytes, keratin, and lipids. Nodules are described as a dermal phlogistic process, nondelimitable, with suppurative elements with a lot of white cells, keratinic fragments, some lymphoid cells, and histiocytes. Acne cysts are not true cysts in the sense that they are not abnormal dilations of skin structure, but rather nodules of inflammation. Cysts or nodules are blockages of oil glands that have burst open and produced inflammation and pus in the surrounding tissue. These lesions have the potential to produce long-term scarring. Acne scars are associated with a loss of collagen. In superficial and medium derma, we can find a sclerotic connective tissue.

3.8 Prognosis

The beginning of clinical signs is usually associated at puberty, and after 4–5 years, we can have the maximum severity grade, to end up approximately in 20–25-year-old patients. Mild acne could regress without scars signs, while in many cases of moderate or severe acne, we can have pigmented zones or atrophic, hypertrophic, and keloidal scars. Acne lesions are esthetically unacceptable and could have negative effect on the psychological attitude of the younger patients, conditioning their quality of life. For some of them, acne could become a dysmorphophobic disease with social isolation. The patient's perception of his disease seems to influence mostly than the severity of the lesions.

3.9 Treatment

Every one of the pathogenetic factors of acne (androgen stimulation, sebaceous hypersecretion, abnormal keratinization, *P. acnes* infection, and inflammation process) could represent a target for the therapy. Combined therapy for acne represents the best therapeutic approach and the most used by dermatologist. Topical therapy could have a cosmetological or a pharmaceutical approach.

Table 3.2 Tensioactives

Cleansing agents: tensioactives	
Anionics	Sodium lauryl sulfate, sodium laureth sulfate, TEA-lauryl sulfate, ammonium lauryl sulfate, sodium stearate
Cationics	Quaternium 15 quaternium, stearalkonium chloride, quaternium stearalkonium hectorite
Anfoterum	Cocamidopropyl betaine, coco-betaine, disodium cocamphodiacetate, CAP-hydroxisulfataine, disodium lauroamphodipropionate
Nonionics	Polysorbate 20, cocamide DEA, lauramide DEA, polysorbate 60, laureth

3.9.1 Cosmetological Approach

The definition of cosmetic is really changed in the last years: we can now talk of cosmeceuticals. These are cosmetic products that are claimed, primarily by those within the cosmetic industry, to have drug-like benefits. Examples of products typically labeled as cosmeceuticals include antiaging creams and moisturizers. The word is a portmanteau of the words "cosmetic" and "pharmaceutical." A successful cosmeceutical could prevent the outbreak of irritative phenomena, improving the penetration of the active principles alleviating the clinical situation (especially for the prevention of acne scarring) and the quality of life of the patients. An appropriate cosmeceutical for acne patient must observe severe scientific requirement: its structural components should not be comedogenic, with no irritative or allergic capability. They should be easy to use and pleasant to the patient.

The most important cosmetics in acne are: cleansing agents, moisturizers, sebum regulator, and keratolytics.

3.9.1.1 Cleansing Agents

A successful detersion in acne patients is very important because it favors the removal of the excess of sebum and of desquamated corneocytes, helping in containing the presence of bacteria on the skin. All this process must respect skin's physiological and structural equilibrium. Nevertheless, often detersion is made with no control both on the typology and the quantity of the product to use. Dermatologist has to value singularly the detersion process, helping patients to understand how to make it and about the frequency of washing. So, choosing a cleanser, the dermatologist must value skin type, pharmaceutical prescription regimen, atmospherical season (temperature, wetness), washing frequency, and its modality. There are many types of cleansing agents: tensioactives, solubilization agents, absorbing agents, and abrasive cleanser. Tensioactives (Table 3.2) remove impurities utilizing their chemical features, able to link both on lipidic skin border and to hydrophilic one, reducing the interfacial tension. There are many cosmetic formulations to choose (liquids, gel, foams, solids). Solubilization cleansing agents remove impurities through formation of micelles. These cosmetics are the common cleansing milks, tonics, and water solutions. Absorbing agents are made up of astringents and siccative masks and of inorganic absorbing powders. Mechanical agents remove solid particles, keratin residues favoring comedolysis. These are scrub agents and twitch masks.

Table 3.3 Cosmetic agents in acne

Cosmetic agents	
Moisturizing	Zinc, aloe, thermal water, glycerine, camomile, hamamelis, bardana, azulene, calendula
Keratolytics	Glycolic acid, Pyruvic acid, salicylic acid, malic acid
Sebum regulators	Piroctone olamine, nicotinamide, Serenoa repens, zinc, phytosphingosine, lactic acids, liposomes

3.9.1.2 Moisturizing Agents

In acne patients, hyperseborrhea slows cutaneous water loss. So, dryness seems to be a secondary problem. But the use of aggressive topical product, as antibiotics and keratolytics, could induce a massive skin water loss damaging skin structures and hydrolipidic film. The most damageable topical agents are tensioactives, salicylic and glycolic acid, benzoyl peroxide, and topical and systemic retinoids. There are a lot of cosmetic moisturizing formulations (Table 3.3): emulsions are the favorite ones by the patients. In emulsions, the oil is dispersed as liquid droplets through the continuous phase, usually but not necessarily water. Water in oil emulsion is commonly named emollients: unfortunately, they offer an occlusive effect (to force skin water retention) and are not very appreciated by the patients. Emollients are often used in association with systemic retinoids. Oil in water emulsions is commonly named humectants: they had not occlusive effect due to the presence of highly hygroscopic agents in their formulation. They are used in association with hydroalcoholic solutions, benzoyl peroxide, and α-/β-hydroxy acids. The ideal moment to use a moisturizing emulsion is after detersion, not as an additional help but as an inalienable support.

3.9.1.3 Sebum Regulators

These agents (Table 3.3) can regulate sebaceous secretion. The sebaceous glands are under the control of gonadic and surrenalic androgens. The target of the sebum regulators is not yet well known, but it is surely linked to a biologic action on 5-alpha reductase or on a superficial sebum oxidation, to obtain an opaque effect. They can be used as emulsions, gel, and lotions. Piroctone olamine, nicotinamide [42], Serenoa repens, zinc [43], phytosphingosine [44], lactic acids, and liposomes [45] are the most important sebum regulators.

3.9.1.4 Keratolytics

In comedogenic acne, dermatologist uses cosmetic products to remove follicular obstruction and enhance cell turnover (Table 3.3). AHAs (alpha hydroxy acids: glycolic acid, malic acid) are the prototype of keratolytics and are used both in active acne and in the reduction of postacneic scars. Pyruvic acid [46], an alpha keto acid, has sebostatic, antimicrobial, and keratolytic activity. Salicylic acid [47], a beta hydroxyl acid, has anti-inflammatory and keratolytic activity. These products can be used in patients that are allergic to topical tretinoin.

3.9.1.5 Photoprotection

A lot of acneic patients associate a better clinical situation to the sun, probably linked to a less anxiety level and a masklike effect due to tan. It is important to recommend a specific photoprotection for all the acne patients, with specific products for acneic and seborrheic skin. These products, rigorously oil-free, containing sebum regulator agents, are gel or spray with physical-chemical filters.

3.9.2 Medical Treatment

Acne treatment is essentially based on pharmaceutical prescription. We can distinguish a topical and a systemic therapy.

3.9.2.1 Topical Medical Treatment

Retinoids

The retinoids [48] are a class of chemical compounds that are related chemically to vitamin A. There are first-generation retinoids which include retinol, retinal, tretinoin, isotretinoin, and alitretinoin, second-generation retinoids which include etretinate and its metabolite acitretin, and third-generation retinoids which include tazarotene, bexarotene, and adapalene. All the retinoids have the keratolytic effect and indirect anti-inflammatory properties inhibiting comedogenesis, preventing the transformation of microcomedo in comedo and the sprouting of inflammatory lesions. Most used topical retinoids are tretinoin, adapalene, tazarotene, and isotretinoin. Tretinoin has a great comedolytic and anticomedogenic action, an indirect antimicrobial action, and a weak anti-inflammatory effect. Adapalene is a third-generation retinoid with a better therapeutic profile than tretinoin: it has a huge anti-inflammatory action with less adverse effect (irritative dermatitis). Tazarotene has been introduced as a drug for the treatment of psoriasis, but for the high price, the strong cutaneous irritative process and the potential teratogenicity have become a second choice drug in acne. Topical isotretinoin has tretinoin similar properties with a stronger anti-inflammatory effect and less possibility of skin irritation (Fig. 3.3a, b).

Antibiotics

Most common topical antibiotics are clindamycin and erythromycin [49]. Topical antibiotics have a bacteriostatic and bactericide effect, reducing *P. acnes* colonization of the sebaceous follicle. Topical antibiotics have an indirect anti-inflammatory action too. Unfortunately, topical antibiotics, compared to systemics, have a slower and weaker action. The most important adverse effect of these drugs is the bacteria resistance induction. Topical antibiotics are not to be used in monotherapy. Associative schemes with zinc (anti-inflammatory activity), benzoyl peroxide (battericid agent with high anticomedogenic and anti-inflammatory properties), and azelaic acid (anticomedogenic and antimicrobial effect) enhance the bactericide effect reducing the risk of drug resistance. Less important adverse effects liked to topical antibiotics are erythema, itching, and xerosis.

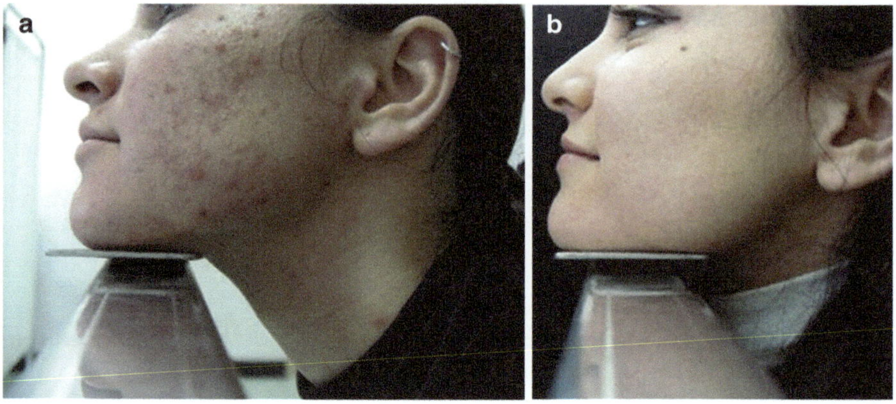

Fig. 3.3 (**a**) Patient pretreatment with topical retinoids. (**b**) Patient posttreatment with topical retinoids

Table 3.4 Superficial peeling

Peeling agents	Concentration %
Glycolic acid	30–70
Salicylic acid	15–25
TCA	10–25
Resorcin	20–30
Pyruvic acid	40 mild, 40 strong

Alpha Hydroxy Acids (AHAs)

Alpha hydroxy acids [50] are a group of compounds derived from food products including glycolic (from sugarcane), lactic (from sour milk), malic (from apples), citric (from fruits), and tartaric acid (from grape wine) For any topical compound, including AHA, it must penetrate into the skin where it can act on living cells. Small molecular size is one characteristic that is important in determining compound's ability to penetrate the top layer of the skin. AHA favors the desquamation of corneous layer and is very useful in comedogenic acne. Associative combination glycolic acid-azelaic acid could represent a real alternative in mild and moderate acne forms.

Chemical Peels

Chemical peel [51] uses a chemical solution to improve and smooth the texture of the facial skin by removing its damaged outer layers. On the skin layer, these substances could decrease keratinocyte binding, removing the corneous layer and enhancing cell turnover. Chemical peel results depend on the depth: the traditional classification subdivides chemical peels in superficial peels (Table 3.4; reaching epidermidis), medium peels (Table 3.5; superficial derma), and deep peels (Table 3.6; medium derma). So, adverse effects too depends on depth of chemical damage. Among the most common adverse effects, we can find bacterial, viral, and fungal infections (*Staphylococcus*, *Streptococcus*, herpes simplex, and *Candida* spp.); acne-like eruptions; and post inflammatory pigmentations. Less common adverse

Table 3.5 Medium peeling

Peeling agents	Concentration %
Glycolic acid + TCA	70/35
Pyruvic acid	50–60
TCA	30–50

Table 3.6 Deep peeling

Peeling agents	Concentration %
TCA	50–100
Phenol	88

effects are allergic reaction, persistent erythema, and dermatitis. Chemical peels are useful for acne scarring and cutaneous dyschromia as chloasma and melasma.

Camouflage

Corrective camouflage [52] uses covering water-resistant correctors to minimize and/or cover cutaneous esthetic disease as vitiligo, melasma, chloasma, couperose, rosacea, or surgical scars. In acne patients, dermatologist uses anallergic, noncomedogenic correctors with sunscreen. Camouflage is a two-step methodology: first a preliminary visit to the patient and then the corrective procedure.

3.9.2.2 Systemic Medical Treatment

Oral Antibiotics

Oral antibiotic represents the first choice in the treatment of intermediate acne and the second choice in severe acne treatment. Now the most used antibiotics are tetracycline, macrolides, and clindamycin.

Tetracycline

Tetracycline [53] is an antibiotic approach that is used to suppress the symptoms of acne, with general success. Doxyclycine, limecycline, and minocycline are the most used. These antibiotics have a bacteriostatic and bacteriocidal activity, reducing inflammatory and noninflammatory lesions. The most important adverse effects are photosensibility, serious gastric intestinal problems, enterocolitis, headaches, and, above all, a bacterial resistance. Women who are pregnant or breast feeding should not take tetracyclines as they can stain teeth permanently and inhibit bone growth, leading to skeletal defects in a fetus. They are also contraindicated for children under 12, for the same reasons.

Macrolides and Clindamycin

Erythromycin [53] represents macrolide prototypes. With azithromycin and roxithromycin are some of the common antibiotics used in acne. They offer a bacteriostatic effect linked to the action on bacterial ribosomes, blocking protein synthesis. At high doses, they can offer a bactericide action too. Clindamycin is used especially as topical antibiotics and could give diarrhea, pseudomembranous colitis, and exanthematic reactions. Women who are pregnant or breast feeding should not take it.

Oral Isotretinoin

Isotretinoin [54] is a retinoid, related chemically to vitamin A. Isotretinoin basically helps the sebaceous gland to mature; it can act in several ways. Testosterone drives this oil gland to produce a number of different oils that influence the lining of the hair follicle. Isotretinoin brings the amount of oils to a more normal level and helps to change the composition of the oil so that it does not allow the pores to clog up. It prevents an excess of keratin from being produced, which means that comedones are not so readily formed. Isotretinoin is used to treat severe acne. It is considered the first choice in acne fulminans and in gram-related folliculitis. When a patient is in oral isotretinoin treatment for acne, he must be followed with an accurate anamnesis, objective examination, and laboratory analysis. Oral isotretinoin could have possible harm to a developing fetus. For sexually active women, a pregnancy test before the start of therapy with isotretinoin is required and at monthly intervals during use of the drug plus use of two forms of contraception or sexual abstinence, beginning 1 month before the drug is started, continued during drug use, and for 1 month after stopping the drug. It requires blood tests to check for effect on blood cells, liver, and fat levels. An associative treatment of oral isotretinoin and salicylic acid could be toxic for the muscles. Systemic adverse effect is headache, and it has been associated with depression, suicidal thoughts, attempted suicide, and (rarely) completed suicide. The cutaneous adverse effect comprehends dry eyes, chapped lips, and drying of the mucous membranes. These are dose-dependent effects, reduced by lower doses or suspending the drug.

Hormonal Therapy

The target of hormonal therapy [55] is to reduce the effect of androgen on sebaceous glands and, probably, on follicular keratinocytes. This effect could be obtained through the use of estrogen, antiandrogen agents (spironolactone, acetate cyproterone, flutamide), oral contraceptives, and low-dose glucocorticoids.

References

1. Aristotle (1605) Historia animalium, 556b, 29; Problemata, 36, 3; in edn. Casaubon p 654B, 639E
2. Hippocritus (1826) De Morbis Vulgaribus; in edn. Loeb Classical Library, Hippocrates, 1, 188. De Internus Affectionibus; in edn. Kuhn Medicorum Grecorum Opera, 22, 427
3. Pliny (1897) Historia naturalis, Lib. 23; in edn. Mayhoff, Lipsiae 4, p 7, 8, 27, 28
4. Celsus (1831) De Medicina, Lib. 6, Cap. 5; Lugduni p. 552; in edn. Lee, London, p. 136
5. Niemeier V, Kupfer J, Gieler U (2006) Acne vulgaris – psychosomatic aspects. Dtsch Dermatol Ges 4(12):1027–1036
6. Goulden V, Stables GI, Cunliffe WJ (1999) Prevalence of facial acne in adults. J Am Acad Dermatol 41:577–580
7. White GM (1998) Recent findings in the epidemiologic evidence, classification, and subtypes of acne vulgaris. J Am Acad Dermatol 39:S34–S37
8. Katsambas AD, Katoulis AC, Stavropoulos P (1999) Acne neonatorum: a study of 22 cases. Int J Dermatol 38(2):128–130
9. Van Praag MC, Van Rooij RW, Folkers E et al (1997) Diagnosis and treatment of pustular disorders in the neonate. Pediatr Dermatol 14(2):131–143

10. Barnes CJ, Eichenfield LF, Lee J et al (2005) A practical approach for the use of oral isotretinoin for infantile acne. Pediatr Dermatol 22(2):166–169
11. Sarazin F, Dompmartin A, Nivot S et al (2004) Treatment of an infantile acne with oral isotretinoin. Eur J Dermatol 14(1):71–72
12. Capitanio B, Sinagra JL, Ottaviani M et al (2007) 'Smoker's acne': a new clinical entity? Br J Dermatol 157:1070–1071
13. Schäfer T, Nienhaus A, Vieluf D et al (2001) Epidemiology of acne in the general population: the risk of smoking. Br J Dermatol 145:100–104
14. Gary M, White MD (1998) Recent findings in the epidemiologic evidence, classification, and subtypes of acne vulgaris. J Am Acad Dermatol 39(2 Pt 3):S34–S37
15. Church JM, Fazio VW, Lavery IC et al (1993) The differential diagnosis and comorbidity of hidradenitis suppurativa and perianal Crohn's disease. Int J Colorectal Dis 8(3):117–119
16. Anderson P (1971) Foods as a cause of acne. Am J Fam Pract 3:102–103
17. Kalminster LH (1978) Acne, what friends or patients ask about. J Am Med Assoc 239:2171–2172
18. Rasmussen J (1977) Diet and acne. Int J Dermatol 16:488–492
19. Aizawa H, Niimura M (1995) Elevated serum insulin-like growth factor-1 (IGF-1) levels in women with postadolescent acne. J Dermatol 22:249–252
20. Cordain L, Eades MR, Eades MD (2003) Hyperinsulinemic diseases of civilization: more than just Syndrome X. Comp Biochem Physiol A Mol Integr Physiol 136:95–112
21. Melnik B (2009) Milk consumption: aggravating factor of acne and promoter of chronic diseases of Western societies. J Dtsch Dermatol Ges 7(4):364–370
22. Del Prete M, Mauriello MC et al (2012) Insulin resistance and acne: a new risk factor for men? Endocrine
23. Gfesser M, Worret WI (1996) Seasonal variations in the severity of acne vulgaris. Int J Dermatol 35:116–117
24. Allen HB, LoPresti PJ (1980) Acne vulgaris aggravated by sunlight. Cutis 26:254–256
25. Papageorgiou P, Katsambas A, Chu A (2000) Phototherapy with blue (415 nm) and red (660 nm) light in the treatment of acne vulgaris. Br J Dermatol 142:973–978
26. Kawada A, Aragane Y, Kameyama H et al (2002) Acne phototherapy with a high intensity, enhanced, narrow band, blue light source: an open study and in vitro investigation. J Dermatol Sci 30:129–135
27. Hongcharu W, Taylor CR, Chang Y et al (2000) Topical ALA-photodynamic therapy for the treatment of acne vulgaris. J Invest Dermatol 115:183–192
28. Fabbrocini G, Cacciapuoti S et al (2009) The effect of ALA PDT on microcomedons and macrocomedons. Dermatology 219(4):322–328
29. Fulton JE Jr, Pay SR, Fulton JE (1984) Comedogenicity of current therapeutic products, cosmetics, and ingredients in the rabbit ear. J Am Acad Dermatol 10:96–105
30. Levy SB (1984) Comedogenicity of cosmetics. J Am Acad Dermatol 10:1072
31. Fulton JE Jr, Bradley S, Aqundez A et al (1976) Non-comedogenic cosmetics. Cutis 17:344–345, 349–51
32. Norris JF, Cunliffe WJ (1988) A histological and immunocytochemical study of early acne lesions. Br J Dermatol 118:651–659
33. Jeremy AHT, Holland DB, Roberts SG et al (2003) Inflammatory events are involved in acne lesion initiation. J Invest Dermatol 121:20–27
34. Zouboulis CC (2001) Is acne vulgaris a genuine inflammatory disease? Dermatology 203:277–279
35. Walton S, Wyatt EH, Cunliffe WJ (1988) Genetic control of sebum excretion and acne – a twin study. Br J Dermatol 118(3):393–396
36. Bekaert C, Song M, Delvigne A (1998) Acne neonatorum and familial hyperandrogenism. Dermatology 196:453–454
37. Ostlere LS, Rumsby G, Holownia P et al (1998) Carrier status for steroid 21-hydroxylase deficiency is only one factor in the variable phenotype of acne. Clin Endocrinol 48:209–215
38. Pochi PE, Strauss JS (1969) Sebaceous gland response in man to the administration of testosterone, delta-4-androstenedione, and dehydroisoandrosterone. J Invest Dermatol 52:32–36

39. Cunliffe W, Forster R (1987) Androgen control of the pilosebaceous duct? Br J Dermatol 116:449
40. Thiboutot D, Knaggs H, Gilliland K et al (1998) Activity of 5α reductase and 17 β hydroxysteroid dehydrogenase in the infrainfundibulum of subjects with and without acne vulgaris. Dermatology 196:38–42
41. Toyoda M, Nakamura M, Makino T et al (2002) Sebaceous glands in acne patients express high levels of neutral endopeptidase. Exp Dermatol 11:241–247
42. Draelos ZD, Matsubara A, Smiles K (2006) The effect of 2 % niacinamide on facial sebum production. J Cosmet Laser Ther 8(2):96–101
43. Bibi Nitzan Y, Cohen AD (2006) Zinc in skin pathology and care. J Dermatolog Treat 17(4): 205–210
44. Pavicic T, Wollenweber U, Farwick M et al (2007) Anti-microbial and -inflammatory activity and efficacy of phytosphingosine: an in vitro and in vivo study addressing acne vulgaris. Int J Cosmet Sci 29(3):181–190
45. Taglietti M, Hawkins CN, Rao J (2008) Novel topical drug delivery systems and their potential use in acne vulgaris. Skin Therapy Lett 13(5):6–8
46. Cotellessa C, Manunta T, Ghersetich I et al (2004) The use of pyruvic acid in the treatment of acne. J Eur Acad Dermatol Venereol 18(3):275–278
47. Bari AU, Iqbal Z, Rahman SB (2007) Superficial chemical peeling with salicylic acid in facial dermatoses. J Coll Physicians Surg Pak 17(4):187–190
48. Thielitz A, Gollnick H (2008) Topical retinoids in acne vulgaris: update on efficacy and safety. Am J Clin Dermatol 9(6):369–381
49. Adişen E, Kaymak Y, Gurer MA (2008) Topical tetracycline in the treatment of acne vulgaris. J Drugs Dermatol 7(10):953–955
50. Fabbrocini G, Annunziata MC, D'Arco V et al (2010) Acne scars: pathogenesis, classification and treatment. Dermatology Research and Practice article ID 893080, 13 pages
51. Fabbrocini G, De Padova MP, Tosti A (2009) Chemical peels: what's new and what isn't new but still works well. Facial Plastic Surgery 25(5):329–336
52. Rayner VL (1995) Camouflage therapy. Dermatol Clin 13(2):467–472
53. Ochsendorf F (2006) Systemic antibiotic therapy of acne vulgaris. J Dtsch Dermatol Ges 4(10):828–841
54. Bener A, Lestringant GG, Ehlayel MS et al (2009) Treatment outcome of acne vulgaris with oral isotretinoin. J Coll Physicians Surg Pak 19(1):49–51
55. George R, Clarke S, Thiboutot D (2008) Hormonal therapy for acne. Semin Cutan Med Surg 27(3):188–196

Subcision®

4

Mariana Soirefmann and Rosemari Mazzuco

Core Messages

- Subcision® is a surgical technique used for the treatment of cutaneous depressions, including cellulite depressed lesions and liposuction depressed sequelae.
- Patients with cellulite must be examinated in standing position. The examination site should have a vertically incident light, in order to provide a better visualization of relief alterations of cellulite.
- Subcision® is not suitable for low degree of cellulite nor localized adiposity and laxity/flaccidity.
- Subcision® should only be performed in depressions smaller than 30 mm in diameter. Larger depressions should be treated in multiple sessions.
- Subcision® is a simple, low cost and very efficacious technique for the treatment of cellulite and other depressions of the skin surface of different causes.

4.1 Introduction

Subcision® is a simple surgical technique used for the treatment of cutaneous depressions. This technique was originally described by Orentreich and Orentreich for the treatment of cutaneous scars and wrinkles in 1995 [17]. Two years later, Subcision®

M. Soirefmann, M.D. (✉)
Department of Dermatology, Pontifícia Universidade Catolica do Rio Grande do Sul (PUC-RS), Porto Alegre, RS, Brazil

Brazilian Center for Studies in Dermatology,
782 Dr. Timoteo, St., Porto Alegre, RS ZIP: 90570-040, Brazil
e-mail: msoirefmann@terra.com.br

R. Mazzuco, M.D.
Brazilian Society of Dermatology and Brazilian Society of Dermatologic Surgery, São Paulo, SP, Brazil
e-mail: rosemazzuco@hotmail.com.br

A. Tosti, D. Hexsel (eds.), *Update in Cosmetic Dermatology*,
DOI 10.1007/978-3-642-34029-1_4,

was reported for the treatment of cellulite and liposuction sequelae by Hexsel and Mazzuco in two series of cases with 46 [5] and 232 [6] patients. Subcision® has also been reported for the treatment of atrophic depressed scars, acne scars, stretch marks, and auricular deformities in rabbits [8].

This chapter describes Subcision® for the treatment of cellulite.

4.2 Relevant Anatomy

Cellulite is considered a noninflammatory degenerative phenomenon that provokes alterations in the subcutis, producing irregular depressions in the skin overlying affected areas when compared to normal skin [2]. Different morphological patterns may be seen in cellulite patients. Usually, cellulite lesions are mainly depressed compared to the normal adjacent skin, but raised areas can also be seen. Lesions of cellulite can give to the skin surface an orange peel [3, 19], cottage cheese [2], or mattress appearance [3]. Cellulite usually occurs on buttocks and thighs, although other areas of the body may also be affected, such as the abdomen, arms, and back [3, 19]. This condition may be found in all ages and in both sexes, but it occurs mainly in women and after puberty. It may also be aggravated by localized fat, obesity, aging, and progressive skin laxity [4].

Depressed lesions of this condition are due to the presence of fibrous septa that pull the skin surface down [3, 7]. Recently, a study demonstrated the presence of significantly thicker subcutaneous fibrous septa, in areas with cellulite depressions compared to areas without cellulite [7]. On the other hand, raised areas are actually the projection of underlying fat to the skin surface [3].

4.3 Classification of Cellulite

Two classifications of cellulite are currently used. The first is made on clinical basis (Box 4.1) [6].

Box 4.1 Classification of Cellulite Based on Clinical Criteria [16]

Grade or stage	Clinical characteristics
0 (zero)	There is no alteration to the skin surface.
I	The skin of the affected area is smooth while the subject is standing or lying, but the alterations to the skin surface can be seen by pinching the skin or with muscle contraction.
II	The orange skin or mattress appearance is evident when standing, without the use of any manipulation (skin pinching or muscle contraction).
III	The alterations described in grade or stage II are present together with raised areas and nodules.

Although this classification is useful, it does not attend to important additional morphological aspects of cellulite (i.e., laxity) and is not the ideal for assessing treatment response. Hexsel, Dal'Forno, and Hexsel published a new cellulite classification, based on a new scale in which important clinical and morphological aspects of cellulite are assessed. The scale is called *Hexsel, Dal'Forno, and Hexsel cellulite severity scale* [9] and is shown in Box 4.2. It is an alpha-photonumeric

Box 4.2 Hexsel, Hexsel, and Dal'Forno Cellulite Severity Scale (CSS)

(A) Number of evident depressions

This item refers to the total number of evident depressions by visual inspection in the area to be examined. The scores are expressed as:

ZERO = None/no depressions

1 = A small amount: 1–4 depressions are visible

2 = A moderate amount: 5–9 depressions are visible

3 = A large amount: 10 or more depressions are visible

(B) Depth of depressions

This item evaluates the depth of depressions by visual inspection of the affected areas; comparison to the pictures of CSS is recommended.

ZERO = No depressions

1 = Superficial depressions

2 = Medium depth depressions

3 = Deep depressions

(C) Morphological appearance of skin surface alterations

Item C assesses the different morphological patterns of skin surface alterations; comparison with the pictures of CSS is recommended.

ZERO = No raised areas

1 = "Orange peel" appearance

2 = "Cottage cheese" appearance

3 = "Mattress" appearance

(D) Grade of laxity, flaccidity, or sagging skin

Laxity, flaccidity, or sagging skin confers the affected skin a draped appearance. This effect aggravates the appearance of cellulite. Item D assesses the grade of flaccidity, and comparison to the pictures of CSS is recommended.

ZERO = Absence of laxity, flaccidity, or sagging skin

1 = Slight draped appearance

2 = Moderate draped appearance

3 = Severe draped appearance

(E) First cellulite classification described by Nürnberger and Müller [16]

This item incorporates the first classification of cellulite, shown in the Box 4.1. Patients should be evaluated in the standing position with relaxed gluteus muscles. However, if the patient has no evident depressions, they should be asked to contract their gluteus muscles or the pinch test should be applied (by pinching the skin between the thumb and the index finger) in order to differentiate between scores zero and 1.

ZERO = Zero grade

1 = First grade

2 = Second grade

3 = Third grade

scale that grades cellulite on basis of five items: (A) number of evident depressed lesions, (B) depth of depressions, (C) morphological appearance of skin surface alterations, (D) grade of flaccidity or sagging skin, and (E) grade of cellulite. Each of these items is graded from zero to three. The sum of these scores will lead to a new classification of the cellulite as mild, moderate, or severe, as shown in Box 4.3.

Box 4.3 New Classification of Cellulite Based on the Results of Scores of Cellulite Severity Scale

Points	New classification of cellulite
1–5	Mild
6–10	Moderate
11–15	Severe

4.4 Indications and Patient Selection

The candidates for Subcision® are healthy patients who present one or more evident depressed lesions of cellulite on the buttocks and/or upper thighs. According to the first classification of cellulite, ideal candidates are those presenting 2nd and/or 3rd grade of cellulite [6]. Candidates for this procedure are also those presenting high scores in the first three letters of the new *Hexsel, Dal' Forno, and Hexsel* CSS.

Patients should be evaluated in standing position with relaxed muscles in order to correctly identify depressions of cellulite that are clearly apparent independently of pinch test or muscular contraction. Lesions up to 3 cm in diameter, or even parts of larger lesions, are eligible for this treatment [6]. Adequate illumination of the exam room is very important, in order to facilitate the correct identification of depressed lesions. Therefore, a light source in a downward position is helpful to visualize and mark the lesions to be treated [8].

The authors also emphasize that Subcision® is an useful technique to correct some "cellulite-like" lesions, such as some scars on the body and liposuction depressed sequelae [6] (Fig. 4.1).

4.5 Contraindications

This technique is not suitable for low degree of cellulite nor localized adiposity and laxity/flaccidity [6]. Therefore, depressed lesions that are only visible with muscular contraction and the usual conditions associated with cellulite may not be indicated for Subcision®. For these conditions, other therapeutic options may be recommended, including lasers, radiofrequency, mechanical massage with or without vacuum, and other specific devices.

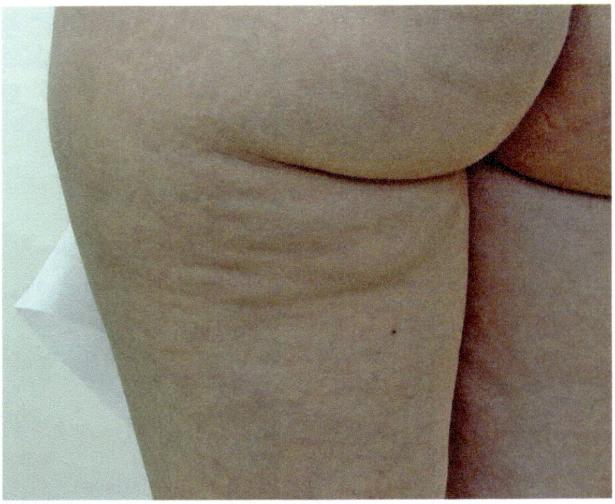

Fig. 4.1 Liposuction depressed sequelae

Contraindications are shown in Box 4.4.

Box 4.4 Relative and Absolute Contraindications to Subcision®

Relative contraindications: history of hypertrophic or keloid scars, active local or systemic infections, and use of drugs that interfere with coagulation or with local anesthetics.

Absolute contraindications: pregnancy, low degree of cellulite, *cottage cheese* or *orange peel* lesions, coagulation disorders, severe illnesses, and patients who are unable to follow postoperatory recommendations or with unrealistic expectations [6].

4.6 Mechanism of Action

Subcision® is indicated for the treatment of evident depressed lesions of cellulite, by a multistep process based in three action mechanisms. The first action mechanism is the section of the fibrous dermal and subcutaneous septa, in order to release their traction applied to the skin [17]. The second is due to the subsequent hematoma formation, followed by secondary connective tissue deposition, which fills the depressions of cellulite [17]. Additionally, a third action mechanism that improves the skin irregularities of the affected areas is due to the redistribution of the traction forces exerted by the fibrous septa and the tension forces exerted by the fat to the skin surface [6].

4.7 Preoperative Recommendations

As any other outpatient surgical procedure, previous medical evaluation and laboratory tests are required for Subcision® candidates, according to specific patient's needs [5, 6].

Medical history should include the following items:

- Onset of cellulite
- Associated clinical diseases
- Associated cellulite conditions (laxity, liposuction sequelae)
- Previous surgical procedures
- Previous cellulite treatments
- History of vascular diseases
- History of pregnancy and/or miscarriage
- Allergies
- Tendency for keloids and hypertrophy scars
- Drugs (regular use and occasional use)
- Dietary habits
- Physical exercises
- Family history of cellulite

Physical exam should focus on:

- Characteristics of cellulite lesions (grade of cellulite, number and distribution of depressed lesions)
- Body weight, height and blood pressure

Preoperative laboratory exams include coagulation tests, as follows:

- PT (prothrombin time)
- PTT (partial thromboplastin time)
- INR (international normalized ratio)

The following recommendations are also given to patients undergoing to Subcision® (Box 4.5):

Box 4.5 Preoperative Recommendations for Subcision®

1. To discontinue any drugs that may interfere with blood coagulation, such as anticoagulants, analgesics, and anti-inflammatory agents, 7 days prior to the procedure.
2. To discontinue iron supplements 1 month prior to the procedure; patients are also encouraged to diminish iron intake in food 1 month before.
3. To use prophylactic antimicrobial therapy with ciprofloxacin 500 mg, twice daily, beginning 6 h before the procedure.
4. To discontinue any drugs that may interfere with the safety and/or results of the procedure (e.g., beta-blockers, immunosuppressants, neuroleptics, and oral isotretinoin).
5. To treat local infections on the surgical areas, if pertinent.

4.8 Procedure Technique

The patient must be examined in standing position. The examination site should have a vertically incident light in order to provide a better visualization of relief alterations of cellulite [6].

The depressions that are easily detected with the patient in a standing position and relaxed muscles are marked [6]. The patient can be asked to contract the muscles to show the full extent and shape of these depressions. However, the depressions that are visible only during muscle contraction (grade I cellulitis) are not suitable for treatment with Subcision®. The number of lesions treated during each session will depend on the available doses of anesthetic, calculated according to the patient's body weight, as described below.

Antisepsis, with iodinated alcohol or chlorhexidine, should be strict and broad, as usual in any surgical procedure [1]. The use of surgical drapes and sterile gowns is recommended, as well as performing the procedure in a surgical environment [11].

Since it is a painful procedure, the patient is submitted to infiltrative local anesthesia, at the sites where Subcision® will be performed. The anesthesia needle must be inserted 1–2 cm outside the cutaneous marking, and the anesthetic should be applied with retrograde injections at the subcutaneous level. An anesthetic button is made at the puncture site, to introduce the scalpel. A vasoconstrictor drug together with the local anesthetic is helpful to control bleeding and to increase the safe doses and the duration of the anesthetic effect [14], a major factor, especially when extensive depressions are treated. Furthermore, with less intra- and postoperative bleeding, the size of the postoperative hematomas is more easily controlled [10]. One or 2 % lidocaine with norepinephrine of phenylephrine can be used. The dose of the lidocaine conventionally considered the maximum by the textbooks [11] and the manufacturers is 7 mg/kg. Some authors suggest that the total dose should not be greater than 500 mg per session [12]. One can also choose tumescent anesthesia [13], when there are many depressions that need to be treated in a single session. In the latter type of anesthesia, the lidocaine dose can be higher [15, 18] .

The 18-gauge BD Nokor® needle (which has a cutting blade tip), connected to a Luer-Lok syringe, is the most used instrument for off-face Subcision® [6]. Other options include a special scalpel that has the same cutting blade or 18-G common needles. The needle or the scalpel should be inserted at the site of the anesthetic button (1–2 cm before the beginning of the depression marking), 1–2 cm below the cutaneous surface. The BD Nokor needle is inserted with the cutting edge toward the left. When the needle is at the subcutaneous level, the needle is pressed against the connective tissue septa, which are sectioned with movements from right to left, at the same time as the needle is pulled firmly toward the exit. The unilateral movement of the needle creates a more precise cut, helping minimize pain during the postoperative period. A slight pinch test is useful to research residual septa pulling the skin surface down or areas that are still retracted [6] (Figs. 4.2 and 4.3).

It should be highlighted that Subcision® should not be performed in large areas, avoiding the creation of large dissection planes. This is because there is a risk of

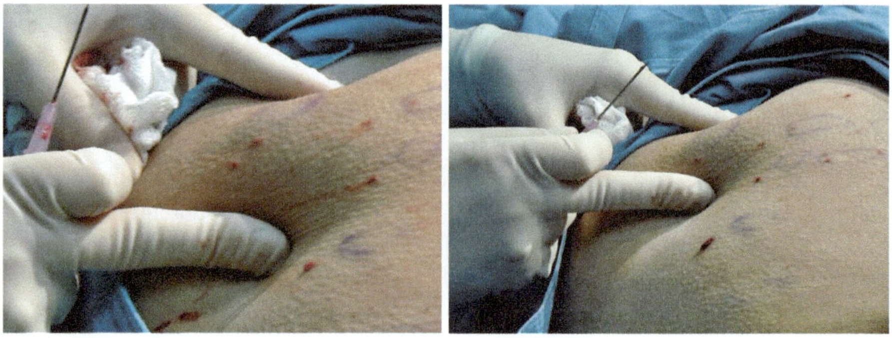

Figs. 4.2 and 4.3 Slight pinch test to check residual septa pulling the skin down

extensive hematomas and skin necrosis. An easy way to avoid excessive undermining is to perform Subcision® only in depressions smaller than 30 mm in diameter. Larger depressions should be treated in multiple sessions.

Immediately after treating each depression, vigorous compression for 5–10 min is applied in the treated areas, reaching to quick hemostasis and promoting an appropriate size of the hematomas. For this purpose, sandbags wrapped in sterilized tissue [6] help achieve more uniform compression than the manual one. These bags weigh approximately 5 kg.

The use of compressive dressings in all the depressions treated, with sterile gauze and micropore, is also helpful to prevent large hematomas. This will be removed 3–5 days after the procedure, during which time the patient should avoid getting them wet. Over the dressing, the patient wears the compressive clothes (elastic pants or walking shorts), which will be used from the time she leaves the surgical room until 30 days after the procedure.

4.9 Postoperative Recommendations

When Subcision® is performed by experienced physicians and using the proper technique, the postoperative period is well tolerated.

Analgesics (acetaminophen or dipyrone) are prescribed for all patients during the first two postoperative days. Prophylactic antibiotic should be maintained until the third day.

The first postoperative revision is done after 3–5 days, when the compressive dressings are removed and the use of antibiotics is stopped [6].

In order to control the extent of the hematomas, the patient must follow recommendation of relative rest during the first week and avoid moderate-to-intense physical exercises during 15 days. The use of compressive clothes should be maintained for 30 days.

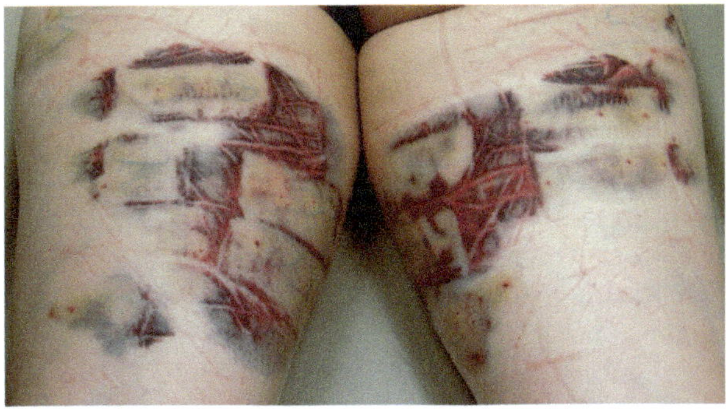

Fig. 4.4 Extensive hematomas

The clinical and photographic evaluation of the results should be performed after spontaneous resolution of the hematomas, which occurs between 20 and 40 days after the Subcision®.

4.10 Complications

The most common complications are easy to handle and almost always resolve spontaneously [6].

Hematomas and ecchymoses are expected in all patients [17]. Extensive and sometimes painful hematomas may occur when the large caliber vessels are sectioned or when some technical details have not been followed (Fig. 4.4). Erythema, edema, and local sensitivity may be seen immediately after the procedure and tend to regress in the first hours.

Seromas are characterized by pain and subcutaneous nodules with hard consistency at palpation. Seromas can occur in a few treated areas, and they are relatively common under areas that had been extensively treated or presented large hematomas [6]. They usually resolve spontaneously in a period of 3–6 months, but the intralesional injections of triamcinolone speed up the regression process.

Hemosiderosis is caused by the deposition of hemosiderin, characterized by brownish pigmentation of the skin in the areas where the hematomas have been reabsorbed. It is observed in variable degrees in all patients and resolves spontaneously, but tends to be persistent in patients undertaking medications with iron or high intake of iron-containing food, or those who had large hematomas in the early postoperative period. As long as hemosiderosis persists, it is important that the patient avoids sun exposure, and further Subcision® sessions are contraindicated at these sites.

Postinflammatory hyperpigmentation is rare but may occur in patients with higher skin phototypes or those prone to develop it.

Variations in the response to Subcision® depend on technical factors, the treated areas, the extension and depth of the depressions, and the personal tendency to respond with more or less neocollagenesis. A suboptimal response is relatively common after Subcision® in very deep or extensive depressions. In such cases, one or more later sessions are needed to achieve the final result. Less common, but more difficult to treat, is a false excessive response, which is characterized by bulging in the areas where Subcision® was performed, due to a fat herniation. This is more common in the lower part of the buttocks and in the upper and posterior part of the thighs. This complication does not respond adequately to intralesional infiltration of steroids, and more favorable results can be obtained by aspiration of the herniated fat through microcannulae. The true excessive response is due to the excessive production of connective tissue, which may be related to personal factors, surgical trauma, and/or the intensity of the inflammatory response. There is no spontaneous regression, and the treatment consists of the infiltration of triamcinolone into the lesion, which is usually effective in most cases [6].

Conclusion

Subcision® is a simple, low cost, and very efficacious technique for the treatment of cellulite and other depressions of the skin surface of different causes (Figs. 4.5, 4.6, 4.7, 4.8, 4.9, and 4.10).

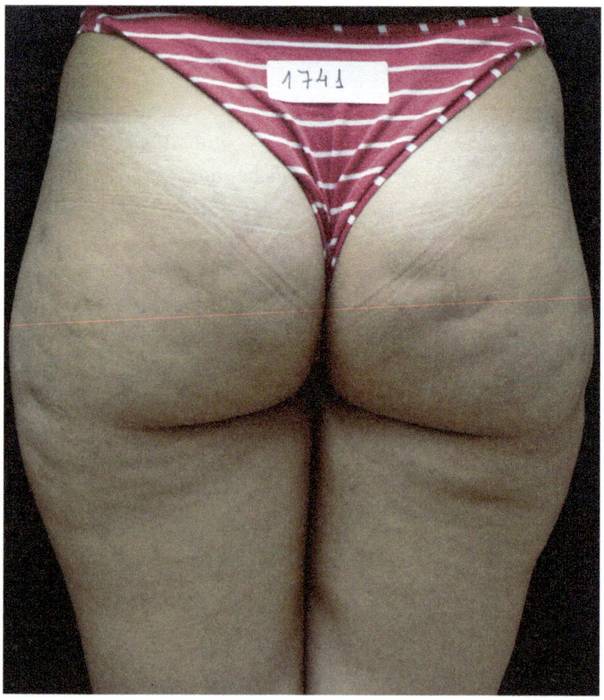

Fig. 4.5 Patient showing cellulite depression on buttocks before Subcision®

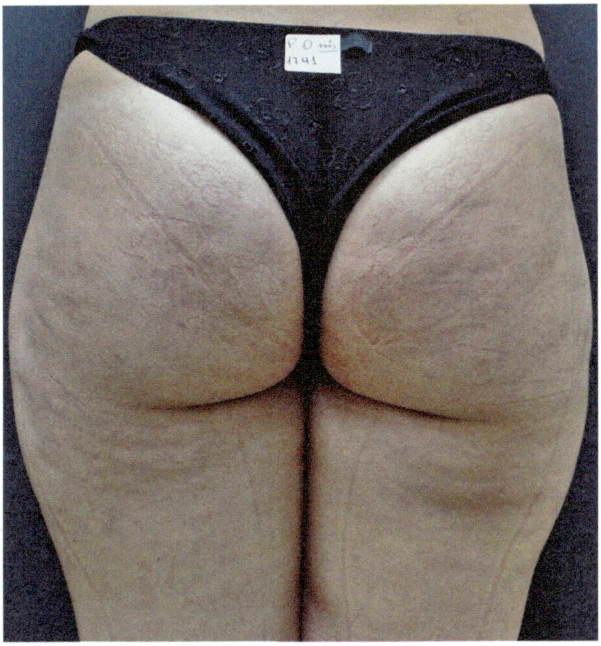

Fig. 4.6 Same patient as in Fig. 4.5, 1 month after Subcision®

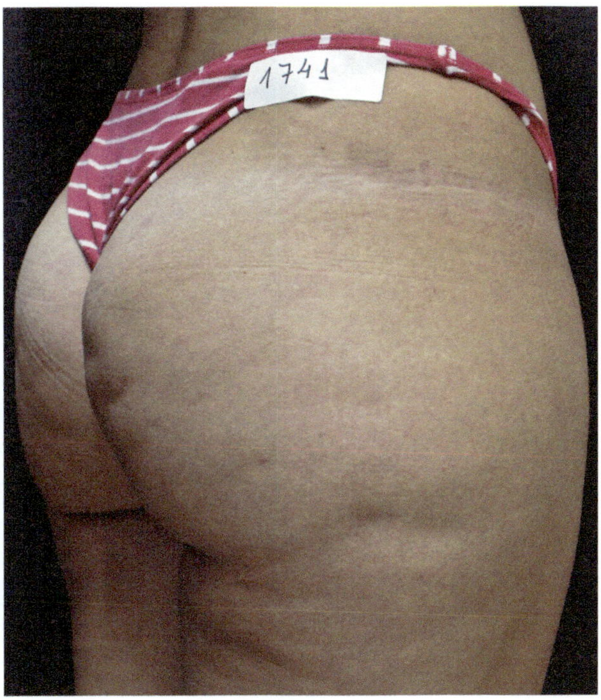

Fig. 4.7 Same patient as in Fig. 4.5, showing cellulite depression on buttocks before Subcision®

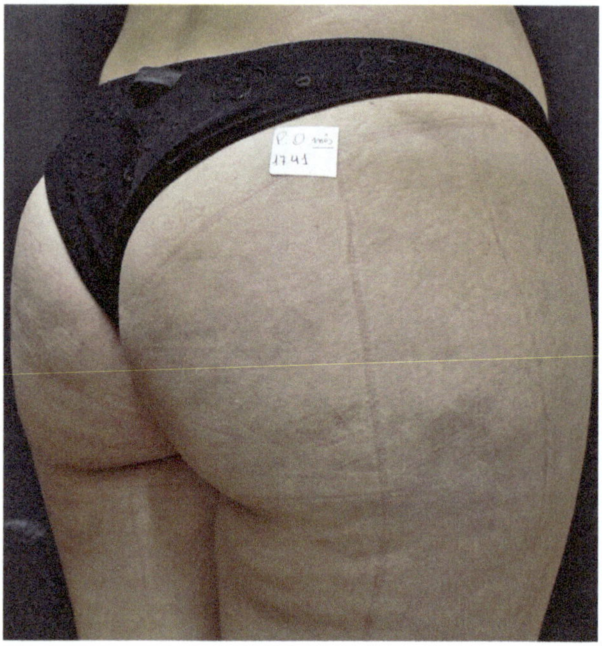

Fig. 4.8 Same patient as in Fig. 4.5, 1 month after Subcision® (lateral view)

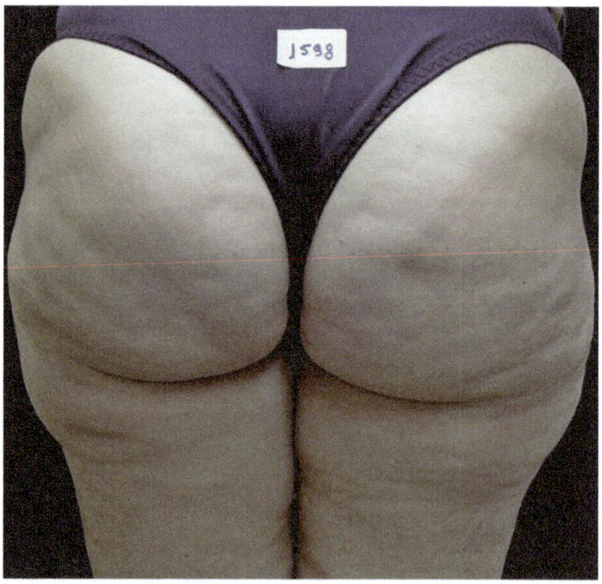

Fig. 4.9 Patient showing cellulite depression on buttocks before Subcision®

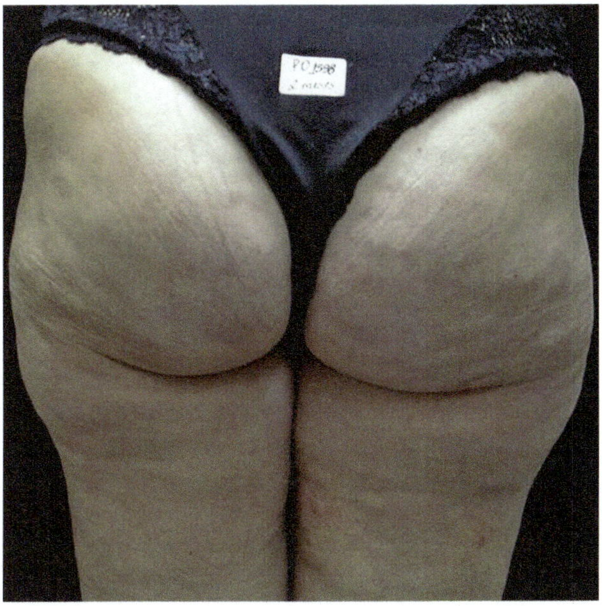

Fig. 4.10 Same patient as in Fig. 4.9, 2 months after Subcision®

References

1. Barie PS (2002) Surgical site infections: epidemiology and prevention. Surg Infect (Larchmt) 3(Suppl 1):S9–S21
2. Draelos ZD (1997) Cellulite. Etiology and purposed treatment. Dermatol Surg 23:1177–1181
3. Hexsel DM (2001) Body repair. In: Parish LC, Brenner S, Ramos e Silva M (eds) Women's dermatology: from infancy to maturity. Parthenon Publishing, New York, pp 586–595
4. Hexsel D (2009) Cellulite. In: Baumann L (ed) Cosmetic dermatology: principles and practice. McGraw-Hill Companies, New York
5. Hexsel DM, Mazzuco R (1997) Subcision: Uma alternativa cirúrgica para a lipodistrofia ginoide ("celulite") e outras alterações do relevo corporal. An Bras Dermatol 72:27–32
6. Hexsel DM, Mazzuco R (2000) Subcision: a treatment for cellulite. Int J Dermatol 39(7):539–544
7. Hexsel DM, Abreu M, Rodrigues TC, Soirefmann M et al (2009) Side-by-side comparison of areas with and without cellulite depressions using magnetic resonance imaging. Dermatol Surg 35(10):1471–1477
8. Hexsel D, Dal'Forno T, Soirefmann M, Hexsel C (2010) Reduction of cellulite with subcision. In: Murad A, Pongprutthipan M (eds) Body rejuvenation. Taylor and Francis, New York, pp 167–172
9. Hexsel D, Hexsel CL, Dal'Forno TO (2009) A validated photonumeric cellulite severity scale. J Eur Acad Dermatol Venereol 23:523–528
10. Hexsel D, Mazzuco R, Dal'Forno T, Hexsel CL (2004) Simple technique provides option for treating scars and other skin depressions. J Cosmet Dermatol 17(1):35–41
11. Hexsel D, Mazzuco R, Soirefmann M (2010) Subcision. In: Goldman M, Hexsel D (eds) Cellulite: pathophysiology and treatment, 2nd edn. Informa Health Care, London, pp 174–179

12. McCalmont TH, Leshin B (1996) Preoperative evaluation of the cutaneous surgery patient. In: Lask GP, Moy RL (eds) Principles and techniques of cutaneous surgery. McGraw-Hill, New York, pp 101–112
13. Namias A, Kaplan B (1998) Tumescent anesthesia for dermatologic surgery, cosmetic and noncosmetic procedures. Dermatol Surg 24(7):755–758
14. Niemi G (2005) Advantages and disadvantages of adrenaline in regional anaesthesia. Best Pract Res Clin Anaesthesiol 19(2):229–245
15. Nordström H, Stånge K (2005) Plasma lidocaine levels and risks after liposuction with tumescent anaesthesia. Acta Anaesthesiol Scand 49(10):1487–1490
16. Nürnberger F, Müller G (1978) So-called cellulite: an invented disease. J Dermatol Surg Oncol 4(3):221–229
17. Orentreich DS, Orentreich N (1995) Subcutaneous incisionless (subcision) surgery for the correction of depressed scars and wrinkles. Dermatol Surg 21(6):543–549
18. Ostad A, Kageyama N, Moy RL (1996) Tumescent anesthesia with a lidocaine dose of 55 mg/kg is safe for liposuction. Dermatol Surg 22(11):921–927
19. Rossi ABR, Vergnanini AL (2000) Cellulite: a review. J Eur Acad Dermatol Venerol 14:251–262

Hirsutism

5

Ticiana C. Rodrigues and Poli Mara Spritzer

Core Messages

- Hirsutism can be a manifestation of an endocrine disease.
- For diagnosis is necessary laboratory evaluation.
- The aims of treatment are to normalize the androgen overproduction, to suppress the androgen action, to identify patients with higher risk of metabolic disorders and to identify patients with reproductive tract neoplasm, as well as to promote aesthetical improvement.

5.1 Introduction

Hirsutism is an excessive terminal hair that appears with a male pattern in women [1]. It is a common report among women that see endocrinologists, dermatologists, and gynecologists.

Hirsutism can be the only manifestation or can be part of hyperandrogenism like acne, menses irregularity, alopecia, seborrhea, and other clinical characteristics. In addition, according with the severity of hirsutism and individual psychological background, patients may present emotional perturbations and social embarrassing that can seriously impact their quality of life [18].

T.C. Rodrigues, M.D. (✉)
Department of Internal Medicine, Universidade Federal do Rio Grande do Sul, Porto Alegre, RS, Brazil

Endocrine Division, Hospital de Clínicas de Porto Alegre, 2350, Ramiro Barcelos Street – Building 12, 4th Floor, ZIP 90035-003 Porto Alegre, RS, Brazil
e-mail: ticianacr@yahoo.com.br

P.M. Spritzer
Endocrine Division, Hospital de Clínicas de Porto Alegre, 2350, Ramiro Barcelos Street – Building 12, 4th Floor, ZIP 90035-003 Porto Alegre, RS, Brazil

Department of Physiology, Universidade Federal do Rio Grande do Sul, Porto Alegre, RS, Brazil

A. Tosti, D. Hexsel (eds.), *Update in Cosmetic Dermatology*,
DOI 10.1007/978-3-642-34029-1_5, © Springer-Verlag Berlin Heidelberg 2013

5.2 Etiology

Hirsutism results from an interaction between the plasma androgens and the apparent sensitivity of the hair follicle to androgen [17]. The sensitivity of the hair follicle is determined in part by the local metabolism of androgens, particularly by conversion of testosterone to dihydrotestosterone (DHT) by 5α-reductase and subsequent binding of these molecules to the androgen receptor. Hirsutism is classified as being produced by an excess of androgens from ovaries and/or adrenals, by an increased sensitivity of the pilosebaceous unit by androgens, or by the use of medications or changes in sex hormone-binding globulin (SHBG) secretion [28].

5.2.1 Idiopathic

Women who present an isolated hirsutism, in the presence of ovulatory menstrual cycles and normal circulating levels of testosterone, androstenedione, and adrenal androgens, have idiopathic or simple hirsutism. These patients have an increased sensibility of the pilosebaceous unit to normal plasma levels of androgen, and this fact could explain the excessive body hair.

5.2.2 Polycystic Ovary Syndrome

Polycystic ovary syndrome (PCOS) is the most frequent cause of hyperandrogenism and oligoanovulation [7, 23], and it is the most important reason for excess androgen production causing hirsutism [38]. The prevalence of PCOS is around 7 % of women in reproductive age. While the etiopathogenesis is still not well recognized, three key features of PCOS have been proposed with various degrees of emphasis to firm the diagnosis. These features are hyperandrogenism and/or hyperandrogenemia, chronic anovulation, and polycystic ovaries on ultrasonography [24]. Recent consensus propose specific criteria for defining PCOS; the 1990 National Institutes of Health (NIH) consensus requires the presence of chronic anovulation plus clinical or biochemical signs of hyperandrogenism, and the 2003 Rotterdam consensus requires the presence of at least two of the following criteria: chronic anovulation, clinical or biochemical signs of hyperandrogenism, and polycystic ovaries [24, 25]. Both definitions emphasize that PCOS should only be considered after exclusion of other known conditions associated with androgen excess. Although obesity, insulin resistance, and metabolic syndrome are frequently present in women with PCOS, they are not regarded as intrinsic disturbances of the disorder [20]. Women with hirsutism and PCOS should also be informed about other problems related to the syndrome such as anovulatory infertility and long-term health consequences including the risk of type 2 diabetes as well as the potential risks of cardiovascular disease and of endometrial cancer. Impaired glucose tolerance or type 2 diabetes are observed in up to 40 % of patients with PCOS, and the rate of undiagnosed diabetes among patients with PCOS is 10 % [36, 37].

5.2.3 Nonclassical 21-Hydroxylase Deficiency

Congenital adrenal hyperplasia (CAH) refers to a family of inherited disorders in which defects occur in one of the five enzymatic steps required to synthesize cortisol from cholesterol in the adrenal gland [18]. The mild form of adrenal steroid 21-hydroxylase deficiency (CYP21) is named nonclassical steroid 21-hydroxylase deficiency (NC-CAH) [19]. In these cases, there is a partial deficiency of 21-hydroxylation, in the absence of ambiguous genitalia at birth. However, a postnatal androgen excess may occur later in life, mainly during puberty, leading to a heterogeneous clinical presentation of hyperandrogenism (acne and/or hirsutism alone or with alopecia, menses irregularity, and infertility). The prevalence is less than 5 % among hirsute women [14, 15] but should be higher in special ethnic groups. Clinical diagnosis of NC-CAH is confirmed by the ACTH-stimulation test which measures the serum concentrations of 17-hydroxyprogesterone (17-OHP) at 0 and 60 min after ACTH administration (Cortrosyn 0.25 mg). Stimulated 17-OHP levels equal or higher than 1,000–1,200 ng/dL are diagnostic of NC-CAH [2, 14, 18].

5.2.4 Androgen-Secreting Tumors

They are present in about 0.2 % of hirsute women; over half are malignant [15] and may occur in any age. The onset of hirsutism is more abrupt than in patients with PCOS as well as testosterone levels, which may be greater than 150 ng/dL. In most cases, there is a palpable mass or they may be detected by ultrasonography or MRI scans. Ovarian tumors that cause virilization are derived from sex cord or stromal cells [26]. Adrenal tumors are a rare cause of androgen excess in women; the symptoms and clinical signs have an abrupt onset and progress rapidly, features that aid in making the diagnosis. High serum levels of dehydroepiandrosterone sulfate – DHEA-S – (>8,000 ng/mL) are highly suggestive of adrenal tumor, and they can be detected by CT or MRI scan.

5.2.5 Medications

Use of androgens or androgenic medications, such as anabolic steroids, danazol, valproic acid, phenytoin, diazoxide, or progestins, must be considered.

5.2.6 Others Causes

Hyperprolactinemia, Cushing's syndrome, acromegaly, menopause, and thyroid dysfunction must be considered as causes of androgen excess, but these patients normally present with the more common clinical manifestation of these disorders.

5.3 Diagnosis

Hirsutism is a clinical diagnosis. It is present when the modified Ferriman–Gallwey hirsutism score is at least 8 [9]. Recently, the Endocrine Society published a practice guideline for hirsutism approach, based on systematic reviews of available evidence about this point [15]. In this report, the evaluation of androgen levels is discouraged when the patients have isolated mild hirsutism. The lab evaluation should be performed when there the following clinical characteristics are present: sudden and/or rapidly progressive hirsutism or hirsutism of any degree with menstrual irregularity or infertility, central obesity, acanthosis nigricans, or clitoromegaly [15].

According to the clinical presentation, the following tests should be usually done, during the follicular phase, for the diagnostic evaluation of hirsutism:

- Testosterone and SHBG levels
- Basal and ACTH-stimulated 17-hydroyprogesterone levels
- If oligomenorrhea or amenorrhea is present: β-hCG, prolactin, and thyroid function tests
- Transvaginal or pelvic ultrasonography to screen for PCOS or ovarian neoplasia
- In case of suspicion, screen for Cushing's syndrome or acromegalia
- Computed tomography or MRI scan if there is suspicion of adrenal tumor
- Androstenedione and DHEA-S levels.

5.4 Treatment

The aims of treatment are to normalize the androgen overproduction, to suppress the androgen action, to identify patients with higher risk of metabolic disorders, and to identify patients with reproductive tract neoplasm as well as to promote aesthetical improvement.

The treatment is surgery for ovary or adrenal neoplasms. Hirsute patients with other endocrine disorder such as thyroid dysfunction, Cushing's syndrome, and hyperprolactinemia should receive specific treatment for the corresponding condition. In cases of hirsutism induced by medications, interruption, substitution, or dosage, changes should be tried according to clinical relevance of these treatments.

There are two main approaches to the management of hirsutism, which may be used either individually or in combination: firstly, pharmacological therapies that target androgen production and action and, secondly, direct methods to reduce and remove hair, including cosmetic approaches like electrolysis and photoepilation. Patients should be informed that the effect of treatment will only be observed after 6 months or more and that the achievement of optimal results will require 12–24 months.

5.4.1 Oral Contraceptives

It reduces the hyperandrogenism via a number of mechanisms including suppression of LH secretion and therefore ovarian androgen secretion [4] and stimulation of hepatic production of SHBG, thereby increasing androgen binding in serum and reducing serum-free androgen concentrations. Besides, it provides the benefit of contraception and menses' regularity. The use of an oral contraceptive is contraindicated in certain clinical conditions, including heavy smoking, uncontrolled hypertension, and history of thrombosis or ischemic heart disease [21]. Recently, a trial compared the effects of oral contraceptive pills containing desogestrel, cyproterone acetate, and drospirenone in polycystic ovary syndrome (PCOS) therapy [3]. No difference in effects after 6 months was observed. At 12 months, cyproterone acetate showed the strongest antiandrogen activities. Effects on metabolic parameters were identical.

5.4.2 Insulin-Lowering Drugs

Insulin-lowering drugs are effective in the management of metabolic disturbances in PCOS patients. However, this class of drugs has a limited and controversial role in hirsutism, especially when there are no menstrual and metabolic disturbs. Imprecise and inconsistent evidence of low to very low quality suggest that insulin sensitizers provide limited or no important benefit for women with hirsutism [10, 16].

5.4.3 Antiandrogens

It is an important strategy to treat hirsutism, especially for moderate or severe cases. Antiandrogens more directly address this concept by competitively inhibiting androgen binding to the androgen receptor or by inhibiting 5α-reductase [23]. Once these drugs suppress the sexual differentiation in male fetus, patients should be using a contraceptive method together. Spironolactone, cyproterone acetate, flutamide, and finasteride are the major antiandrogen drugs usually used and studied for the treatment of hirsutism. Liver function tests should be performed before the prescription of oral contraceptives and antiandrogens. Kidney function and serum potassium levels should be assessed when spironolactone is used, especially in patients with diabetes or hypertension.

Spironolactone: It competes with DHT for binding to the androgen receptor, has inhibitory effects on 5α-reductase, competes for binding to SHBG, and inhibits enzymes involved in androgen biosynthesis [1].

Cyproterone acetate is a 17-hydroxyprogesterone acetate derivative that competes with DHT for binding to the androgen receptor and reduces LH levels with consequent decrease of ovarian secretion of testosterone and androstenedione [1]. In patients with previous regular cycles, both spironolactone and cyproterone acetate may produce irregular menses or spotting. These effects can be reduced with the addition of an oral contraceptive to the antiandrogen treatment. Flutamide is a nonsteroidal androgen receptor blocker. It also may reduce the synthesis of androgens or increase their metabolism [1] and present a higher incidence of liver toxicity. For this reason, flutamide is not recommended as first-line treatment of hirsutism [15]. Finasteride is usually considered an antiandrogen because it competitively inhibits type 2 5α-reductase, which inhibits the conversion of testosterone to DHT [1].

All these medications have similar results in improving hirsutism [6, 8, 11, 30, 32, 34, 35].

A systematic review [31] shows that the antiandrogens seem to be mildly effective agents for the treatment of hirsutism. They appear more efficacious than placebo and metformin, and some antiandrogens appear to demonstrate additional improvements when added to oral contraceptive or metformin.

5.4.4 Glucocorticoid Monotherapy

Glucocorticoids are used long-term to suppress adrenal androgens in women with classic congenital adrenal hyperplasia due to 21-hydroxylase deficiency. In these patients, glucocorticoids help to prevent and manage hirsutism, and they are effective for maintaining normal ovulatory cycles. In women with the NC-CAH, glucocorticoids are effective for ovulation induction, but their role in the management of hirsutism is less clear [28, 29].

5.4.5 GnRH Agonists

The action of chronic GnRH agonist therapy is to inhibit LH and to a lesser extent FSH secretion, thereby leading to a decline in ovarian function and consequently decreased ovarian androgen production. There are weak evidences suggesting that GnRH agonist therapy is more effective than placebo or no therapy for hirsutism. It appears to have no therapeutic advantages when compared with oral contraceptives and antiandrogens [5]. Furthermore, this therapy is expensive, requires injections, and results in severe estrogen deficiency.

5.4.6 Direct Methods

5.4.6.1 Temporary Methods of Hair Removal

Epilation methods, such as plucking or waxing, or other methods that extract hairs to above the bulb are relatively safe and inexpensive, but it can produce some discomforts: scarring, folliculitis, and hyperpigmentation may occur. Depilation is the removal of the hair shaft from the skin surface. The effect usually lasts just for a maximum of a few days.

Shaving is a popular depilation method that removes hair down to just below the surface of the skin. Shaving does not affect the rate or duration of the anagen phase or diameter of hair.

5.4.7 Long-Term Methods of Hair Removal

5.4.7.1 Electrolysis

A fine needle is inserted into the hair follicle and an electrical current is applied. The galvanic electrolysis causes chemical destruction and thermolysis causes thermal destruction. The electrolysis is effective to reduce the hirsutism [22, 33] and is a cost-effective method of treatment for small areas of hirsutism.

5.4.7.2 Photoepilation

It is a method widely used. It includes laser and nonlaser light sources, such as intense pulsed light (IPL). Different laser types and changes in energy fluence and pulse duration allow a wide range of treatment modalities for specific skin types. The most commonly used lasers include alexandrite, neodymium:yttrium-aluminum-garnet (Nd:YAG), and ruby lasers. Laser therapy has been superior to electrolysis, being faster and less painful [12].

5.4.8 Topical Treatment

Eflornithine is an irreversible inhibitor of ornithine decarboxylase, an enzyme that catalyzes the rate-limiting step for follicular polyamine synthesis, which is necessary for hair growth. A topical preparation, cream 13.9 % is approved in many countries for the treatment of facial hair in women. It does not remove the hair, but acts to reduce hair growth. There are studies showing the benefit of eflornithine when added to laser therapy [13, 27].

References

1. Azziz R, Carmina E, Sawaya ME (2000) Idiopathic hirsutism. Endocr Rev 21:347–362
2. Azziz R, Zacur A (1989) 21-hydroxylase deficiency in female hyperandrogenism; screening and diagnosis. J Clin Endocrinol Metab 69:569–577
3. Bhattacharya SM, Jha A (2012) Comparative study of the therapeutic effects of oral contraceptive pills containing desogestrel, cyproterone acetate, and drospirenone in patients with polycystic ovary syndrome. Fertil Steril 98:1053–1059, Epub 2012 Jul 13
4. Cosma M, Swiglo BA, Flynn DN, Kurtz DM, LaBella ML, Mullan RJ, Elamin MB, Erwin PJ, Montori VM (2008) Insulin sensitizers for the treatment of hirsutism: a systematic review and metaanalyses of randomized controlled trials. J Clin Endocrinol Metab 93:1135–1142
5. Couzinet B, Le Strat N, Brilly S, Schaison G (1986) Comparative effects of cyproterone acetate or a long-acting gonadotropin-releasing hormone agonist in polycystic ovarian disease. J Clin Endocrinol Metab 63:1031–1035
6. Cusan L, Dupont A, Gomez J-L (1994) Comparison of flutamide and spironolactone in the treatment of hirsutism: a randomized controlled trial. Fertil Steril 61:281–287
7. Ehrmann DA (2005) Polycystic ovary syndrome. N Engl J Med 352:1223–1236
8. Erenus M, Gurbuz O, Durmusoglu F, Demircay Z (1994) Comparison of the efficacy of spironolactone versus flutamide in the treatment of hirsutism. Fertil Steril 61:613–616
9. Ferriman D, Gallwey JD (1961) Clinical assessment of body hair growth in women. J Clin Endocrinol Metab 21:1140–1148
10. Fitzgerald C, Elstein M, Spona J (1999) Effect of age on the response of the hypothalamo-pituitary-ovarian axis to a combined oral contraceptive. Fertil Steril 71:1079–1084
11. Fruzzetti F, De Lorenzo D, Parrini D, Ricci C (1994) Effects of finasteride, a 5α-reductase inhibitor, on circulating androgens and gonadotropin secretion in hirsute women. J Clin Endocrinol Metab 79:831–835

12. Gorgu M, Aslan G, Akoz T, Endogan B (2000) Comparison of alexandrite laser and electrolysis for hair removal. Dermatol Surg 26:37–41
13. Hamzavi I, Tan E, Shapiro J, Luis H (2007) A randomized bilateral vehicle-controlled study of eflornithine cream combined with laser treatment versus laser treatment alone for facial hirsutism in women. J Am Acad Dermatol 57:54–59
14. Kuttenn F, Couillin P, Girard F, Billaud L, Vincens M, Boucekkine C, Thalabard JC, Maudelonde T, Spritzer P, Mowszowicz I, Mauvais-Jarvis P (1985) Late-onset adrenal hyperplasia in hirsutism. N Eng J Med 313:224–231
15. Martin KA, Chang RJ, Ehrmann DA, Ibanez L, Lobo RA, Rosenfield RL, Shapiro J, Montori VM, Swiglo BA (2008) Evaluation and treatment of hirsutism in premenopausal women: an endocrine society clinical practice guideline. J Clin Endocrinol Metab 93:1105–1120
16. Mercurio MG (2001) Hirsutism: diagnosis and management. J Gend Specif Med 4:29–34
17. Mowszowicz I, Melanitou E, Doukani A, Wright F, Kuttenn F, Mauvais-Jarvis P (1983) Androgen binding capacity and 5 alpha-reductase activity in pubic skin fibroblasts from hirsute patients. J Clin Endocrinol Metab 56:1209–1213
18. New MI (2006) Nonclassical 21-hydroxylase deficiency. J Clin Endocrinol Metab 91:4205–4214
19. New MI, Lorenzen F, Pang S, Gunczler P, Dupont B, Levine LS (1979) Acquired adrenal hyperplasia with 21-hydroxylase deficiency is not the same genetic disorders as congenital adrenal hyperplasia. J Clin Endocrinol Metab 48:356–359
20. Norman RJ, Dewailly D, Legro RS, Hickey TE (2007) Polycystic ovary syndrome. Lancet 370:685–697
21. Petitti DB (2003) Combination estrogen-progestin oral contraceptives. N Engl J Med 349:1443–1450
22. Richards RN, Mcharg GE (1995) Electrolysis: observations from 13 years and 140.000 hours of experience. J Am Acad Dermatol 33:662–666
23. Rosenfield RL (2005) Clinical practice. Hirsutism. N Engl J Med 353:2578–2588
24. Rotterdam ESHRE/ASRM-Sponsored PCOS Consensus Workshop Group (2004) Revised 2003 consensus on diagnosis criteria and long-term health risks related to polycystic ovary syndrome. Fertile Steril 81:19–125
25. Rotterdam ESHRE/ASRM-Sponsored PCOS Consensus Workshop Group (2004) Revised 2003 consensus on diagnosis criteria and long-term health risks related to polycystic ovary syndrome (PCOS). Hum Reprod 19:41–47
26. Scully RE (1989) Ovarian tumors with endocrine manifestations. In: DeGroot LJ, Besser GM, Cahill GF (eds) Endocrinology, 2nd edn. WB Saunders, Philadelphia, pp 1994–2008
27. Smith SR, Piacquado DJ, Beger B, Littler C (2006) Eflornithine cream combined with laser therapy in the management of unwanted facial hair is growth in women: a randomized trial. Dermatol Surg 32:1237–1243
28. Spritzer PM (2002) Hirsutism revisited. Arq Bras Endocrinol Metab 46:127–136
29. Spritzer PM, Billaud L, Thalabard JC, Birman P, Mowszowicz I, Raux-Demay MC, Clair F, Kuttenn F, Mauvais-Jarvis P (1990) Cyproterone acetate versus hydrocortisone treatment in late-onset adrenal hyperplasia. J Clin Endocrinol Metab 70:642–646
30. Spritzer PM, Oppermann-Lisboa K, Mattiello S, Lhulier F (2000) Spironolactone as a single agent for long-term therapy of hirsute patients. Clin Endocrinol 52:587–594
31. Swiglo BA, Cosma M, Flynn DN, Kurtz DN, LaBella ML, Mullan RJ, Erwin PJ, Montori VM (2008) Antiandrogens for the treatment of hirsutism: a systematic review and metaanalyses of randomized controlled trials. J Clin Endocrinol Metab 93:1153–1160
32. Tolino A, Petrone A, Sarnacchiaro F, Cirillo D, Ronsini S, Lombardi G, Nappi C (1996) Finasteride in the treatment of hirsutism: new therapeutic perspectives. Fertil Steril 66:61–65
33. Urushibata O, Kase K (1995) A comparative study of axillar hair removal in women: plucking versus the blend method. J Dermatol 22:738–742
34. Venturoli S, Marescalchi O, Colombo FM, Macrelli S, Ravaioli B, Bagnoli A, Paradisi R, Flamigni C (1999) A prospective randomized trial comparing low dose flutamide, finasteride,

ketoconazole and cyproterone acetate-estrogen regimens in the treatment of hirsutism. J Clin Endocrinol Metab 84:1304–1310

35. Wong IL, Morris RS, Chang L, Spahn MA, Stanczyk FZ, Lobo RA (1995) A prospective randomized trial comparing finasteride to spironolactone in the treatment of hirsute women. J Clin Endocrinol Metab 80:233–238
36. Yildiz BO (2004) Recent advances in the treatment of polycystic ovary syndrome. Expert Opin Investig Drugs 13:1295–1305
37. Yildiz BO (2008) Assessment, diagnosis and treatment of a patient with hirsutism. Nat Clin Pract Endocrinol Metab 4:294–300
38. Zawadski JK, Dunaif A (1990) Diagnostic criteria for polycystic ovary syndrome: towards a rational approach. In: Evans JR, Hersaltine S, Marriam GR (eds) Polycystic ovary syndrome. Blackwell, Boston, pp 377–384

Striae Distensae

6

Taciana Dal'Forno

Core Messages

- Striae Distensae are linear atrophic lesions of the skin that are formed in areas of dermal damage. They are usually multiple, well-defined linear atrophic lesions.
- Many factors including hormones, mechanical stress, and genetic predisposition, seem to play a role in the onset of Striae Distensae.
- For clinical, histological and therapeutic purposes, the Striae Distensae can be divided in early striae distensae and old striae distensae.
- The treatment can be based on single or associated therapeutic modalities, according to the clinical evaluation. Fractional photothermolysis appears as one of the most promising methods for both early and old striae distensae.

6.1 General Aspects

Striae distensae (SD) are also known as stretch marks and striae atrophicans. They are visible as linear scars which are formed in areas of dermal damage produced by stretching of the skin [10]. They are associated with various physiologic states including puberty, pregnancy, grown spurts, rapid weight gain, obesity, and states leading to excess of cortisol [29, 48].

The factors which rule the development of SD are poorly understood. Many authors have suggested that SD develop as a result of stress rupture of the connective tissue framework, but others disagree. It has been suggested that they develop more easily in skin which has a critical proportion of rigid cross-linked collagen, as

T. Dal'Forno, M.D., Ph.D.
Department of Dermatology, Pontifícia Universidade Catolica do Rio Grande do Sul (PUC-RS), Brazilian Center for Studies in Dermatology
782 Dr. Timoteo, St., ZIP: 90570-040 Porto Alegre, RS, Brazil
e-mail: tacianad@terra.com.br

A. Tosti, D. Hexsel (eds.), *Update in Cosmetic Dermatology*,
DOI 10.1007/978-3-642-34029-1_6, © Springer-Verlag Berlin Heidelberg 2013

they occur in early adult life [10]. Many factors including hormones (particularly corticosteroids), mechanical stress, and genetic predisposition also seem to play a role in the onset of SD [29].

A recent study shows an increased estrogen, androgen, and glucocorticoid receptors in the SD skin. These findings indicate that under certain conditions, there is an increase in hormonal receptor expression, suggesting that regions that undergo greater mechanical stretching of the skin may express greater hormonal receptor activity. This activity may influence the metabolism of the extracellular matrix, causing the formation of SD [11].

In adolescence, some factors are directly related to the increase in local volume in risky areas, causing acute distention of the skin, with the consequent appearance of SD. Factors of particular note in this age range are the greater accumulation of fat in certain areas of the body, making the body lines more curved, mainly in women, as well as weight gain and the increase in the 17-ketosteroids [37].

In pregnant women, a combination of hormonal factors (e.g., adrenocortical hormones, estrogen, relaxin) associated with increased lateral stress on the connective tissue due to increased size of the various portions of the body is thought to be important [20, 26]. An observational analysis of 324 primiparae observed SD in 52 % at delivery and concluded that the most significant risk factor was low maternal age [6]. Another study evaluated the risk factors for the development of SD in 112 primiparae, showing that women who developed SD were significantly younger and had gained significantly more weight during pregnancy. Moderate and severe SD were associated with lower maternal age, higher birth weight, more advanced gestational age at delivery, and family history of SD [34].

Striae distensae are a feature of Cushing's disease, and they may be induced by local or systemic steroid therapy [10]. Topical corticosteroids, especially when used in larger areas and under occlusion, favor the appearance of SD in the area or even at some distance [8]. Striae distensae have been reported in human immunodeficiency virus (HIV)-positive patients receiving the protease inhibitor indinavir [10].

6.2 Diagnosis and Differential Diagnosis

Striae distensae occur in areas of reduced skin resistance and greatest accumulation of adipose tissue. They are linear atrophic depressions of the skin that are formed in areas of dermal damage. Striae distensae are usually multiple, well-defined linear atrophic lesions that follow the lines of cleavage. Initially, they appear as red-to-violaceous elevated lines that can be mildly pruritic and are called striae rubra (Fig. 6.1). Over time, the color gradually fades, and the lesions become atrophic, with the skin surface exhibiting a fine wrinkled appearance, the striae alba (Fig. 6.2) [29]. These characteristics of atrophy are permanent in SD [19].

Striae distensae are common during adolescence and seem to be associated with rapid increase in volume of a particular region [10]. Women are most commonly affected, occurring initially and predominantly on breasts and some areas also affected by cellulite, like hips and abdomen. In males, they more frequently occur on the back,

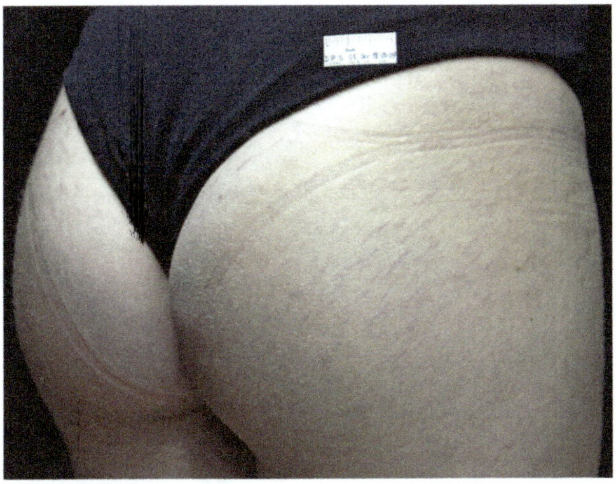

Fig. 6.1 Clinical aspect of striae rubra on the buttocks in a 14-year-old female patient

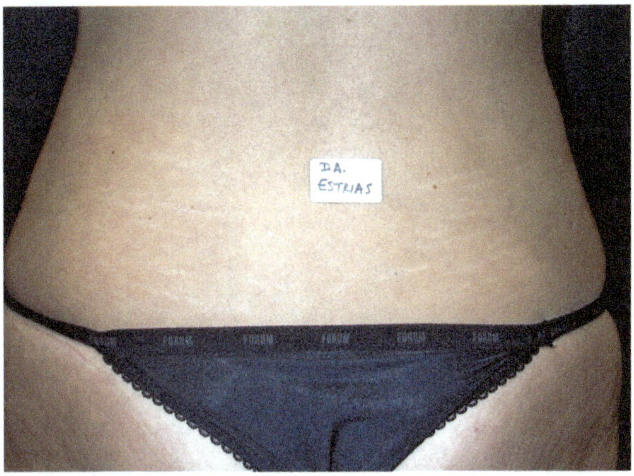

Fig. 6.2 Clinical aspect of multiple striae alba on the lower back in a 26-year-old female patient

lower back, and outer edge of the thighs [15, 19]. They may develop on the shoulders in young male weight lifters, when their muscle mass rapidly increases [10].

Striae distensae occur in up to 90 % of pregnant women. They are very common over the abdomen and breasts in pregnancy, but they can occur on hips, buttocks, thighs, and flanks. The SD associated with systemic corticosteroid therapy and Cushing's syndrome can be larger and more violaceous and widely distributed (Fig. 6.3) [29].

From a clinical and histological point of view, there are no significant differences between SD of different etiology or localization or between striae of patients of different sex or age group. Basically, they differ according to the time of evolution and may be divided in early or old. Therefore, for clinical, histological, and therapeutic purposes, the very simple classification was suggested [19]:

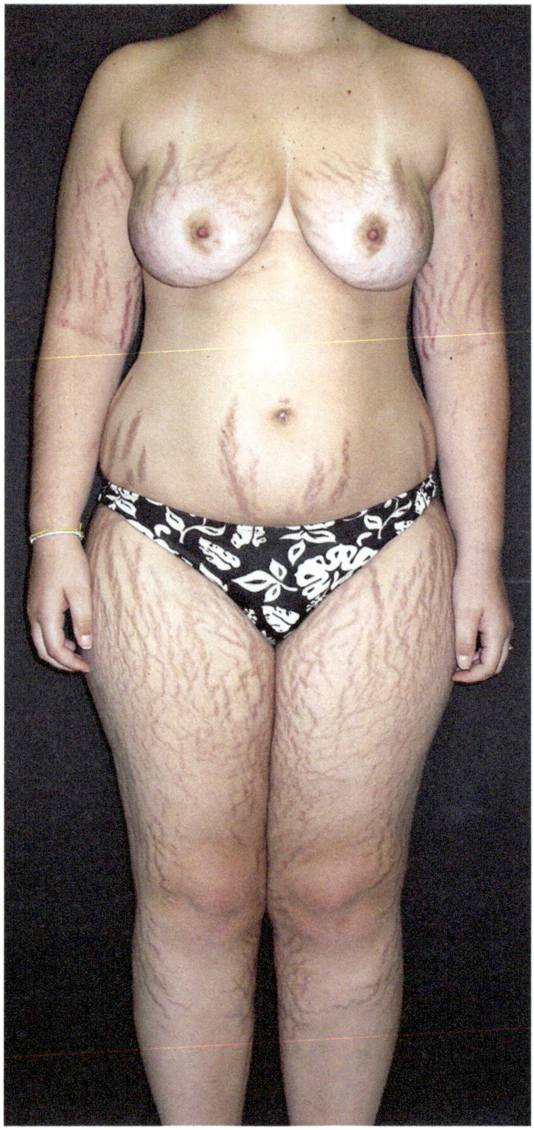

Fig. 6.3 Clinical aspect and large distribution of striae distensae in a 21-year-old female patient posttreatment with high oral doses of dexamethasone

Early striae distensae (Fig. 6.2) may be narrow (up to 5 mm) or wide (>5 mm), onset up to 6–12 months, usually pink, erythematous, and sometimes hyperpigmented. Old striae distensae (Fig. 6.3) may also be narrow (up to 5 mm) or wide (>5 mm), onset more than 6–12 months, and usually hypochromic or same color as nonaffected skin.

The histology of SD is that of a scar, and the development of SD has been likened to that of wound healing or scar formation [6]. In the early stages, inflammatory changes may be conspicuous, but later the epidermis is thin and flattened. Early SD show a deep and superficial perivascular lymphocytic infiltrate around the venules [4]. Collagen bands on the upper third of the reticular dermis are stretched and aligned parallel to the surface of the skin. In the latter stages, there is thinning of the epidermis due to flattening of the rete ridges and loss of collagen and elastin [36].

Striae distensae must be differentiated from linear focal elastosis that is characterized by rows of yellow palpable striae-like bands on the lower back. Unlike striae, these lesions are raised and yellow rather than depressed and white. Elderly men are most commonly affected, although cases in teenagers have been described. Histologically, there is a focal increase in the number of elongated or fragmented elastic fibers and a thickened dermis [29]. From the clinical and histologic point of view, as mentioned above, SD must be differentiated from linear scars.

6.3 Treatment

Different treatments may be indicated for early (rubra) or old (alba) striae distensae. As these lesions tend to become better in cosmetic aspect spontaneously over time, the usefulness of treatments that have been tried without case controls was not well established [29]. Early therapeutic interventions may guarantee better and more successful results by preventing or at least minimizing the structural alterations in the epidermis [19].

6.3.1 Topical Treatments

6.3.1.1 Moisturizers

The application of natural oils on the skin, such as cocoa butter, sweet almond oil and avocado oil are used to keep skin hydrated and soft. Despite its widespread use, there is no scientific evidence of its efficacy in the treatment and prevention of SD.

Two multicenter, double-blind, randomized, and placebo-controlled trial evaluated the effect of daily application of cocoa butter (*Theobroma cacao*) lotion on 175 and 150 women, respectively, since first or second trimester until delivery, showing no difference in the development or severity of SD in pregnant women [9, 35] Another study does not show statistical difference between women that use or not an olive oil cream at the third trimester of pregnancy [43].

6.3.1.2 Tretinoin

Some studies have shown that treatment with the 0.1 % tretinoin cream, with or without other active ingredients, can improve the clinical appearance as well as the length and width of early SD [23, 38, 5]. Despite presenting a considerable incidence of adverse effects such as erythema and scaling, improved clinical appearance of early SD with topical tretinoin appears to be evident and has been demonstrated.

Although few studies have shown positive results, the use of tretinoin for treating SD remains controversial, and the optimal concentration of this active ingredient in the formulations has not been established [37]. Tretinoin is contraindicated during pregnancy and lactation and therefore should not be used for prevention and treatment of early SD in pregnant women.

6.3.1.3 Other Active Cosmeceuticals

Other active cosmeceuticals such as glycolic acid, ascorbic acid, hyaluronic acid, Centella asiatica, wheat (Triticum vulgare), and onion (Allium cepa) extracts have been evaluated in some studies for the treatment and prevention of SD, especially in pregnant women. However, these cosmeceuticals were not generally evaluated alone, making it difficult to analyze the results [12, 46].

A recent study, published by Draelos et al., evaluated the effect of an onion extract cream with Centella asiatica and hyaluronic acid in improving the appearance of recent SD. The treated thigh demonstrated a statistically significant difference in the mean change in participant and investigator evaluations in overall appearance, texture, color, and softness compared with the untreated thigh after 3 months [13].

6.3.2 Surgical Treatments

Evidences show better results in the treatment of SD with surgical procedures, which can be associated or not to topical treatment. Many surgical procedures are used to treat SD, but just those with some scientific evidence will be referred in this chapter.

6.3.2.1 Lasers, Light Devices, and Radiofrequency

Treatment with the 585-nm pulsed dye laser at low-energy densities seems to improve the appearance of old SD. The use of the 10-mm spot size with fluence of 3.0 J/cm^2 improved the appearance of striae better than the other parameters. Apparent increased dermal elastin was also observed 8 weeks post-therapy [31]. Nonetheless, another study only showed moderate beneficial effect in reducing the degree of erythema in early SD and no apparent clinical change in old SD, recommending this laser only for early SD in patient skin types II to IV [22].

A study that evaluated the effects of 585-nm pulse dye laser and the short-pulsed CO_2 laser in old striae in patients with types IV, V, and VI skin showed no improvement, hyperpigmentation, and persistent erythema. This study concluded that in patients with higher skin phototypes, laser treatment of striae should be avoided or used with great caution [33].

Intense pulsed light (IPL) is a noncoherent, nonlaser, filtered flashlamp, emitting a broadband visible light. Its efficacy has been reported recently in the treatment of photodamaged facial skin, promoting the production of neocollagen and ordering of elastic fibers. Because of the stimulation of collagen production, one study evaluated the effect of IPL in the treatment of old striae. Fifteen women with old striae were treated with five sessions of IPL, showing a statistically significative difference ($p<0.01$) in the posttreatment dermal thickness. A clinical and microscopical improvement was obtained in all patients [18].

Treatment with the 308-nm excimer laser seems to be safe and effective in pigment correction of hypopigmented scars and old striae. Final averages of pigment correction rates relative to control sites were approximately 60–70 % by visual assessment and 100 % by colorimetric analysis after nine treatments administered biweekly. Maintenance treatment every 1–4 months seems to be required to sustain the cosmetic benefit [3]. Light sources emitting ultraviolet B (UVB) and narrowband UVB/UVA1 therapy irradiation also have been shown to repigment old striae [16, 39]. The repigmentation after UVB occurs due to increase in melanin pigment, hypertrophy of melanocytes, and an increase in the number of melanocytes [16].

In a study, a radiofrequency (RF) device in combination with 585-nm pulsed dye laser was used to treat abdominal striae in 37 patients. Almost 90 % of the patients showed overall improvement. All the biopsies of nine patients showed an increase in the amount of collagen fibers, and increased elastic fibers were found in six specimens [42]. Bipolar RF device seems also to be effective with clinical, histological, and immunohistochemical improvement of treated striae [32].

The 1,064-nm long-pulsed Nd:YAG laser has been used to promote an increase in dermal collagen and is known to be a laser that has a high affinity for vascular chromophores. This laser was evaluated in a study with 20 patients presented early SD. The improvements were considered excellent by 55 % of the patients and 40 % of the evaluators, showing that this laser should be effective in early SD [17].

The non-ablative 1,450-nm diode laser has been shown to improve atrophic scars, but, in a study, was ineffective to improve the clinical aspect of early or old SD in Asian patients with skin types IV to VI. A high percentage of patients (64 %) had post-inflammatory hyperpigmentation [45].

Many recent studies have shown that non-ablative fractional photothermolysis with 1,550-nm erbium-doped fiber laser seems to be safe and effective in the treatment of early and old SD [24, 25, 41, 44]. One study evaluated 22 women with SD treated with two sessions of fractional photothermolysis each at a pulse energy of 30 mJ, a density level of 6, and eight passes at intervals of 4 weeks showed good to excellent clinical improvement from baseline in 27 %. Most of the lesions with excellent results were white in color and of long duration. Skin biopsy revealed that average epidermal thickness and dermal thickness were greater than at baseline. The immunoreactivity of procollagen type 1 increased after treatment. There were no significant side effects except erythema and mild pigmentation [7]. Figures 6.4 and 6.5 show the results with fractional photothermolysis with 1,550-nm erbium-doped fiber laser after 3 sessions on old SD.

Ablative fractional photothermolysis with 10,600-nm carbon dioxide laser to treat old SD was evaluated in a recent study with 27 participants. The authors performed a single session and obtained some improvement of cosmetic appearance in all patients. However, 7.4 % of the patients were unsatisfied despite the results [27].

A randomized controlled study compared the results of CO_2 ablative fractional photothermolysis versus non-ablative 1,550-nm fractional erbium in the treatment

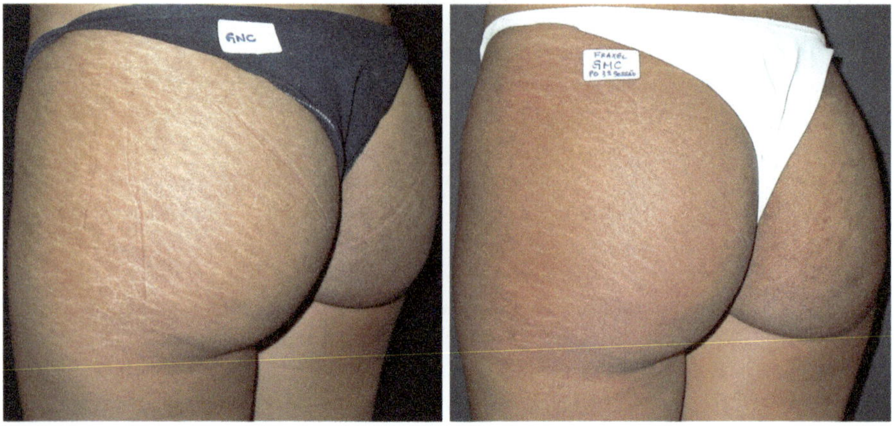

Figs. 6.4 and 6.5 Old stretch marks' aspect before and after three sessions of fractional photothermolysis with 1,550-nm erbium-doped fiber laser (Fraxel™) on the left buttock in a 28-year-old female patient

of old abdominal SD, after three sessions. Both treatments showed good clinical and histologic results, without statistically significant difference between them. However, patients treated with ablative method reported more severe pain and had more post-inflammatory hyperpigmentation [47].

6.3.3 Subcision®

Subcision® may be useful when the striae surface is very depressed, because it favors the formation of neocollagen, when performed in the dermis. However, this procedure is not very effective as an isolated method, because it does not structurally alter the epidermis [19]. In a preliminary study, there was necrosis in a high percentage of SD treated with Subcision. The authors considered subjective the results in the majority of the patients [28].

6.3.4 Microdermabrasion, Sand Abrasion, and Serial Superficial Dermabrasion

The microdermabrasion was described also to treat early and old SD, but further studies on a larger scale are needed to identify the efficacy of using such technique for SD [40]. Mahuzier in his textbook on microdermabrasion stated that 10–20 sessions of microdermabrasion at an interval of not less than 1 month, each session resulting in bleeding points, provide satisfactory improvement in SD [30]. A more recent controlled study on the clinical and molecular evaluation of treating SD with microdermabrasion in 20 patients that received five microdermabrasion treatments at

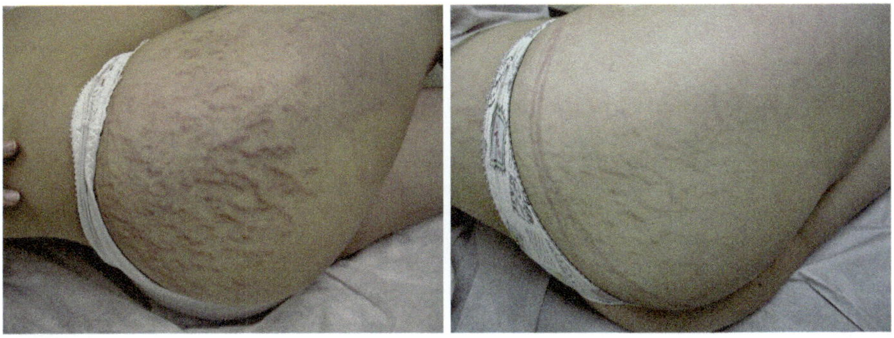

Figs. 6.6 and 6.7 Recent stretch marks' aspect before and after serial superficial dermabrasion in a pregnant woman

weekly intervals on half of the body demonstrated overall good to excellent response in more than half of the subjects, with improvement more marked in striae rubra, and upregulation of type I procollagen mRNA was found in all treated SD samples [1].

A report of a series of cases treated by a combination treatment (sand abrasion and a patent mixture containing 15 % trichloroacetic acid) followed by 6–24 h of a patent cream under plastic occlusion in the striae of 69 patients showed clinical improvement by 70 % [2].

Superficial dermabrasion gives good results on early narrow SD. In a study, 28 patients, with mean ages of 16 years and multiple early SD on the abdomen, hips, tights or breasts, underwent to a weekly serial superficial dermabrasion treatment with a dermabrasion device (10,000 rpm) with 3-mm round diamond fraises. On the dermatologic evaluation, all patients had some clinical improvement of the early SD, but those that had just or in the majority narrow SD improved more (82.1 % had moderate to accentuate improvement) (Figs. 6.6 and 6.7) [21]. As it is only a mechanical treatment, it may also be useful in pregnant women.

Conclusion

The complete evaluation of a patient with striae distensae should include consideration of the stage and of the skin type. Expectations must be realistic, and the optimal treatment modality should be carefully selected to avoid any exaggeration of the problem or complications [14].

The therapeutic modalities are numerous and may be associated and individualized regarding the clinical evaluation. Topical treatment seems to be more useful when associated with surgical dermatologic procedures. Fractional photothermolysis appears as one of the most promising methods for both early and old striae distensae, but more researches and clinical trials are needed to improve the results of these new promising treatments aiming to treat this very common, sometimes disfiguring, cosmetic problem.

References

1. Abdel-Latif AM, Elbendary AS (2008) Treatment of striae distensae with microdermabrasion: a clinical and molecular study. JEWDS 5:24–30
2. Adatto MA, Deprez P (2003) Striae treated by a novel combination treatment–sand abrasion and a patent mixture containing 15 % trichloroacetic acid followed by 6–24 hrs of a patent cream under plastic occlusion. J Cosmet Dermatol 2(2):61–67
3. Alexiades-Armenakas MR, Bernstein LJ, Friedman PM, Geronemus RG (2004) The safety and efficacy of the 308-nm excimer laser for pigment correction of hypopigmented scars and striae alba. Arch Dermatol 140(8):955–960
4. Arem AJ, Kischer CW (1980) Analysis of striae. Palst Reconstr Surg 65:22–29
5. Ash K, Lord J, Zukowski M, McDaniel DH (1998) Comparison of topical therapy for striae alba (20 % glycolic acid/0.05 % tretinoin versus 20 % glycolic acid/10 % L-ascorbic acid). Dermatol Surg 24(8):849–856
6. Atwal GS, Manku LK, Griffiths CE, Polson DW (2006) Striae gravidarum in primiparae. Br J Dermatol 155(5):965–969
7. Bak H, Kim BJ, Lee WJ, Bang JS, Lee SY, Choi JH, Chang SE (2009) Treatment of striae distensae with fractional photothermolysis. Dermatol Surg 35(8):1215–1220
8. Beer K, Downie J (2007) Sequelae from inadvertent long-term use of potent topical steroids. J Drugs Dermatol 6(5):550–551
9. Buchanan K, Fletcher HM, Reid M (2010) Prevention of striae gravidarum with cocoa butter cream. Int J Gynecol Obstet 68(1):65–68
10. Burrows NP, Lovell CR (2004) Disorders of connective tissue. In: Champion RH, Burton JL, Ebling FJG (eds) Rook's textbook of dermatology, vol 46, 7th edn. Blackwell, Oxford, pp 1–71
11. Cordeiro RC, Zecchin KG, de Moraes AM (2010) Expression of estrogen, androgen, and glucocorticoid receptors in recent striae distensae. Int J Dermatol 49(1):30–32
12. De-Bauman M, Walther M, de-Weck R (1987) Effectiveness of alphastria cream in the prevention of pregnancy stretch marks (striae distensae). results of a double-blind study. Gynakol Rundsch 27:79–84
13. Draelos ZD, Gold MH, Kaur M, Olayinka B, Grundy SL, Pappert JL et al (2010) Evaluation of an onion extract, centella asiatica, and hyaluronic acid cream in the appearance of striae rubra. Skinmed 8(2):80–86
14. Elsaie ML, Baumann LS, Elsaaiee LT (2009) Striae distensae (stretch marks) and different modalities of therapy: an update. Dermatol Surg 35(4):563–573
15. Fredérique H, Piérard FC et al (1997) Striae distensae of pregnancy: in vivo biomechanical evaluation. Int J Dermatol 36:506–508
16. Goldberg DJ, Marmur ES, Schmults C, Hussain M, Phelps R (2005) Histologic and ultrastructural analysis of ultraviolet B laser and light source treatment of leukoderma in striae distensae. Dermatol Surg 31(4):385–387
17. Goldman A, Rossato F, Prati C (2008) Stretch marks: treatment using the 1,064-nm Nd:YAG laser. Dermatol Surg 34(5):686–691
18. Hernández-Pérez E, Colombo-Charrier E, Valencia-Ibiett E (2002) Intense pulsed light in the treatment of striae distensae. Dermatol Surg 28(12):1124–1130
19. Hexsel D (2001) Body repair. In: Parish LC, Brenner S, Ramos-e-Silva M (eds) Women's dermatology. From infancy to maturity. Parthenon, London, pp 586–595
20. Hexsel D, Costa A, Soirefmann M, Dal'Forno T (2009) Estrias gestacionais. In: Costa A, Alves G, Azulay L (eds) Dermatologia e Gravidez. Elsevier, Rio de Janeiro, pp 165–171
21. Hexsel DM, Dal'Forno T, Mazzuco R (2009) Superficial dermabrasion in the treatment of recent stretch marks (striae rubra). Poster 350. 67th annual meeting of the American Academy of Dermatology, San Francisco, 6–10 Mar 2009
22. Jiménez GP, Flores F, Berman B, Gunja-Smith Z (2003) Treatment of striae rubra and striae alba with the 585-nm pulsed-dye laser. Dermatol Surg 29(4):362–365

23. Kang S (1998) Topical tretinoin therapy for management of early striae. J Am Acad Dermatol 39(2 Pt 3):S90–S92
24. Katz TM, Goldberg LH, Friedman PM (2009) Nonablative fractional photothermolysis for the treatment of striae rubra. Dermatol Surg 35(9):1430–1433
25. Kim BJ, Lee DH, Kim MN et al (2008) Fractional photothermolysis for the treatment of striae distensae in Asian skin. Am J Clin Dermatol 9(1):33–37
26. Lawley TJ, Yancey KB (2003) Skin changes and diseases in pregnancy. In: Freedberg IM, Eisen AZ, Wolff K (eds) Fitzpatrick's dermatology in general medicine, 6th edn. McGraw Hill, New York, pp 1361–1366
27. Lee SE, Kim JH, Lee SJ et al (2010) Treatment of striae distensae using an ablative 10,600-nm carbon dioxide fractional laser: a retrospective review of 27 participants. Dermatol Surg 36(11):1683–1690
28. Luis-Montoya P, Pichardo-Velázquez P, Hojyo-Tomoka MT, Domínguez-Cherit J (2005) Evaluation of subcision as a treatment for cutaneous striae. J Drugs Dermatol 4(3):346–350
29. Maari C, Powell J (2003) Atrophies of connective tissue. In: Bologna JL, Jorizzo JL, Rapini RP (eds) Dermatology. Mosby, London, pp 1539–1548
30. Mahuzier F (1999) Microdermabrasion of stretch marks. In: Mahuzeier F (ed) Microdermabrasion or Parisian peel in practice. Solal, Marseille, pp 25–65
31. McDaniel DH, Ash K, Zukowski M (1996) Treatment of stretch marks with the 585-nm flashlamp-pumped pulsed dye laser. Dermatol Surg 22(4):332–337
32. Montesi G, Calvieri S, Balzani A, Gold MH (2007) Bipolar radiofrequency in the treatment of dermatologic imperfections: clinicopathological and immunohistochemical aspects. J Drugs Dermatol 6(9):890–896
33. Nouri K, Romagosa R, Chartier T et al (1999) Comparison of the 585 nm pulse dye laser and the short pulsed CO2 laser in the treatment of striae distensae in skin types IV and VI. Dermatol Surg 25(5):368–370
34. Osman H, Rubeiz N, Tamim H, Nassar AH (2007) Risk factors for the development of striae gravidarum. Am J Obstet Gynecol 196(1):62.e1–62.e5
35. Osman H, Usta IM, Rubeiz N et al (2008) Cocoa prevention of striae gravidarum: a double-blind, randomised and placebo controlled trial. BJOG 115(9):1138–1142
36. Pierard GE, Nizet JL, Adant JP et al (1999) Tensile properties of relaxed excised skin exhibiting striae distensae. J Med Eng Technol 23:69–72
37. Pribanich S, Simpson FG, Held B et al (1994) Low-dose tretinoin does not improve striae distensae: a double-blind, placebo-controlled study. Cutis 54:121–124
38. Rangel O, Arias I, García E, Lopez-Padilla S (2001) Topical tretinoin 0.1 % for pregnancy-related abdominal striae: an open-label, multicenter, prospective study. Adv Ther 18(4): 181–186
39. Sadick NS, Magro C, Hoenig A (2007) Prospective clinical and histological study to evaluate the efficacy and safety of a targeted high-intensity narrow band UVB/UVA1 therapy for striae alba. J Cosmet Laser Ther 9(2):79–83
40. Spencer JM (2005) Microdermabrasion. Am J Clin Dermatol 6(2):89–92
41. Stotland M, Chapas AM, Brightman L et al (2008) The safety and efficacy of fractional photothermolysis for the correction of striae distensae. J Drugs Dermatol 7(9):857–861
42. Suh DH, Chang KY, Son HC et al (2007) Radiofrequency and 585-nm pulsed dye laser treatment of striae distensae: a report of 37 Asian patients. Dermatol Surg 33(1):29–34
43. Taavoni S, Soltanipour F, Haghani H et al (2011) Effects of olive oil on striae gravidarum in the second trimester of pregnancy. Complement Ther Clin Pract 17:167–169, Epub 2010 Nov 23
44. Taub AF (2007) Fractionated delivery systems for difficult to treat clinical applications: acne scarring, melasma, atrophic scarring, striae distensae, and deep rhytides. J Drugs Dermatol 6(11):1120–1128
45. Tay YK, Kwok C, Tan E (2006) Non-ablative 1,450-nm diode laser treatment of striae distensae. Lasers Surg Med 38(3):196–199

46. Wierrani F, Kozak W, Schramm W, Grünberger W (1992) Attempt of preventive treatment of striae gravidarum using preventive massage ointment administration. Wien Klin Wochenschr 104(2):42–44
47. Yang YJ, Lee GY (2011) Treatment of striae distensae with nonablative fractional laser versus ablative CO_2 fractional laser: a randomized controlled trial. Ann Dermatol 23(4):481–489
48. Yosipovitch G, DeVore A, Dawn A (2007) Obesity and the skin: skin physiology and skin manifestations of obesity. J Am Acad Dermatol 56(6):901–916; quiz 917–920

Cosmeceuticals in Dermatology

7

Aurora Tedeschi, Lee E. West, Laura Guzzardi, Karishma H. Bhatt, Erika E. Reid, Giovanni Scapagnini, and Giuseppe Micali

Core Messages

- The term "cosmeceuticals" refers to a new category of products considered as having both pharmaceutical and cosmetic properties. The aim of this review is to discuss about the common systemic and topical cosmeceutic agents with potential use in dermatology.

7.1 Cosmeceuticals

The term "cosmeceuticals", suggested by Kligman more than 20 years ago, refers to topical products that lie in a gray zone where they are viewed as having both pharmaceutical and cosmetic properties [1]. Although the neologism was innovative and relevant, it was rejected from the US Food, Drug, and Cosmetic Act that, according to the 1938s US Congress, labels as drug every substance for use in the diagnosis,

A. Tedeschi, M.D., Ph.D. (✉) • L. Guzzardi, M.D. • G. Micali, M.D.
Department of Dermatology, Dermatologic Clinic, University of Catania, Catania, Italy
e-mail: auroratedeschi@gmail.com

L.E. West, B.S. Pharm • K.H. Bhatt, B.S.
Department of Pharmacology, Northwestern Memorial Hospital, Chicago, IL, USA

E.E. Reid, B.S.
Department of Dermatology, Northwestern University, Feinberg School of Medicine, Chicago, IL, USA

G. Scapagnini, M.D., Ph.D.
Department of Health Science, University of Molise, Campobasso, Italy

A. Tosti, D. Hexsel (eds.), *Update in Cosmetic Dermatology*,
DOI 10.1007/978-3-642-34029-1_7, © Springer-Verlag Berlin Heidelberg 2013

cure, treatment or prevention of disease, and as cosmetic any product intended for beautifying and promoting attractiveness. In spite of this, the term cosmeceuticals has recently been gaining increasing popularity, as the term cosmetic seems to be restrictive for those substances that have druglike beneficial effects. On the other hand, the "cosmeceuticals" concept has caused a lot of confusion, because of similar neologisms such as neutraceuticals and/or neoceuticals. Actually, in USA and Canada, most cosmeceuticals are regulated as over the counter (OTC) products, while in Europe they are considered as cosmetics. Only in Japan, a new class of products, called quasi-drugs, has been created [2].

The cosmeceutical market represents a fast-growing segment of industry, and it continues to grow as the demand for youthful skin by both men and women increases with the general population's median age. Although cosmeceuticals have the potential to provide both therapeutic and cosmetic benefits, they are perceived to produce little or no systemic biological effect and are therefore not usually subject to rigorous testing and regulation as required of pharmaceuticals by the FDA and EMEA [3]. Excipients in cosmeceuticals are typically identified in product packaging similar to that of cosmetics, i.e., in descending order of ingredient concentration and with no distinction of any ingredient over another ingredient so that no "active" ingredient is identifiable and no medical claim is made. This overview is aimed to identify cosmeceuticals currently in use and their "active" ingredients.

Cosmeceuticals are often used to improve skin appearance. There is a wide range of available products, such as prescription only and nonprescription topical products, as well as some so-called dietary supplements. This review will focus only on topical nonprescription ones and on their correspective oral supplement, excluding prescription pharmaceuticals with cosmetic benefits. Cosmeceuticals classification category includes: antioxidants, growth factors, peptides, anti-inflammatory agents, botanicals, polysaccharides and hypopigmenting agents (Table 7.1) [3, 4]. Because there is relatively less regulation applicable to the marketing of cosmeceuticals, consumers may be easily led to believe these products are safe and that their advertisements are supported by the level of evidence required for pharmaceuticals. The potential or unwanted side effects of cosmeceutical agents, as well as the investigational evidence, should be considered to support their indications and use. Guidance for use of cosmeceuticals according to age, skin type, gender, and skin disorder is provided as part of this review. Furthermore, side effects, if reported in the literature, will be discussed.

7.2 Antioxidants

Free radicals are highly reactive molecules formed by endogenous and exogenous damaging agents such as UV radiation, drugs, air pollutions, and cigarette smoke. They are reactive oxygen intermediates which include singlet oxygen, superoxides, peroxides, hydroxyl radical, and hypochlorous acid. They are characterized by unpaired electrons that can cause serious damage to cell membranes, lipids, proteins, and DNA. Free radicals are implicated in the development of inflammation, photodamage, and carcinogenesis. In a biological context,

Table 7.1 Common cosmeceutic agents (listed by category), with potential use in dermatology

Category	Agent
Antioxidants	Non prescription retinoids and vitamin A derivatives[a]
	Vitamin B (niacinamide[a,b], panthenol[a])
	Vitamin C (L-ascorbic acid)[a]
	Vitamin E (alpha-tocopherol)[a,b]
	Alpha-lipoic acid (ALA)[a,b]
	Coenzyme Q10 (ubiquinone[a,b], idebenone[a])
	Selenium[a], EPA[a,b]
	Polyphenols[a,b]
	Kinetin (N-6-furfuryladenine)[a]
Growth factors	Epidermal growth factor (EGF)[a]
	Transforming growth factor (TGF)[a]
Peptides	Signal peptides[a]
	Carrier peptides[a]
	Neurotransmitter-modulating peptides (argireline[a], dimethylaminoethanol[a])
Antiinflammatories/ botanicals	Propolis[a]
	Oatmeal[a]
	Olive oil[a,b]
	Botanicals with high levels of polyphenols (grape seed[a,b], *Coffea arabica* and cofeeberry extracts[a,b], green tea[a,b], pomegranade[a,b])
	Polyphenols (resveratrol[a,b], soy isoflavones[a,b], ferulic acid[a,b], silymarin[a,b], quercetin[a,b], curcumin[a])
	Arnica[a,b]
	Chamomile[a,b]
	Aloe vera[a]
	Allantoin[a]
	Bromelain[a,b]
	Feverfew[a,b]
	Licorice extracts[a,b]
	Lycopene[a]
	Sulforaphane[a,b]
	Others (rosemary, polypodium leucotomas, prickly pears, witch hazel, papaya, date, garlic, echinacea, saw palmetto, ginseng, noni, hypericum, Melaleuca alternifolia, lavender, willow bark, black cohosh, ginkgo biloba, mushroom, capparis and horse chestnut)
Hydroxy acid	Alpha hydroxy acids (glycolic, lactic and malic, citric acid)[a]
	Beta-hydroxy acids (salicylic acid)[a]
	Poly-hydroxy acids (gluconolactone, lactobionic acid)[a]
Depigmenting agents	Hydroquinone[a]
	Licorice extracts[a]
	Kojic acid[a]
	Arbutin[a]
	Aloesin[a]
	Ellagic acid[a]

[a]Topical application
[b]Oral assumption

antioxidant compounds protect against oxidative damage through four main mechanisms: (a) preventing ROS formation by sequestering transition metal ions into complexes; (b) scavenging or quenching free radicals and other reactive species; (c) breaking chain reactions initiated by free radicals; and (d) inducing antioxidants and repair systems.

7.2.1 Nonprescription Retinoids and Vitamin A Derivates

Retinoids are part of a class of substances derived from vitamin A and its natural and synthetic derivatives. Derivatives of vitamin A are found in various concentrations in cosmeceuticals and include vitamin A alcohol (retinol), vitamin A esters (retinyl palmitate, retinyl acetate), vitamin A aldehyde (retinal) and retinoic acid (tretinoin). As lipophilic molecules, they can diffuse through phospholipidic membranes. Inside the cells, they bind specific to nuclear receptors (RAR-α, -β, -γ and RXR-α, -β, -γ), forming ligand receptor complexes which modulate the expression of genes involved in cellular differentiation and proliferation [5]. The cosmeceutical benefits from vitamin A and its derivates lie in their ability as retinoids to regulate epithelial cell growth and differentiation and, finally, to normalize keratinization. Retinoids have been shown to have receptor-specific effects on the skin, resulting in decreased roughness, facial wrinkling and fine lines [6] allowed for the synthesis of novel pharmacologic classes of compounds that have broader structural diversity with greater variance of pharmacological properties than natural retinoids. Topical use of retinoids has shown to be effective in the treatment of acne, photodamage, and psoriasis. Irritation is the most common side effect associated with topical retinoids; however teratogenicity is often the major concern.

Vitamin A belongs to the retinoid family, whose prototype is tretinoin, a prescription drug, useful in increasing collagen and successfully used to treat wrinkles and photodamage. Although the use of tretinoin is well documented in acne and photoaging treatment, retinol is a cosmeceutical which is not as irritating nor as potent as tretinoin. However, retinol is reported to increase water content and collagen synthesis [6, 7], as well as inhibit melanogenesis and matrix metalloproteinases (MMPs) involved in collagen disruption, thus improving skin texture and reducing the visibility of skin lines and wrinkles. *Retinol* is a nonprescription cosmeceutical product, particularly used as an alternative approach for sensitive skin that does not tolerate tretinoin. The two retinyl esters of vitamin A, *retinyl propionate* and *retinyl palmitate*, are also used in the cosmeceutical marketplace. They both have better tolerance profiles among topical retinoids [8]. *Retinaldehyde* (RAL) an intermediate form in the conversion of retinol to retinoic acid, is a well-tolerated retinoid that may also alleviate the vascular component of rosacea symptoms [9]. Moreover, 0.1 % retinaldehyde in association with 6 % glycolic acid (GA) has shown a significant decreasing in both inflammatory and retentional lesions in acne patients [10]. Also, this combination seems to be effective to prevent and treat acne scars [11].

7.2.2 B Vitamins

This group of vitamins, including niacinamide (vitamin B3) and panthenol (vitamin B5), has been evaluated topically in the treatment of acne, wounds, bullous pemphigoid, and also as chemopreventive agents.

7.2.2.1 Niacinamide

Niacinamide, or nicotinamide, is a water-soluble, stable, low molecular weight substance that is a precursor of nicotinamide adenine dinucleotide phosphate (NADP) as well as of its reduced form (NADPH), both of them are considered as antioxidants. Topical nicotinamide decreases transepidermal water loss (TEWL), improving skin barrier function; for these reasons it is indicated in atopic dermatitis and rosacea. It also decreases hyperpigmentation by inhibiting melanosome transfer from melanocytes to keratinocytes. Because of its effects on sebum production, on follicular ostia diameter and of its anti-inflammatory properties (inhibition of Propionibacterium acnes-induced IL-8 production in keratinocytes through the NF-κB and MAPK pathways), it is often used in the treatment of acne [12, 13]. Smoother skin texture and little but significant wrinkle reduction may be observed after chronic topical treatment, as a result of its stimulation on collagen production [12]. Moreover, topical niacinamide seems to prevent UV immunosuppression [14]. Mild side effects, such as erythema, pruritus and burning are sometimes reported after topical application [15]. Oral supplementation of nicotinamide seems to be useful in the treatment of several inflammatory skin conditions, including acne, rosacea, [16] dermatitis herpetiformis, generalized granuloma annulare, necrobiosis lipoidica, and bullous pemphigoid. The association of oral nicotinamide and tetracycline in the treatment of erythema elevatum diutinum, linear IgA dermatosis, pemphigus, cicatricial pemphigoid, and lichen planus pemphigoides has also been reported [12]. At both high and low doses, oral nicotinamide reduces the degree of UV-induced immunosuppression [17].

Panthenol (provitamin B5, also pantothenyl alcohol) is a water-soluble, stable, low molecular weight cosmeceutical that easily penetrates the stratum corneum. It is a humectant, a lipid synthesis promoter, that improves skin barrier function. Panthenol also contributes to fibroblast proliferation and epidermal re-epithelization and, because of this, has been used in the treatment of wound healing, photoaging, hyperpigmentation, pruritus, and various inflammatory skin disorders [18, 19].

7.2.3 Vitamin C

Vitamin C (ascorbic acid) is a naturally occurring antioxidant used for the prevention and treatment of sun-damaged skin and an essential ingredient for collagen biosynthesis, acting as a cofactor for prolyl and lysyl hydroxylases, enzymes that stabilize and cross-link collagen. For topical use it is primarily available in three formulations: *L-ascorbic acid* and its more stable esterified derivatives, including *ascorbyl-6-palmitate* and *magnesium ascorbyl phosphate*, all used in cosmeceutical formulations.

L-ascorbic acid is one of the most potent antioxidants in human skin. It is able to reduce reactive oxygen species (ROS), including superoxide anion, peroxide, and singlet oxygen, all of which are known to contribute to skin aging effects. The role in photodamage is related to the improvement in both collagen and elastic tissue repair. Moreover, L-ascorbic acid assists vitamin E oxidative regeneration, producing synergistic repair of photodamage [20]. Further, vitamin C decreases melanogenesis by inhibiting tyrosinase activity and may also enhance skin lightening [21].

7.2.4 E Vitamins

Commonly, the term "vitamin E" includes eight naturally occurring molecules (four tocopherols and four tocotrienols) [22]. In humans, α-tocopherol is the main form of vitamin E homologue, followed by γ-tocopherol. Alpha-tocopherol is a lipid soluble molecule present in soy, nuts, whole-wheat flour and oils.

Topical application of vitamin E significantly reduces acute skin response to UV exposure (erythema and edema) [23].

It is also effective in some skin conditions resulting from both acute and chronic UV exposure, such as wrinkles [24] and skin cancers [25]. Topical combination with vitamin C enhances its antioxidant and photoprotective effects, as well as its stability [3]. This combination is successful used to treat melasma and post inflammatory hyperpigmentation occurring in the setting of chronic contact dermatitis [22]. Vitamin E esters, especially vitamin E acetate, seem to be able to reduce UVR-induced skin damage; however, their photoprotective effect is lower with respect to vitamin E itself [22]. Finally, topical vitamin E seems to improve some dermatologic conditions, such as xerosis, allergic and inflammatory dermatitis, psoriasis, annular granulomas, ulcers, onychoschizia, trichorrhexis nodosa, cheilitis, aftosis, lichen sclerosus, inflammatory balanitis, and vaginitis [24]. Rare side effects are reported for topical application of vitamin E such as local and generalized contact dermatitis, contact urticaria, and erythema multiforme-like lesions [22].

When taken orally, it seems to protect membrane lipids from peroxidation [3] and for these reasons, benefic effects on cardiovascular system and eyes are reported [26]. Oral supplementation with vitamin E, especially if combined with topical vitamin C, may enhance photoprotection due to their synergistic relationship. It has also been used to treat various conditions, such as atopic dermatitis, yellow nail syndrome, epidermolysis bullosa, cancer prevention, cutaneous ulcers, wound healing, claudication, and vibration disease [22]. Vitamin E supplementation, at high or lower doses (pregnancy), is usually well tolerated with no or poor side effects. Since tocopherol and their oxidation products inhibit platelet aggregation, the concurrent use of vitamin E and anticoagulants is not recommended [22].

7.2.5 Alpha Lipoic Acid (ALA)

ALA is a lipoamide synthesized in the mitochondria of plants and animals. It is a scavenger of reactive oxygen species (ROS) and a metal chelating agent. Additionally, it regenerates several endogenous antioxidant molecules such as vitamins C and E, glutathione, and ubiquinol. The topical use of ALA as cosmeceutical is based on its antioxidant, anti-inflammatory and exfoliant properties, and there are some evidence about its role in improving skin quality, decreasing skin roughness and on solar lentigines and fine wrinkles [3]. The role of ALA against UV-induced damage is still controversial since it is easily photodegraded [3, 27].

7.2.6 Ubiquinone

Ubiquinone (coenzyme Q-10, CoQ-10) is a lipid-soluble quinone derivative found in the mitochondrial membrane. It is involved in the synthesis of adenosine triphosphate (ATP) and it also has antioxidant properties, including reduction of low-density lipoproteins peroxidation, regeneration of vitamin E and protection against oxidative injury from UVR [28]. Topical application of ubiquinone improves skin appearance of periorbital wrinkles [20]. Oral supplementation with coenzyme Q-10, alone or combined with other compounds, such as, vitamin E, selenium, and methionine, seems to boost post laser and peeling re-epithelization as well healing of viral-induced mucocutaneous lesions [29].

7.2.7 Idebenone

Idebenone, hydroxydecyl ubiquinone, is a synthetic analog of CoQ-10 and a powerful antioxidant [1]. It downregulates (MMP) expression, repairs damaged mitochondrial DNA and decreases nuclear thymine dimer photoproducts. Clinical studies support the ability of idebenone to decrease skin roughness, dryness, and fine lines, and to increase hydration [30]. The possibility of allergic contact dermatitis should be noted [31, 32].

7.2.8 Selenium

It is an essential micronutrient for animals and a component of two amino acids: selenocysteine and selenomethionine. In humans, selenium is a trace element nutrient that plays as cofactor for reduction of antioxidant enzymes, such as glutathione peroxidases and certain forms of thioredoxin reductase, found in animals and some plants. It is also a cofactor of vitamin E regeneration. Selenium sulfide and L-seleniomethionine represent the main topical delivery forms. Especially, L-seleniomethionine seems to have major transepidermal delivery and, when it is used topically, increases the minimal erythemal dose in humans. Furthermore, in vitro studies have shown that topical L-seleniomethionine combined with topical and oral vitamin E plays an important role as photoprotective agent, reducing UV-induced blistering, pigmentations and skin tumors [33].

7.2.9 Eicosapentaenoic Acid

Eicosapentaenoic acid (EPA) is a ω-3 fatty acid with anti-oxidant properties. Topical application of EPA inhibits UV-induced collagen decrease and reduces MMP-1 and MMP-9 expression, caused by UV exposure, preventing photoaging damage [34]. Krill oil (KO), extracted from Antarctic krill (Euphausia superba), is a compound rich in both EPA and docosahexaenoic acid (DHA). In contrast to traditional oral ω-3 bound to triglycerides or cod liver oil and fish oil, as well ethyl esters, KO contains a high percentage of ω-3 fatty acids bound to phospholipids, that are better absorbed [35]. Oral KO supplementation seems to decrease transepidermal water loss (TEWL), improving skin barrier function. For these reasons, it has been used to treat aging in pre-and menopausal women [36]. Recent studies on KO supplementation has shown a significant reduction in hepatomegaly, hepatic steatosis, and hypercholesterolemia, as well as fasting blood glucose in mice fed a high-fat diet, showing a beneficial effect on lipid and glucose metabolism [37]. Also, KO supplements, administered (2 g/day) in overweight and obese men and women, has shown to significantly increase levels of EPA with respect to menhaden oil and a control (olive) oil [38]. EPA and DHA acids show a metabolic and cardiovascular effect, decreasing both triglyceride and very low density lipoproteins cholesterol levels. They also improve vascular reactivity and have antithrombotic and antiarrhythmic properties [38]. Furthermore, mice fed on a KO diet showed a significant decrease of inflammatory cells into the joint and synovial layer hyperplasia, when compared to control group treated with fish oil. Therefore, KO supplementation seems to be able to inhibit the development of arthritis in experimental mice [39].

7.2.10 Polyphenols

Polyphenols are produced by plants, in order to protect themselves from biotic and abiotic stress such as UVR, temperature changes, infections, wounding and herbivores. These xenobiotics possess potent anti-inflammatory, antioxidant, photoprotective, and anticarcinogenic properties. They appear to have a number of different molecular targets, including components of the nuclear factor kB (NF-kB) pathway and the transcription factor nuclear factor E2-related factor 2 (Nrf2) pathway. Healing activity of polyphenols may be due to their apparent ability to induce expression of a number of protective genes involved in the cellular stress response [40]. Polyphenols, along with flavonoids (a subgroup of polyphenols), will be discussed in the anti-inflammatory/botanical section.

7.2.11 Kinetin

Kinetin (N6–furfuryladenine) is a botanical-derived synthetic growth hormone with both antioxidant properties and photoprotective effects. In plants, kinetin regulates cellular differentiation by an endocrine pathway with unknown mechanism. Its molecular effects and mechanism of action in humans are also still unclear, but topical application of kinetin has been shown to improve the appearance of fine wrinkles, as well as to increase skin firmness, texture and lightening [41].

7.3 Growth Factors

Growth factors (GF) include a large group of regulatory proteins able to mediate inter and intracellular signaling pathways [3]. The most commonly used GF include *epidermal growth factor* (EGF) and *transforming growth factor* (TGF). GF play a relevant role in wound healing [42], inducing collagen, elastin, and glycosaminoglycan formation and mediating angiogenesis [3, 43]. Cosmeceuticals containing GF are reported to improve the appearance of photodamaged skin, decreasing wrinkles and roughness [44]. Usually, no side effects are reported for GF. Possible allergic reactions in hypersensitive patients should be taken into account [43].

7.3.1 Epidermal Growth Factor (EGF)

EGF is normally present in many biological secretions, including plasma, sweat, urine, and saliva. After its binding to the epidermal growth factor receptor (EGFR), it stimulates epidermal growth and differentiation. It has been reported to be useful as a re-epithelization agent in the treatment of burns and excision wounds [45, 46].

7.3.2 Transforming Growth Factor (TGF)

TGF stimulates physiological skin growth, cellular growth, and skin repair. It promotes re-epithelization and mediates fibrosis. TGF is involved in tissue repair and angiogenesis. It may increase the risk for hypertrophic scarring, because of its function in activating fibroblasts [43].

7.4 Peptides

Peptides, short-chain sequences of amino acids, primarily comprise three types that are used in cosmeceuticals: signal, carrier, and neurotransmitter-modulating peptides. The role of peptides in cosmeceuticals, as well as their efficacy and safety, are relatively undefined.

7.4.1 Signal Peptides

Signal peptides, that increase fibroblast production of collagen and decrease collagenase activity, were first described in wound healing research about human skin fibroblast growth stimulation [47]. These peptides are topically used to improve wrinkles and lines in both aging and photoaging. Signal peptides include an *esapeptide* (valine-lysine-valine-alanine-proline-glycine peptide [VGVAPG]), an *eptapeptide* (tyrosine-tyrosine-arginine-alanine-aspartame-aspartame-alanine [YYRADDA]) and a *pentapeptide* (lysine-threonine-threonine-lysine-serine peptide [KTTKS]) found on type 1 procollagen [48].

7.4.2 Carrier Peptides

Carrier peptides are necessary to stabilize and delivery essential metals for wound healing and several enzymatic processes. Copper, the most well-known metal involved with carrier peptides, [48] is an essential cofactor for collagen stimulation. Moreover, carrier peptides increase levels of both MMP-2 and MMP-2 m-RNA as well as tissue inhibitors metalloproteinases (TIMP) 1 and 2 and, for these reasons, they allow dermal tissue remodeling [48, 49]. The *tripeptide* glycyl-L-histidyl-L-lysine (GHK) is used as a copper vehicle. Copper peptide, as a cosmeceutical, is reported to improve skin firmness and texture, and to decrease fine lines and to improve hyperpigmentation [49, 50].

7.4.3 Neurotransmitter-Modulating Peptides

Neurotransmitter-modulating peptides currently used in cosmeceutical products were developed as topical mimics of botulinum neurotoxin [51–53]. *Acetyl hexapeptide-3* (argireline) is the prototype of this group of peptides, which is supposed to inhibit acetylcholine release at the neuromuscular junction. This hypothesis, however, should be confirmed by proofs that the topical compound penetrates down to the neuromuscular junction [54]. *Dimethylaminoethanol* (DMAE), an analog of choline (a B vitamin), is another compound belonging to this category. It is a membrane stabilizer which, in topical formulations, seems to improve skin firming. Oral administration of dimethylaminoethanol has been used as homeopathic remedy to enhance mental and physical performance [55].

7.5 Botanicals

There has been a growing interest in the purported beneficial effects of several commonly used plant-derived products as topical cosmeceuticals. Many of these botanicals have been used for years in traditional or folk medicine and are now being studied for use in the prevention of various age-related pathologic conditions, including skin disorders. Botanicals are derivatives of leaves, barks, roots, and flowers that undergo processing to produce essential oils or other derivatives that are then incorporated into cosmeceutical products. Active substances found in spices and herbs, including polyphenols or alkaloids, may possess potent antioxidative and chemopreventive properties. Some of these compounds may be useful in a variety of skin disorders, including non-melanoma skin cancers.

7.5.1 Propolis

Propolis is an anti-inflammatory and antibacterial remedy derived from the bark of conifer trees and carried by honeybees to their hives. In dermatology it is used to assist wounds and herpes simplex type 1 and 2 lesions. Among its components, caffeic acid phenethyl ester (CAPE) is an electrophilic polyphenol that has a broad spectrum of biological activities, including anti-inflammatory, antioxidant, and immunomodulatory effects [56–58]. Propolis is contained in several products such as creams, shampoos, toothpastes and lipsticks [59].

7.5.2 Oatmeal

Evidence supports the primary role of colloidal oatmeal suspension in protecting and repairing skin and hair damage against a wide range of inflammatory triggers, such as UVR, free radicals, cigarette smoke, and air pollution [60]. Colloidal oatmeal is commonly used in many dermatological disorders and pruritic conditions that include insect bites, varicella, atopic dermatitis, diaper dermatitis, sunburn, xerosis, psoriasis, and epidermolysis bullosa. Oatmeal is indicated for daily gentle cleansing and moisturizing, especially for sensitive dry skin [61]. Oatmeal is contained in various topical formulations, although, the most popular typical oatmeal products are represented by colloidal baths. Colloidal oatmeal suspensions have been found to be safe, physically stable, and well-tolerated by sensitive skin.

7.5.3 Olive Oil

Olive oil contains polyphenolic compounds with reported anti-inflammatory effects [59]. Olive oil products include soaps, lip balms, shampoos and moisturizers that, combined with other ingredients, such as honey and beeswax, may be useful to treat various skin disorders such as diaper dermatitis, psoriasis, atopic dermatitis, rosacea, superficial fungal infection, hemorrhoids and anal fissures [62–64]. *Oleocanthal*, a potent anti-inflammatory compound found in extra-virgin olive oil, has been found to inhibit cyclooxygenase enzymes in the prostaglandin-biosynthesis pathway in a manner strikingly similar to the NSAID ibuprofen [65]. Hydroxytyrosol, the major antioxidant polyphenol present in olive oil, has recently been shown to protect human keratinocytes against UV-induced damages [66].

7.5.4 Grape Seed

Grape seed extract (*Vitis vinifera*), contains high levels of polyphenols, including tannins, flavonoids and resveratrol. Among these, *oligomeric proanthocyanidins* (OPCs) have been reported to be the most potent antioxidants. OPCs belong to the flavonoid family and are also found in bilberries, cranberries, black currants, green tea, and black tea [59]. Anecdotal evidence only supports the use of grape seed oil for hair growth, wound healing, UV protection as well elastin and collagen stabilization. It also demonstrated to enhance vascular endothelial growth factor and tenascin in wound edge tissue [67]. Its topical use in combination with other botanical extracts is also reported to improve skin firmness in postmenopausal women [68]. Oral administration of grape seed extract has shown to be effective in reducing hyperpigmentation due to chloasma [69].

7.5.5 *Coffea arabica* and Cofeeberry Extract

The antioxidant activity of *Coffea arabica's* extract is apparently related to several polyphenols (chlorogenic acid, proanthocyanidins, quinic acid and ferulic acid) contained in its fruit. Coffea arabica, extracted from the leaves and not from the berries, is used in several topical formulations for cellulite, because of its ability to cause dehydration of fat cells, temporarily improving the appearance of cellulite [59, 70]. The anticarcinogenic and antioxidant properties of topically applied caffeine have been studied and caffeine has been found to induce apoptosis of UVR-damaged cells and to reduce the risk of epithelial cancer development [71].

7.5.6 Green Tea

The use of green tea has recently attracted scientific attention as a potential nutritional approach in the prevention of several age-related chronic disorders. A number of epidemiological studies have suggested that consuming green tea on a daily basis may improve longevity [72, 73]. The health-promoting effects of green tea consumption are mainly attributed to polyphenol content [74]. Compared to black tea, green tea is particularly rich in catechins that include (–)-*epigallocatechin-3-gallate* (EGCG), (–)-*epicatechin-3-gallate*, (–)-*epigallocatechin*, and *epicatechin*. EGCG is the most active and abundant compound in green tea, representing approximately 43 % of the total polyphenols. EGCG possesses antioxidant and anti-inflammatory properties that include the ability to inhibit overexpression of cyclooxygenase-2 and nitric oxide synthase [75]. It has also been shown to have photoprotective and anticarcinogenic activities [72, 73]. It induces apoptosis in several types of cancer cells by inactivating transcription factors such as NF-kB, AP-1, and STAT-1 [76]. EGCG also inhibits cancer cell invasion, angiogenesis, and metastasis by downregulating expression of MMPs and by inhibiting cell adhesion [77]. Several reports have also shown the ability of EGCG to induce a general xenobiotic response in target cells, thereby activating multiple defense genes [78]. The role of EGCG in decreasing UVB-DNA damage and erythema has been well established [79, 80], while its role in increasing epidermal thickness by inducing keratinocyte proliferation remains unconfirmed. It should be noted that it is not the amount of green tea per se, but the amount of green polyphenols contained that contribute to the antioxidant effects [59].

7.5.7 Pomegranate

Pomegranate (*Purnica granatum*) is rich in polyphenols with antioxidant and antiviral effects, as well as chemopreventive activity, possibly against non-melanoma skin cancers [81]. Potential effects also include promotion of both dermal and epidermal regeneration [82]. Ellagic acid, ascorbic acid, niacin, antocyanins potassium and piperidine alkaloids represent its major constituents [83].

7.5.8 Resveratrol

Resveratrol is a polyphenolic agent found in grape, red wine and peanuts, although the main natural source for commercial use is the medical plant *Polygonum cuspidatum*. It has antioxidant, anti-inflammatory and antitumorigenic activity. When used topically, antifungal and antibacterial properties are reported as well wound healing improvement. Also, it is potentially useful for the management of diabetic ulcers, [84] to treat comedonal and inflammatory acne, to improve skin damaged by UV exposure and to promote healing in herpes simplex virus 1 infection in mice [85–87]. Recently, a double blind, placebo controlled study has shown that supplementation with a specific grape extract containing 8 mg of resveratrol, is effective in reducing skin wrinkling and oxidative damage [88].

7.5.9 Soy Isoflavones

Soy isoflavones, genistein and daidzein are phytoestrogens that exhibit anti-inflammatory and anticarcinogenic properties. When used topically, they increase skin thickness and reduce fine wrinkles [89]. Genistein is thought to be a scavenger of free radicals and an inhibitor of lipid peroxidation [89, 90]. Different studies support its oral use in the prevention of cardiovascular diseases, post-menopausal syndrome, as well breast and prostate cancer. Moreover, oral isoflavones also inhibit UV-induced carcinogenesis and photodamage in both humans and mice, [91] as well improve aged skin in adult women [92]. In vitro studies also reported the potential role of genistein in decreasing hypertrophic scars [93].

7.5.10 Ferulic Acid

Ferulic acid is a polyphenolic compound and a hydroxycinnamic acid capable of absorbing UVR. It is derived from the seeds of a wide variety of plants (grains, fruits and vegetables) and functions mainly as an antioxidant and photoprotective agent [94]. It is used in some sunscreen products [95].

7.5.11 Silymarin

Silymarin is a polyphenolic flavonoid compound able to inhibit UVB-induced sunburn, apoptotic cell formation and edema. It has anti-inflammatory effects due to cyclooxygenase type 2 (COX-2) and interleukin 1α (IL-1α) inhibition [3]. Topical application of silymarin seems to reduce erythema of rosacea [3] as well as chemical induced irritant contact dermatitis in mice [96]. Moreover it also decreases UV-induced skin tumors in mice model [97].

7.5.12 Quercetin

Quercetin is a flavonoid, found naturally in various fruits and vegetables, that is reported to have topical anti-inflammatory, antioxidant and anticarcinogenic effects [98]. It inhibits lypoxygenase and cyclooxygenase type 2 (COX-2) as well histamine release from basophils and mast cells [3]. Quercetin in w/o microemulsion has been evaluated in vitro and in vivo against UVB-induced skin damages [99].

7.5.13 Curcumin

Curcumin is a phytochemical compound extracted from the rhizome of *Curcuma longa*. Also known as turmeric, it is the pigment responsible for the characteristic yellow color of curry. It has been used for centuries as a food preservative and in Indian traditional medicine as a topical remedy for wound healing and treatment of various skin disorders and infections [100]. A standard burn wound-healing rat model reported positive results [101]. An antioxidant effect of curcumin may reduce the production of free radicals and improve cell viability under conditions of enhanced oxidative stress [102]. Moreover, curcumin has anti-inflammatory properties that include the capacity to inhibit 5- and 8-lipoxygenases, cyclooxygenases and MMPs as demonstrated in a study of skin exposed to sulfur mustard [103, 104]. Finally, curcumin exhibits a possible anticancer activity, [105] perhaps related to its ability to induce multiple defense genes and apoptosis [106]. It also inhibits enzymes involved in aging, such as collagenase, elastase and hyaluronidase, thereby potentially improving skin thickness and firmness [107]. Curcumin' s color, lack of water solubility and relatively low in vivo solubility are limiting factors in its cosmetic acceptability [108].

7.5.14 Arnica

Topical *Arnica montana* has been shown to have anti-inflammatory properties, to reduce bruising and to help healing of chronic wounds. Its anti-inflammatory effect may be due to *sesquiterpene lactones* [109] that are concentrated in the dried flower heads of the plant. Its topical use may assist healing after cosmetic dermatology procedures, [110] whereas its oral use has been reported to minimize ecchymosis when used before and after surgery. Finally its use has been evaluated in the treatment of androgenetic alopecia [111].

7.5.15 Chamomile

Chamomile has been used for its therapeutic properties since the time of Hippocrates. The most common type of chamomile found in topical cosmeceutical products is *German chamomile* (*Matricaria recutita* or *Chamomilla recutita*). It is reported to have anti-inflammatory effects, potentially improving skin texture and elasticity and decreasing pruritus and photoaging [112]. It may alleviate xerosis, atopic dermatitis, allergic contact dermatitis and sunburn. Numerous cosmeceuticals contain chamomile, and they are typically reported to be useful for sensitive skin. Several hair products containing chamomile are used to enhance blond color hair [59].

7.5.16 Aloe vera

Aloe vera botanical extract has anti-inflammatory properties. It is reported to enhance wound healing and to exert antibacterial, antifungal and antiviral effects [113].

7.5.17 Allantoin

Allantoin is present in botanical extracts of the comfrey plant and is recognized as having potential wound healing properties by stimulating healthy tissue growth and debriding necrotic tissue. Allantoin (5 % allantoin in petrolatum) has also been found to reduce pain in bilateral ulcers compared to petrolatum alone and appeared to stimulate granulation tissue formation. None of the ulcer subjects became sensitive to allantoin [114]. Allantoin has been classified by the FDA as an over-the-counter Category 1 (safe and effective) skin protectant active ingredient when used in concentrations of 0.1–2.0 % [4].

Wound healing is improved by allantoin, due to the regulation of the inflammatory process that induces fibroblastic proliferation and extracellular matrix synthesis. Histological studies in rats has shown that allantoin is able to ameliorate and fasten the reestablishment of the normal skin during wound healing [115]. Comfrey may contain hepatotoxic pyrrolizidine alkaloids; they may be carcinogenic and are contraindicated in pregnancy and lactation [4].

7.5.18 Bromelain

The active compound derived from the stem of the pineapple plant (*Ananas comosus*) is typically known as bromelain. Its efficacy to aid digestion, when taken orally, is well known, although bromelain has also been used topically and systemically for its anti-inflammatory effects, considered similar to non-steroidal anti-inflammatory drug [116]. Moreover, bromelain contains proteolytic enzymes and, when used orally, it seems to stimulate wound-healing, and to reduce edema, bruising and local pain [117].

7.5.19 Feverfew

Feverfew (*Tanacetum parthenium*) is a traditional medical remedy historically used to treat fever and inflammation. Its ingredients include: volatile oils, flavonoids and *parthenolide*, a sesquiterpene lactone, found in plant leaves. The anti-inflammatory effects of topical feverfew may be related to inhibition of NF-κB, similar to the effect of corticosteroids. It may also have an anticarcinogenic effect [118] and has been shown in vitro to inhibit UVB-induced skin cancer [59, 119]. Parthenolide may be associated with allergic contact dermatitis [120]. For these reasons this molecule has been removed so that all products are parthenolide-free [59].

7.5.20 Lycorice

Glycyrrhiza glabra and *Glycyrrhiza inflata* are the most popular licorice species used in medicine. *Glycyrrhiza glabra* has anti-inflammatory effects that have been used in herbal medicine to treat atopic dermatitis, dermatitis, pruritus and cysts [59]. One of its derivatives, *liquiritin*, has also been used to treat melasma. *Glycyrrhiza inflata's* extract is licochalcone A, a bioactive ingredient that also has anti-inflammatory effects thought to be due to inhibition of both cyclooxygenase and lipoxygenase [121]. Licochalcone A is reported to be useful in topical formulations for erythema reduction in rosacea-prone skin [122].

7.5.21 Lycopene

The characteristic color of red tomatoes is related to lycopene, a carotenoid compound, that demonstrates antioxidant and antitumorigenic properties. Topically applied, it inhibits UV-induced apoptotic cell death, thereby exerting a photoprotective activity. Topical application of lycopene may also inhibit UV-induced erythema [123]. Oral assumption of lycopene has been also reported to be photoprotective [124, 125] and a recent randomized controlled study on healthy women assuming tomato paste (16 mg lycopene/day) for 12 weeks showed that lycopene provides protection against acute and potentially longer-term aspects of photodamage [126].

7.5.22 Sulforaphane

Sulforaphane, a dietary isothiocyanate derived from broccoli sprouts, exhibits chemopreventive effects through the induction of antioxidant enzymes via the transcription factor nuclear factor E2-related factor 2 (Nrf2) [127]. Topical application of sulforaphane-rich extract of broccoli sprouts upregulates phase 2 enzymes in human skin, thereby protecting against UVR-induced inflammation and edema. Moreover, topical use reduces susceptibility to erythema arising from narrow-band 311-nm UVB radiation [128]. There is also reported anti-tumor activity in multiple myeloma [129].

7.5.23 Other Botanicals

Other botanicals with anti-inflammatory and antioxidant effects are represented by rosemary, Polypodium leucotomos, prickly pears, witch hazel, papaya, date, garlic, Echinacea, saw palmetto, ginseng, noni, hypericum, Melaleuca alternifolia, lavender, willow bark, black cohosh, Ginkgo biloba, mushroom, capparis and horse chestnut [59, 83, 89].

7.6 Polysaccharides

Hydroxy acids are polysaccharides that include *alpha hydroxy acids* (AHA), *beta hydroxy acids* (BHA), and *polyhydroxy acids* (PHA). Depending on their formulation, vehicle, pH, concentration, and body area treated, these acids provide a spectrum of possible skin benefits.

7.6.1 Alpha Hydroxy Acids (AHAs)

The topical AHAs in current clinical use include *glycolic acid, lactic acid, malic acid* and *citric acid.* They work as keratolytic agents by diminishing corneocyte adhesion in the lower levels of the stratum corneum and promoting skin exfoliation with epidermal regeneration. AHAs also work as humectant agents, increasing dermal glycosaminoglycans content and improving stratum corneum barrier function [3]. The exact mechanism of action of AHA remains somewhat controversial.

Although AHAs are endogenous to various plant systems, they are synthetically manufactured and used in low concentration in nonprescription cosmetics able to decrease corneocyte adhesion and reduce scale formation. At, higher concentrations they produce epidermolysis and are used as peeling agents. AHAs are used in several topical formulations for the treatment of dry skin, seborrheic dermatitis, acne scarring, actinic and seborrheic keratoses, common warts, and photodamaged skin. Treated skin shows smoother texture and a thinned epidermis [130].

7.6.2 Beta Hydroxy Acids (BHAs)

BHAs are a group of aromatic compounds of which *salicylic acid* (SA) is a prototype. SA is a keratolytic agent able to diffuse adequately into the pilosebaceous unit. It is used for acne and oil-prone skin as well for common warts and xerotic disorders. Finally, it is used as a peeling agent and is considered safe to treat inflammatory acne, melasma, and photoaged skin [131–133].

7.6.3 Polyhydroxy Acids (PHAs)

PHAs provide similar effects to AHAs [134]. *Gluconolactone* and *lactobionic acid* are prototypes for these polysaccharides. They are stronger humectants and moisturizers than AHAs, and enhance stratum corneum barrier function. PHAs also possess antioxidant properties that may contribute to improving the appearance of aged skin [135].

7.7 Hypopigmenting Agents

Two pathological processes may contribute to hyperpigmenting changes: an increased number of melanocytes (melanocytosis) or an increased melanin content (melanosis). If both of these processes exist and are confined essentially to epidermis, the so called skin-lightening agents should work effectively. A recent review has outlined the various compounds that may be effective hypopigmenting agents [136].

7.7.1 Hydroquinone

Hydroquinone is a phenolic compound that metabolizes to a potentially toxic compound that is currently under FDA review for safety. Its hypopigmenting action is due to local inhibition of tyrosinase, an essential enzyme in the melanin biosynthesis [3]. Hydroquinone is typically available as monotherapy or in combination with other hypopigmenting agents (retinoids, AHAs, vitamin C, topical steroids). Irritant contact dermatitis is the most common side effects [137]. However, chronic use has been rarely associated with ochronosis, characterized by asymptomatic blue-black pigmentation of skin and cartilage [138]. For this reason, its use has been restricted or highly regulated in some countries (Africa, Asia) [137]. Although carcinogenic effects, described in murine models, have not been proved in humans [139], concern exists and it has caused the ban of hydroquinone containing products in Europe and Japan [137].

7.7.2 Licorice Extracts

Topical licorice extracts such as *liquiritin, isoliquertin*, and *glabridin* are used in several topical formulations to induce hypopigmentation. Their mechanism of action is related to melanin dispersion and inhibition of tyrosinase activity [140]. Additionally, glabridin has anti-inflammatory effects due to cyclooxygenase inhibition [141]. Finally, licorice extracts have been found to have anticarcinogenic and tumor suppressive properties in animal models [141], as well as antiparasitic and antibacterial effects [142].

7.7.3 Kojic Acid

Kojic acid is a fungal metabolic product used as a skin care product, in concentrations ranging between 1 and 4 %, as a skin hypopigmenting agent. Kojic acid inhibits tyrosinase activity, possibly due to its ability to chelate the copper required by tyrosinase [143]. Like hydroquinone, it is often combined with other cosmeceutical agents (retinol, AHAs, or vitamin C) to enhance hypopigmenting activity. To reduce its potential irritation it may be combined with topical corticosteroids [136]. Hypersensitivity is also reported during its use [144].

7.7.4 Arbutin

Arbutin is a hydroquinone-beta-D-glucopyranoside, naturally obtained from the leaves of *Vaccinium vitis-idaea* and some other plants, that can inhibit melanogenesis by mimicking tyrosine, the substrate of tyrosinase [145]. Furthermore, arbutin interferes with melanosome maturation to achieve a hypopigmenting effect. It is available in concentration of 1 % in several topical depigmenting cosmeceuticals. Although efficacy correlates with dose, increased dosage is paradoxically associated with hyperpigmentation [146].

7.7.5 Aloesin

Aloesin is a glycoprotein derived from the *Aloe vera* plant. Its mechanism of action is similar to hydroquinone. It is a competitive tyrosinase inhibitor, but, unlike hydroquinone, it is not melanotoxic. Because of its hydrophilic structure, penetrating into the epidermis is difficult. It is usually used, in topical products, in combination with other skin-lightening compounds, such as arbutin, to enhance its efficacy [147]. It is reported that it acts synergistically with arbutin to reduce melanin and may be an alternative to hydroquinone [148].

7.7.6 Ellagic Acid

Ellagic acid is a polyphenol derived from various plants, including pomegranate. Like kojic acid, its skin lightening activity is related to inhibition of tyrosinase activity by chelating copper, thereby inhibiting melanin synthesis. Topical application, especially when combinated with arbutin, is considered as an alternative treatment for melasma [149, 150]. Oral use has been studied for potential hypopigmenting activity [151, 152].

7.7.7 Other Compounds

Several cosmeceuticals, including topical vitamin C [150], vitamin E [153], pycnogenol [154], niacinamide [12], rucinol [155] and soybean trypsin inhibitors [3] also possess hypopigmenting activity and may be used in combination with other hypopigmenting agents.

New promising molecules possessing a potential depigmenting role are represented by paper mulberry melatonin, oleic and linoleic acid, Helix aspersa Muller's extract and tyrostat. For some of them, in vitro studies were performed; in vivo studies, however, are necessary to confirm their efficacy.

Conclusions

Cosmeceuticals represent a growing sector for cosmetic and pharmaceutical industry, due to increasing consumer demand for cosmetics concurrent with an increase in the population's median age and changes in concepts of well-being and beauty.

Selecting the most appropriate cosmetics/cosmeceuticals among a wide range of available products – natural or industrial manufactured – is quite challenging. Knowledge in this field is required in order to identify the most appropriate compound, in consideration of age, gender, skin type and skin characteristics (hypersensitivity, hyperseborrhea, xerosis, etc.) as well anatomic site.

References

1. Kligman AM (1993) Why cosmeceuticals? Cosmet Toilet 108:37–38
2. Comparative study on cosmetics legislation in the EU and other principal markets with special attention to so-called Borderline products. Available at: http://ec.europa.eu/enterprise/newsroom/cf/itemdetail.cfm?item_id=3620. Accessed August 2004, Risk and Policy Analysts Limited. www.rpaltd.co.uk
3. Choi CM, Berson DS (2006) Cosmeceuticals. Semin Cutan Med Surg 25(3):163–168
4. Thornfeldt C (2005) Cosmeceuticals containing herbs: fact, fiction, and future. Dermatol Surg 31(7 Pt 2):873–880
5. Bellemere G, Stamatas GN, Bruere V, Bertin C, Issachar N, Oddos T (2009) Antiaging action of retinol: from molecular to clinical. Skin Pharmacol Physiol 22(4):200–209
6. Sorg O, Kuenzli S, Kaya G, Saurat JH (2005) Proposed mechanisms of action for retinoid derivatives in the treatment of skin aging. J Cosmet Dermatol 4(4):237–244
7. Kafi R, Kwak HS, Schumacher WE et al (2007) Improvement of naturally aged skin with vitamin A (retinol). Arch Dermatol 143(5):606–612
8. Sorg O, Antille C, Kaya G, Saurat JH (2006) Retinoids in cosmeceuticals. Dermatol Ther 19(5):289–296
9. Vienne MP, Ochando N, Borrel MT, Gall Y, Lauze C, Dupuy P (1999) Retinaldehyde alleviates rosacea. Dermatology 199(Suppl 1):53–56

10. Dreno B, Castell A, Tsankov N et al (2009) Interest of the association retinaldehyde/glycolic acid in adult acne. J Eur Acad Dermatol Venereol 23:529–532
11. Dreno B, Katsambas A, Pelfini C, Plantier D, Jancovici E, Ribet V, Nocera T, Morinet P, Khammari A (2007) Combined 0.1 % retinaldehyde/6 % glycolic acid cream in prophylaxis and treatment of acne scarring. Dermatology 214(3):260–267
12. Namazi MR (2007) Nicotinamide in dermatology: a capsule summary. Int J Dermatol 46:1229–1231
13. Veraldi S, Micali G, Barbareschi M, Tedeschi A, Schianchi R (2012) Topical nicotinamide in acne: a critical review. Eur J Acne Relat Dis 3(2):21–26
14. Kim N, Yang A, Kirsner RS (2008) Topical nicotinamide prevents UV immunosuppression. J Invest Dermatol 128:250
15. Navarrete-Solís J, Castanedo-Cázares JP, Torres-Álvarez B et al (2011) A double-blind, randomized clinical trial of niacinamide 4 % versus hydroquinone 4 % in the treatment of melasma. Dermatol Res Pract 2011:379173
16. Niren NM (2006) Pharmacologic doses of nicotinamide in the treatment of inflammatory skin conditions: a review. Cutis 77(1 Suppl):11–16
17. Yiasemides E, Sivapirabu G, Halliday GM, Park J, Damian DL (2009) Oral nicotinamide protects against ultraviolet radiation-induced immunosuppression in humans. Carcinogenesis 30(1):101–105
18. Bissett DL, Miyamoto K, Sun P, Li J, Berge CA (2004) Topical niacinamide reduces yellowing, wrinkling, red blotchiness, and hyperpigmented spots in aging facial skin. Int J Cosmet Sci 26(5):231–238
19. Bissett DL, Oblong JE, Berge CA (2005) Niacinamide: a B vitamin that improves aging facial skin appearance. Dermatol Surg 31:860–865
20. Burke KE (2007) Interaction of vitamins C and E as better cosmeceuticals. Dermatol Ther 20(5):314–321
21. Ando S, Ando O, Suemoto Y, Mishima Y (1993) Tyrosinase gene transcription and its control by melanogenic inhibitors. J Invest Dermatol 100(2 Suppl):150S–155S
22. Thiele JJ, Hsieh SN, Ekanayake-Mudiyanselage S (2005) Vitamin E: critical review of its current use in cosmetic and clinical dermatology. Dermatol Surg 31(7 Pt 2):805–813
23. Darr D, Dunston S, Faust H, Pinnell S (1996) Effectiveness of antioxidants (vitamin C and E) with and without sunscreens as topical photoprotectants. Acta Derm Venereol 76(4):264–268
24. Veraldi S, Romani S (2012) Vitamina E. In: Berardesca E, Celleno L, Manfredini S, Veraldi S (eds) Le vitamine topiche a, C, E: biologia, dermatologia, cosmetologia (I ristampa). Cluster, Torino, pp 63–78
25. Burke KE, Clive J, Combs GF Jr, Commisso J, Keen CL, Nakamura RM (2000) Effects of topical and oral vitamin E on pigmentation and skin cancer induced by ultraviolet irradiation in Skh:2 hairless mice. Nutr Cancer 38(1):87–97
26. Lupo MP (2001) Antioxidants and vitamins in cosmetics. Clin Dermatol 19(4):467–473
27. Wada N, Wakami H, Konishi T, Matsugo S (2009) The degradation and regeneration of alpha-lipoic acid under the irradiation of UV light in the existence of homocysteine. J Clin Biochem Nutr 44(3):218–222
28. Kaikkonen J, Tuomainen TP, Nyyssonen K, Salonen JT (2002) Coenzyme Q10: absorption, antioxidative properties, determinants, and plasma levels. Free Radic Res 36(4):389–397
29. De Luca C, Kharaeva Z, Raskovic D, Pastore P, Luci A, Korkina L (2012) Coenzyme Q(10), vitamin E, selenium, and methionine in the treatment of chronic recurrent viral mucocutaneous infections. Nutrition 28(5):509–514
30. McDaniel D, Neudecker B, Dinardo J, Lewis J 2nd, Maibach H (2005) Clinical efficacy assessment in photodamaged skin of 0.5 % and 1.0 % idebenone. J Cosmet Dermatol 4(3):167–173
31. Natkunarajah J, Ostlere L (2008) Allergic contact dermatitis to idebenone in an over-the-counter anti-ageing cream. Contact Dermatitis 58(4):239
32. Sasseville D, Moreau L, Al-Sowaidi M (2007) Allergic contact dermatitis to idebenone used as an antioxidant in an anti-wrinkle cream. Contact Dermatitis 56(2):117–118

33. Chen L, Judy Y, Steven QW (2012) The role of antioxidants in photoprotections: a critical review. J Am Acad Dermatol 67(5):1013–1024
34. Kim HH, Cho S, Lee S, Kim KH, Cho KH, Eun HC, Chung JH (2006) Photoprotective and anti-skin-aging effects of eicosapentaenoic acid in human skin in vivo. J Lipid Res 47:921–930
35. Winther B, Hoem N, Berge K, Reubsaet L (2011) Elucidation of phosphatidylcholine composition in krill oil extracted from Euphausia superba. Lipids 46(1):25–36
36. Tedeschi A, Umana M, D'Agata O, Dall'Oglio F, Nardone B, Micali G (2007) Valutazione dell'efficacia di un integratore alimentare associato ad una emulsione anti eta' rispetto al solo trattamento topico: studio clinico su 40 donne in pre e/o menopausa. J Plast Dermatol 3:1–7
37. Tandy S, Chung RW, Wat E, Kamili A, Berge K, Griinari M, Cohn JS (2009) Dietary krill oil supplementation reduces hepatic steatosis, glycemia, and hypercholesterolemia in high-fat-fed mice. J Agric Food Chem 57(19):9339–9345
38. Maki KC, Reeves MS, Farmer M, Griinari M, Berge K, Vik H, Hubacher R, Rains TM (2009) Krill oil supplementation increases plasma concentrations of eicosapentaenoic and docosahexaenoic acids in overweight and obese men and women. Nutr Res 29(9):609–615
39. Ierna M, Kerr A, Scales H, Berge K, Griinari M (2010) Supplementation of diet with krill oil protects against experimental rheumatoid arthritis. BMC Musculoskelet Disord 11:136
40. Lin JK, Liang YC, Lin-Shiau SY (1999) Cancer chemoprevention by tea polyphenols through mitotic signal transduction blockade. Biochem Pharmacol 58(6):911–915
41. Chiu PC, Chan CC, Lin HM, Chiu HC (2007) The clinical anti-aging effects of topical kinetin and niacinamide in Asians: a randomized, double-blind, placebo-controlled, split-face comparative trial. J Cosmet Dermatol 6(4):243–249
42. Martinez-Ferrer M, Afshar-Sherif AR, Uwamariya C, de Crombrugghe B, Davidson JM, Bhowmick NA (2009) Dermal transforming growth factor-{beta} responsiveness mediates wound contraction and epithelial closure. Am J Pathol 176:98–107
43. Fitzpatrick RE, Mehta RC (2009) Endogenous growth factors as cosmeceuticals. In: Draelos ZD (ed) Procedures in cosmetic dermatology: cosmeceuticals, 2nd edn. Saunders/Elsevier, Philadelphia, pp 137–143
44. Fitzpatrick RE, Rostan EF (2003) Reversal of photodamage with topical growth factor: a pilot study. J Cosmet Laser Ther 5:25–34
45. Alemdaroglu C, Degim Z, Celebi N, Sengezer M, Alomeroglu M, Nacar A (2008) Investigation of epidermal growth factor containing liposome formulation effects on burn wound healing. J Biomed Mater Res A 85(1):271–283
46. Ryu SH, Moon SY, Yang YJ et al (2009) Recombinant human epidermal growth factor accelerates the proliferation of irradiated human fibroblasts and keratinocytes in vitro and in vivo. J Radiat Res (Tokyo) 50(6):545–552
47. Kamoun A, Landeau JM, Godeau G et al (1995) Growth stimulation of human skin fibroblasts by elastin-derived peptides. Cell Adhes Commun 3(4):273–281
48. Lupo MP, Cole AL (2009) Peptides and proteins. In: Draelos ZD (ed) Procedures in cosmetic dermatology: cosmeceuticals, 2nd edn. Saunders/Elsevier, Philadelphia, pp 121–127
49. Lupo MP (2005) Cosmeceutical peptides. Dermatol Surg 31:832–836
50. Leyden JJ (2002) Skin care benefits of copper peptide containing facial cream. Presented at the American Academy of Dermatology 60th Annual Meeting; New Orleans
51. Gutierrez LM, Canaves JM, Ferrer-Montiel AV, Reig JA, Montal M, Viniegra S (1995) A peptide that mimics the carboxy-terminal domain of SNAP-25 blocks Ca(2+)-dependent exocytosis in chromaffin cells. FEBS Lett 372(1):39–43
52. Gutierrez LM, Viniegra S, Rueda J, Ferrer-Montiel AV, Canaves JM, Montal M (1997) A peptide that mimics the C-terminal sequence of SNAP-25 inhibits secretory vesicle docking in chromaffin cells. J Biol Chem 272(5):2634–2639
53. Blanes-Mira C, Merino JM, Valera E et al (2004) Small peptides patterned after the N-terminus domain of SNAP25 inhibit SNARE complex assembly and regulated exocytosis. J Neurochem 88(1):124–135

54. Blanes-Mira C, Clemente J, Jodas G et al (2002) A synthetic hexapeptide (Argireline) with antiwrinkle activity. Int J Cosmet Sci 24(5):303–310
55. Gao XH, Zhang L, Wei H, Chen HD (2008) Efficacy and safety of innovative cosmeceuticals. Clin Dermatol 26(4):367–374
56. Michaluart P, Masferrer JL, Carothers AM et al (1999) Inhibitory effects of caffeic acid phenethyl ester on the activity and expression of cyclooxygenase-2 in human oral epithelial cells and in a rat model of inflammation. Cancer Res 59(10):2347–2352
57. Chen YJ, Shiao MS, Wang SY (2001) The antioxidant caffeic acid phenethyl ester induces apoptosis associated with selective scavenging of hydrogen peroxide in human leukemic HL-60 cells. Anticancer Drugs 12(2):143–149
58. Huang MT, Ma W, Yen P et al (1996) Inhibitory effects of caffeic acid phenethyl ester (CAPE) on 12-O-tetradecanoylphorbol-13-acetate-induced tumor promotion in mouse skin and the synthesis of DNA, RNA and protein in HeLa cells. Carcinogenesis 17(4):761–765
59. Baumann LS (2007) Less-known botanical cosmeceuticals. Dermatol Ther 20(5):330–342
60. Aries MF, Vaissiere C, Pinelli E, Pipy B, Charveron M (2005) Avena Rhealba inhibits A23187-stimulated arachidonic acid mobilization, eicosanoid release, and cPLA2 expression in human keratinocytes: potential in cutaneous inflammatory disorders. Biol Pharm Bull 28(4):601–606
61. Sur R, Nigam A, Grote D, Liebel F, Southall MD (2008) Avenanthramides, polyphenols from oats, exhibit anti-inflammatory and anti-itch activity. Arch Dermatol Res 300(10):569–574
62. Al-Waili NS (2003) Topical application of natural honey, beeswax and olive oil mixture for atopic dermatitis or psoriasis: partially controlled, single-blinded study. Complement Ther Med 11(4):226–234
63. Al-Waili NS (2005) Clinical and mycological benefits of topical application of honey, olive oil and beeswax in diaper dermatitis. Clin Microbiol Infect 11(2):160–163
64. Al-Waili NS, Saloom KS, Al-Waili TN, Al-Waili AN (2006) The safety and efficacy of a mixture of honey, olive oil, and beeswax for the management of hemorrhoids and anal fissure: a pilot study. ScientificWorldJournal 6:1998–2005
65. Beauchamp GK, Keast RS, Morel D et al (2005) Phytochemistry: ibuprofen-like activity in extra-virgin olive oil. Nature 437(7055):45–46
66. Zwane RE, Parker A, Kudanga T, Davids LM, Burton SG (2012) Novel, biocatalytically produced hydroxytyrosol dimer protects against ultraviolet-induced cell death in human immortalized keratinocytes. J Agric Food Chem 60(46):11509–11517
67. Reddy KK, Grossman L, Rogers GS (2011) Common complementary and alternative therapies with potential use in dermatologic surgery: risks and benefits. J Am Acad Dermatol [Epub ahead of print]
68. Skovgaard GR, Jensen AS, Sigler ML (2006) Effect of a novel dietary supplement on skin aging in post-menopausal women. Eur J Clin Nutr 60(10):1201–1206
69. Yamakoshi J, Sano A, Tokutake S et al (2004) Oral intake of proanthocyanidin-rich extract from grape seeds improves chloasma. Phytother Res 18(11):895–899
70. Lu YP, Lou YR, Li XH et al (2002) Stimulatory effect of topical application of caffeine on UVB-induced apoptosis in mouse skin. Oncol Res 13(2):61–70
71. Song F, Qureshi AA, Han J (2012) Increased caffeine intake is associated with reduced risk of basal cell carcinoma of the skin. Cancer Res 72(13):3282–3289
72. Bouzari N, Romagosa Y, Kirsner RS (2009) Green tea prevents skin cancer by two mechanisms. J Invest Dermatol 129(5):1054
73. Chiu AE, Chan JL, Kern DG, Kohler S, Rehmus WE, Kimball AB (2005) Double-blinded, placebo-controlled trial of green tea extracts in the clinical and histologic appearance of photoaging skin. Dermatol Surg 31(7 Pt 2):855–860
74. Kidd PM (2009) Bioavailability and activity of phytosome complexes from botanical polyphenols: the silymarin, curcumin, green tea, and grape seed extracts. Altern Med Rev 14(3):226–246
75. Ahmed S, Rahman A, Hasnain A, Lalonde M, Goldberg VM, Haqqi TM (2002) Green tea polyphenol epigallocatechin-3-gallate inhibits the IL-1 beta-induced activity and expression of cyclooxygenase-2 and nitric oxide synthase-2 in human chondrocytes. Free Radic Biol Med 33(8):1097–1105

76. Kim SJ, Jeong HJ, Lee KM, Myung NY, An NH, Yang WM, Park SK, Lee HJ, Hong SH, Kim HM, Um JY (2007) Epigallocatechin-3-gallate suppresses NF-kappaB activation and phosphorylation of p38 MAPK and JNK in human astrocytoma U373MG cells. J Nutr Biochem 18(9):587–596
77. Ahmed S, Wang N, Lalonde M, Goldberg VM, Haqqi TM (2004) Green tea polyphenol epigallocatechin-3-gallate (EGCG) differentially inhibits interleukin-1 beta-induced expression of matrix metalloproteinase-1 and −13 in human chondrocytes. J Pharmacol Exp Ther 308(2):767–773
78. Khan N, Mukhtar H (2008) Multitargeted therapy of cancer by green tea polyphenols. Cancer Lett 269(2):269–280
79. Katiyar S, Elmets CA, Katiyar SK (2007) Green tea and skin cancer: photoimmunology, angiogenesis and DNA repair. J Nutr Biochem 18(5):287–296
80. Katiyar SK, Matsui MS, Elmets CA, Mukhtar H (1999) Polyphenolic antioxidant (−)-epigallocatechin-3-gallate from green tea reduces UVB-induced inflammatory responses and infiltration of leukocytes in human skin. Photochem Photobiol 69(2):148–153
81. Afaq F, Zaid MA, Khan N, Dreher M, Mukhtar H (2009) Protective effect of pomegranate-derived products on UVB-mediated damage in human reconstituted skin. Exp Dermatol 18(6):553–561
82. Aslam MN, Lansky EP, Varani J (2006) Pomegranate as a cosmeceutical source: pomegranate fractions promote proliferation and procollagen synthesis and inhibit matrix metalloproteinase-1 production in human skin cells. J Ethnopharmacol 103(3):311–318
83. Thornfeldt CR (2009) Cosmecutical botanical: part 2. In: Draelos ZD (ed) Procedures in cosmetic dermatology: cosmeceuticals, 2nd edn. Saunders/Elsevier, Philadelphia, pp 77–85
84. Khanna S, Venojarvi M, Roy S et al (2002) Dermal wound healing properties of redox-active grape seed proanthocyanidins. Free Radic Biol Med 33(8):1089–1096
85. Docherty JJ, Smith JS, Fu MM, Stoner T, Booth T (2004) Effect of topically applied resveratrol on cutaneous herpes simplex virus infections in hairless mice. Antiviral Res 61(1):19–26
86. Chen ML, Li J, Xiao WR et al (2006) Protective effect of resveratrol against oxidative damage of UVA irradiated HaCaT cells. Zhong Nan Da Xue Xue Bao Yi Xue Ban 31(5):635–639
87. Fabbrocini G, Staibano S, De Rosa G et al (2011) Resveratrol-containing gel for the treatment of acne vulgaris: a single-blind, vehicle-controlled, pilot study. Am J Clin Dermatol 12:133–141
88. Buonocore D, Lazzeretti A, Tocabens P, Nobile V, Cestone E, Santin G, Bottone MG, Marzatico F (2012) Resveratrol-procyanidin blend: nutraceutical and antiaging efficacy evaluated in a placebocontrolled, double-blind study. Clin Cosmet Investig Dermatol 5:159–165
89. Draelos ZD (2009) Comeceutical botanicals: part 1. In: Draelos ZD (ed) Procedures in cosmetic dermatology: cosmeceuticals, 2nd edn. Saunders/Elsevier, Philadelphia, pp 69–75
90. Burke KE (2009) Nutritional antioxidants. In: Draelos ZD (ed) Procedures in cosmetic dermatology: cosmeceuticals, 2nd edn. Saunders/Elsevier, Philadelphia, pp 129–136
91. Sadick NS (2009) Future cosmeceuticals of dermatologic importance. In: Draelos ZD (ed) Procedures in cosmetic dermatology: cosmeceuticals, 2nd edn. Saunders/Elsevier, Philadelphia, pp 203–208
92. Izumi T, Saito M, Obata A, Arii M, Yamaguchi H, Matsuyama A (2007) Oral intake of soy isoflavone aglycone improves the aged skin of adult women. J Nutr Sci Vitaminol (Tokyo) 53(1):57–62
93. Cao C, Li S, Dai X et al (2009) Genistein inhibits proliferation and functions of hypertrophic scar fibroblasts. Burns 35(1):89–97
94. Barone E, Calabrese V, Mancuso C (2009) Ferulic acid and its therapeutic potential as a hormetin for age-related diseases. Biogerontology 10(2):97–108
95. Di Domenico F, Perluigi M, Foppoli C et al (2009) Protective effect of ferulic acid ethyl ester against oxidative stress mediated by UVB irradiation in human epidermal melanocytes. Free Radic Res 43(4):365–375
96. Han MH, Yoon WK, Lee H et al (2007) Topical application of silymarin reduces chemical-induced irritant contact dermatitis in BALB/c mice. Int Immunopharmacol 7(13):1651–1658

97. Katiyar SK, Korman NJ, Mukhtar H, Agarwal R (1997) Protective effects of silymarin against photocarcinogenesis in a mouse skin model. J Natl Cancer Inst 89(8):556–566
98. Bhatia N, Agarwal C, Agarwal R (2001) Differential responses of skin cancer-chemopreventive agents silibinin, quercetin and epigallocatechin 3-gallate on mitogenic signaling and cell cycle regulators in human epidermoid carcinoma A431 cells. Nutr Cancer 39:292–299
99. Vicentini FT, Simi TR, Del Ciampo JO et al (2008) Quercetin in w/o microemulsion: in vitro and in vivo skin penetration and efficacy against UVB-induced skin damages evaluated in vivo. Eur J Pharm Biopharm 69(3):948–957
100. Thangapazham RL, Sharma A, Maheshwari RK (2007) Beneficial role of curcumin in skin diseases. Adv Exp Med Biol 595:343–357
101. Kulac M, Aktas C, Tulubas F, Uygur R, Kanter M, Erboga M, Ceber M, Topcu B, Ozen OA (2013) The effects of topical treatment with curcumin on burn wound healing in rats. J Mol Histol 44:83–90
102. Dinkova-Kostova AT, Massiah MA, Bozak RE, Hicks RJ, Talalay P (2001) Potency of Michael reaction acceptors as inducers of enzymes that protect against carcinogenesis depends on their reactivity with sulfhydryl groups. Proc Natl Acad Sci USA 98(6):3404–3409
103. Kang G, Kong PJ, Yuh YJ et al (2004) Curcumin suppresses lipopolysaccharide-induced cyclooxygenase-2 expression by inhibiting activator protein 1 and nuclear factor kappab bindings in BV2 microglial cells. J Pharmacol Sci 94(3):325–328
104. Panahi Y, Sahebkar A, Parvin S, Saadat A (2012) A randomized controlled trial on the anti-inflammatory effects of curcumin in patients with chronic sulphur mustard-induced cutaneous complications. Ann Clin Biochem 49(Pt 6):580–588
105. Reuter S, Eifes S, Dicato M, Aggarwal BB, Diederich M (2008) Modulation of anti-apoptotic and survival pathways by curcumin as a strategy to induce apoptosis in cancer cells. Biochem Pharmacol 76(11):1340–1351
106. Scapagnini G, Colombrita C, Amadio M et al (2006) Curcumin activates defensive genes and protects neurons against oxidative stress. Antioxid Redox Signal 8(3–4):395–403
107. Joe B, Lokesh BR (1997) Effect of curcumin and capsaicin on arachidonic acid metabolism and lysosomal enzyme secretion by rat peritoneal macrophages. Lipids 32(11):1173–1180
108. Kurien BT, Singh A, Matsumoto H, Scofield RH (2007) Improving the solubility and pharmacological efficacy of curcumin by heat treatment. Assay Drug Dev Technol 5(4):567–576
109. Wagner S, Suter A, Merfort I (2004) Skin penetration studies of Arnica preparations and of their sesquiterpene lactones. Planta Med 70(10):897–903
110. Seeley BM, Denton AB, Ahn MS, Maas CS (2006) Effect of homeopathic Arnica montana on bruising in face-lifts: results of a randomized, double-blind, placebo-controlled clinical trial. Arch Facial Plast Surg 8(1):54–59
111. Sawaya ME, Shapiro J (2000) Androgenetic alopecia. New approved and unapproved treatments. Dermatol Clin 18(1):47–61
112. Srivastava JK, Pandey M, Gupta S (2009) Chamomile, a novel and selective COX-2 inhibitor with anti-inflammatory activity. Life Sci 85(19–20):663–669
113. Vazquez B, Avila G, Segura D, Escalante B (1996) Antiinflammatory activity of extracts from Aloe vera gel. J Ethnopharmacol 55(1):69–75
114. Fisher AA (1981) Allantoin: a non-sensitizing topical medicament. Therapeutic effects of the addition of 5 percent allantoin to Vaseline. Cutis 27(3):230–231, 4, 329
115. Araújo LU, Grabe-Guimarães A, Mosqueira VC, Carneiro CM, Silva-Barcellos NM (2010) Profile of wound healing process induced by allantoin. Acta Cir Bras 25(5):460–466
116. Izaka KI, Yamada M, Kawano T, Suyama T (1972) Gastrointestinal absorption and antiinflammatory effect of bromelain. Jpn J Pharmacol 22(4):519–534
117. Ruhl F, Otto H (1965) On the oral therapy of posttraumatic edema and hematomas with the plant proteolytic enzyme bromelain. Therapiewoche 15(11):555–559
118. Zhang S, Lin ZN, Yang CF, Shi X, Ong CN, Shen HM (2004) Suppressed NF-kappaB and sustained JNK activation contribute to the sensitization effect of parthenolide to TNF-alpha-induced apoptosis in human cancer cells. Carcinogenesis 25(11):2191–2199

119. Lesiak K, Koprowska K, Zalesna I, Nejc D, Duchler M, Czyz M (2010) Parthenolide, a sesquiterpene lactone from the medical herb feverfew, shows anticancer activity against human melanoma cells in vitro. Melanoma Res 20(1):21–34
120. Killoran CE, Crawford GH, Pedvis-Leftick A (2007) Two cases of compositae dermatitis exacerbated by moisturizer containing feverfew. Dermatitis 18(4):225–229
121. Cui Y, Ao M, Li W, Hu J, Yu L (2008) Anti-inflammatory activity of licochalcone A isolated from Glycyrrhiza inflata. Z Naturforsch C 63(5–6):361–365
122. Weber TM, Ceilley RI, Buerger A et al (2006) Skin tolerance, efficacy, and quality of life of patients with red facial skin using a skin care regimen containing Licochalcone A. J Cosmet Dermatol 5(3):227–232
123. Andreassi M, Stanghellini E, Ettorre A, Di Stefano A, Andreassi L (2004) Antioxidant activity of topically applied lycopene. J Eur Acad Dermatol Venereol 18(1):52–55
124. Böhm F, Edge R, Truscott TG (2012) Interactions of dietary carotenoids with singlet oxygen (1O2) and free radicals: potential effects for human health. Acta Biochim Pol 59(1):27–30
125. Böhm F, Edge R, Truscott G (2012) Interactions of dietary carotenoids with activated (singlet) oxygen and free radicals: potential effects for human health. Mol Nutr Food Res 56(2):205–216
126. Rizwan M, Rodriguez-Blanco I, Harbottle A, Birch-Machin MA, Watson RE, Rhodes LE (2011) Tomato paste rich in lycopene protects against cutaneous photodamage in humans in vivo: a randomized controlled trial. Br J Dermatol 164(1):154–162
127. Juge N, Mithen RF, Traka M (2007) Molecular basis for chemoprevention by sulforaphane: a comprehensive review. Cell Mol Life Sci 64(9):1105–1127
128. Talalay P, Fahey JW, Healy ZR et al (2007) Sulforaphane mobilizes cellular defenses that protect skin against damage by UV radiation. Proc Natl Acad Sci USA 104(44):17500–17505
129. Jakubikova J, Cervi D, Ooi M, Kim K, Nahar S, Klippel S, Cholujova D, Leiba M, Daley JF, Delmore J, Negri J, Blotta S, McMillin DW, Hideshima T, Richardson PG, Sedlak J, Anderson KC, Mitsiades CS (2011) Anti-tumor activity and signaling events triggered by the isothiocyanates, sulforaphane and phenethyl isothiocyanate, in multiple myeloma. Haematologica 96(8):1170–1179
130. Van Scott EJ, Yu RJ (1984) Hyperkeratinization, corneocyte cohesion, and alpha hydroxy acids. J Am Acad Dermatol 11(5 Pt 1):867–879
131. Dainichi T, Ueda S, Imayama S, Furue M (2008) Excellent clinical results with a new preparation for chemical peeling in acne: 30 % salicylic acid in polyethylene glycol vehicle. Dermatol Surg 34(7):891–899
132. Ejaz A, Raza N, Iftikhar N, Muzzafar F (2008) Comparison of 30 % salicylic acid with Jessner's solution for superficial chemical peeling in epidermal melasma. J Coll Physicians Surg Pak 18(4):205–208
133. Kligman D, Kligman AM (1998) Salicylic acid peels for the treatment of photoaging. Dermatol Surg 24(3):325–328
134. Edison BL, Green BA, Wildnauer RH, Sigler ML (2004) A polyhydroxy acid skin care regimen provides antiaging effects comparable to an alpha-hydroxyacid regimen. Cutis 73(2 Suppl):14–17
135. Bernstein EF, Brown DB, Schwartz MD, Kaidbey K, Ksenzenko SM (2004) The polyhydroxy acid gluconolactone protects against ultraviolet radiation in an in vitro model of cutaneous photoaging. Dermatol Surg 30(2 Pt 1):189–195; discussion 96
136. Kim H, Choi HR, Kim DS, Park KC (2012) Topical hypopigmenting agents for pigmentary disorders and their mechanisms of action. Ann Dermatol 24(1):1–6
137. Rendon MI, Gavina JI (2009) Skin lightening agents. In: Draelos ZD (ed) Procedures in cosmetic dermatology: cosmeceuticals, 2nd edn. Saunders/Elsevier, Philadelphia, pp 103–111
138. Jordaan HF, Van Niekerk DJ (1991) Transepidermal elimination in exogenous ochronosis. A report of two cases. Am J Dermatopathol 13(4):418–424

139. McGregor D (2007) Hydroquinone: an evaluation of the human risks from its carcinogenic and mutagenic properties. Crit Rev Toxicol 37(10):887–914
140. Nerya O, Vaya J, Musa R, Izrael S, Ben-Arie R, Tamir S (2003) Glabrene and isoliquiritigenin as tyrosinase inhibitors from licorice roots. J Agric Food Chem 51(5):1201–1207
141. Yokota T, Nishio H, Kubota Y, Mizoguchi M (1998) The inhibitory effect of glabridin from licorice extracts on melanogenesis and inflammation. Pigment Cell Res 11(6):355–361
142. Lee JW, Ji YJ, Yu MH et al (2009) Antimicrobial effect and resistant regulation of Glycyrrhiza uralensis on methicillin-resistant Staphylococcus aureus. Nat Prod Res 23(2):101–111
143. Kahn V (1995) Effect of kojic acid on the oxidation of DL-DOPA, norepinephrine, and dopamine by mushroom tyrosinase. Pigment Cell Res 8(5):234–240
144. Nakagawa M, Kawai K (1995) Contact allergy to kojic acidin skin care products. Contact Dermatitis 32:9–13
145. Lim YJ, Lee EH, Kang TH et al (2009) Inhibitory effects of arbutin on melanin biosynthesis of alpha-melanocyte stimulating hormone-induced hyperpigmentation in cultured brownish guinea pig skin tissues. Arch Pharm Res 32(3):367–373
146. Draelos ZD (2008) The cosmeceutical realm. Clin Dermatol 26(6):627–632
147. Jin YH, Lee SJ, Chung MH et al (1999) Aloesin and arbutin inhibit tyrosinase activity in a synergistic manner via a different action mechanism. Arch Pharm Res 22(3):232–236
148. Jin YH, Lee SJ, Chung MH, Park JH, Park YI, Cho TH, Lee SK (1999) Aloesin and arbutin inhibit tyrosinase activity in a synergistic manner via a different action mechanism. Arch Pharm Res 22(3):232–236
149. Ertam I, Mutlu B, Unal I, Alper S, Kivçak B, Ozer O (2008) Efficiency of ellagic acid and arbutin in melasma: a randomized, prospective, open-label study. J Dermatol 35(9):570–574
150. Smith WP (1999) The effects of topical l(+) lactic Acid and ascorbic Acid on skin whitening. Int J Cosmet Sci 21(1):33–40
151. Kasai K, Yoshimura M, Koga T, Arii M, Kawasaki S (2006) Effects of oral administration of ellagic acid-rich pomegranate extract on ultraviolet-induced pigmentation in the human skin. J Nutr Sci Vitaminol (Tokyo) 52(5):383–388
152. Yoshimura M, Watanabe Y, Kasai K, Yamakoshi J, Koga T (2005) Inhibitory effect of an ellagic acid-rich pomegranate extract on tyrosinase activity and ultraviolet-induced pigmentation. Biosci Biotechnol Biochem 69(12):2368–2373
153. Shimizu K, Kondo R, Sakai K, Takeda N, Nagahata T, Oniki T (2001) Novel vitamin E derivative with 4-substituted resorcinol moiety has both antioxidant and tyrosinase inhibitory properties. Lipids 36(12):1321–1326
154. Cho HS, Lee MH, Lee JW et al (2007) Anti-wrinkling effects of the mixture of vitamin C, vitamin E, pycnogenol and evening primrose oil, and molecular mechanisms on hairless mouse skin caused by chronic ultraviolet B irradiation. Photodermatol Photoimmunol Photomed 23(5):155–162
155. Khemis A, Kaiafa A, Queille-Roussel C, Duteil L, Ortonne JP (2007) Evaluation of efficacy and safety of rucinol serum in patients with melasma: a randomized controlled trial. Br J Dermatol 156(5):997–1004

Photodynamic Therapy

8

Mariana Soirefmann, Manoela Porto, and Gislaine Ceccon

Core Messages

- Photodynamic therapy promote selective destruction of targeted abnormal cells, while preserving normal structures.
- The efficacy of photodynamic reaction is dependent on the presence of sufficient quantities of photosensitizer, time between application and light exposure, appropriate light source and tissue oxygen availability.
- Topical PDT is highly effective in the treatment of actinic keratoses, Bowen's disease, superficial and thin nodular basal cell carcinomas.
- Topical PDT has shown to be an effective tool to treat several dermatological conditions such as acne, sebaceous hyperplasia, photoaging and other inflammatory skin disease.

M. Soirefmann (✉)
Department of Dermatology, Pontifícia Universidade Catolica do Rio Grande do Sul (PUC-RS), Porto Alegre, Brazil

Brazilian Center for Studies in Dermatology, Porto Alegre, Brazil

782 Dr. Timoteo, St., 90570-040 Porto Alegre, RS, Brazil
e-mail: msoirefmann@terra.com.br

M. Porto
Brazilian Center for Studies in Dermatology, Porto Alegre, Brazil

G. Ceccon
Brazilian Society of Dermatology,
203 Dona Laura St., Suite 207, Porto Alegre, RS, Brazil
e-mail: ggceccon@gmail.com

A. Tosti, D. Hexsel (eds.), *Update in Cosmetic Dermatology*,
DOI 10.1007/978-3-642-34029-1_8,

8.1 Introduction

Since the beginning of the twentieth century, photodynamic therapy (PDT) has substantially evolved, and it is considered a topical treatment with minimal side effects for a variety of skin conditions.

Topical PDT is based on the principle of targeted tissue destruction using selective photosensitization via topical porphyrin precursor followed by light exposure. It is well established for the treatment of actinic keratosis (AK) and superficial nonmelanoma skin cancers. Some studies have reported good efficacy in several other indications.

8.2 History of Use

Since 1903, topical photosensitizers were studied. In 1904, the term "photodynamic reaction" was first described by Von Tappeiner and Jodblauer as an oxygen-dependent tissue reaction following photosensitization and irradiation with light [8, 21]. In 1948, Figge et al. found that hematoporphyrin would selectively concentrate in neoplastic, embryonic, and traumatized tissue [21].

In 1978, Thomas Dougherty used a purified derivative hematoporphyrin to treat cutaneous and other malignancies by photoactivation with a red light. In 1990, Kennedy et al. introduced 5-aminolevulinic acid (ALA) as a new photosensitizing agent, what was the trigger for the development of PDT in dermatology. In the same period, the methyl aminolevulinate (MAL), a methyl ester of ALA, was also available [8].

8.3 Mechanism of Action

Photodynamic therapy involves irradiation with a visible light to activate a photosensitizer, localized in diseased tissues, resulting in the formation of cytotoxic reactive oxygen species, which cause selective destruction of targeted abnormal cells, while preserving normal structures [7, 8, 32]. Therefore, this photodynamic reaction is dependent on the presence of sufficient quantities of photosensitizer, activating light and oxygen.

The ideal photosensitizer should have the following characteristics: low toxicity, target tissue selective, more rapid clearance in healthy than diseased tissue, ability to penetrate the target tissue, activation at a wavelength that can penetrate the target tissues, and the capacity to produce sufficiently large quantities of cytotoxic molecules to eliminate the target tissue. The most commonly used photosensitizers in dermatology are 5-aminolevulinic acid (5-ALA – Levulan, DUSA Pharmaceuticals, Wilmington, MA, USA) and the methyl ester of 5-ALA (MAL – Metvix, PhotoCure ASA, Oslo, Norway and Galderma, Paris, France) [14].

In fact, aminolevulinic acid itself is not a photosensitizer. It is a prodrug that is metabolized intracellularly to form the photosensizing molecule, protoporphyrin IX (PpIX), which binds with iron to form heme. When Pp IX is activated by light, cytotoxic reactive oxygen species (ROS) and free radicals are generated. This phototoxic effect may cause hyperproliferative tissue (malignant or not) destruction by apoptosis and cell necrosis [8, 24]. The cytotoxic effects result also in immunomodulatory effects, improving inflammatory conditions. The photosensitizers are relatively selective concentrated in the target cells (neoplastic or dysplastic tissue), possibly related to alterations in surface permeability and tumor porphyrin metabolism (relatively iron-deficient tumor cells) [24, 32, 36]. Same applies for cells constituting inflammatory dermatoses [4]. Interestingly, ALA is reported to result in higher PpIX levels than MAL, but with less selectivity for the diseased compared with healthy tissue, in both AK and inflammatory acne lesions [11, 36, 37].

Regarding the activation of light, it is important to choose an appropriate light source for PDT to ensure optimal photosensitizer excitation and tissue penetration [7]. Therefore, the light source necessary to achieve the photodynamic reaction must have two important characteristics: a wavelength that coincides with the peak absorbance of the photosensitizer and that is capable of penetrating deep into the target tissue and distributing evenly so that a ratio is obtained between the concentration in the target tissue and that in the healthy tissue [14].

Retrospective comparison of laser and filtered broadband sources suggests equivalent efficacy in topical PDT [25]. In the last few years, LED sources have shown considerable development, with improvements in design making these relatively inexpensive sources convenient for wide area irradiation and popular for patient use [37]. Although blue light may allow sufficient tissue penetration for the treatment of thin AK lesions, red light penetrates deeper and may be more effective for the treatment of thicker lesions such as BCC [7]. Studies have addressed the possibility of using ambient light for ALA-PDT of AK with two reports of therapeutic benefit but with a randomized ambient light-controlled study using Levulan® (ALA) demonstrating no significant effect on lesion ablation [6, 31, 35]. A randomized right/left intrapatient comparison of conventional MAL-PDT delivered with a LED device versus daylight for the treatment of AK of face and scalp showed an equivalent reduction in AK and significantly less pain with daylight [54]. However, although ambient light exposure might achieve a therapeutically effective dose in certain circumstances, it is unlikely to offer a consistent, practical, and safe approach to the delivery of PDT [37].

After illumination, photoactive porphyrins are excited to their higher energy "triplet" state. Energy is then transferred to oxygen molecules, resulting in the formation of cytotoxic free radicals and singlet oxygen. The precise mechanisms (at a cellular level) underlying the efficacy of topical PDT in the treatment of nonmelanoma skin cancer (NMSC) are not fully known. Both apoptosis and necrosis [16, 33, 39] have been described as occurring after topical PDT, and the importance of each phenomenon may be influenced by intracellular localization of the photosensitizer and illumination parameters [7].

8.4 Indications

8.4.1 Actinic Keratosis and Nonmelanoma Skin Cancer

PDT is a well-established treatment modality for premalignant and superficial nonmelanoma skin lesions, with highly successful rates reported for AK, Bowen's disease, and superficial basal cell carcinoma (BCC) [7]. At present, the use of ALA in

PDT is currently approved by the Food and Drug Administration (FDA) only for the treatment of AKs [51]. On the other hand, the use of MAL in PDT is currently approved for the treatment of AK, Bowen's disease, and superficial and nodular basal cell carcinoma [37].

MAL-PDT is an excellent option for those cases in which surgery may not be feasible, such as patients with multiple comorbidities, large or multiple lesions within a certain area, or lesions in a cosmetically sensitive area [48].

8.4.2 Acne

As acne vulgaris is a disease of pilosebaceous units, and porphyrin accumulates preferentially in sebaceous glands; PDT is a useful tool for the treatment of this frequent condition [44]. When exposed to light, porphyrins cause the formation of singlet oxygen and other potent oxidizers that mediate the benefits of photodynamic therapy [44]. The improvement in acne lesions may be via antibacterial activity, selective damage to sebaceous gland with decreased of sebum excretion, and reduction in follicular obstruction [26, 37]. Topical application of ALA in combination with broadband red light demonstrated that ALA-induced PPIX fluorescence was greater in acne lesions than surrounding normal skin and that PDT with red light was shown to diminish sebaceous gland size [26, 37] (Figs. 8.1 and 8.2).

A study that compared ALA-PDT and MAL-PDT with red light (Aktilite, PhotoCure ASA) showed that there is no significant difference in response rate between ALA-PDT and MAL-PDT for inflammatory acne vulgaris treatment [53]. Therefore, if high-dose conditions (long incubation time, high fluence, and red light exposure) are used, ALA-PDT and MAL-PDT have been shown to produce similar effects for acne treatment [45].

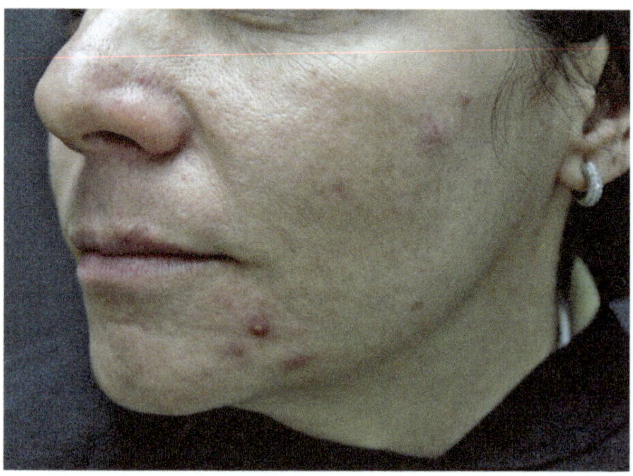

Fig. 8.1 Patient showing inflammatory acne lesions before PDT treatment

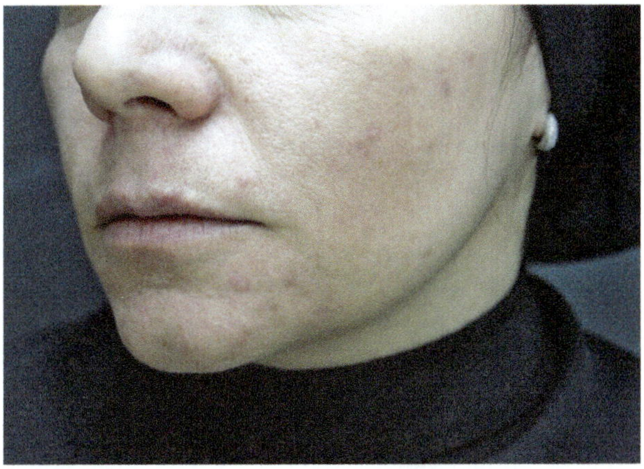

Fig. 8.2 Same patient, as in Fig. 8.1, 1 month after a single-treatment session with ALA-PDT (illumination with Aktilite® light-emitting diode 37 J/cm^2)

There is no consensus about the optimal light dosimetry and irradiance of PDT in acne [45]. However, deeper penetration and continuous and high-intensity red light sources such as lasers and light-emitting diode sources are required to reach and activate porphyrins in sebaceous gland and provide better results [45]. The response to treatment depends on the correct skin preparation, which drug is applied and for how long, whether skin occlusion is used, light source, and light treatment parameters [45].

8.4.3 Photodamage

The use of PDT for photodamaged skin is off-label and has been investigated [20]. Among all the light sources, intense pulsed light (IPL) combined with ALA-PDT has been the most extensively studied for use in photorejuvenation, this largely stemming from the fact that IPL has independently been shown to rejuvenate skin while spanning wavelengths that activate PPIX. Standard PDT and ALA-IPL are effective in photorejuvenation, with improvement in telangiectasias, pigmentary irregularities, and skin texture [13, 22]. A split-face design clinical study comparing ALA-IPL to IPL alone demonstrated greater improvement on the ALA side [22]. However, a controlled investigative study, performed in healthy human skin in vivo following microdermabrasion and acetone scrub, showed that two pulsed light sources, PDL and a broadband flashlamp filtered IPL, produced evidence of minimal activation of photosensitizer, with a dramatically smaller photodynamic reaction than seen with a conventional continuous wave broadband source [50]. And, a split-face randomized placebo-controlled trial observed no statistically significant differences between the use of red versus blue light sources in the treatment of photodamage [40]. The mechanism of improvement in the signs of photoaging may be related to the increase in intense type I collagen production. Other possible mechanisms will be PDT-induced photorejuvenation, which include the activation of specific molecular pathways by photosensitizers and nonspecific immune response [42].

8.4.4 Other Inflammatory/Infective Diseases

The use of PDT for other dermatological inflammatory/infective diseases is off-label and has been investigated [20]. Case reports and small series attest to the potential of PDT in a wide range of inflammatory, proliferative, or angiogenic skin lesions. Topical PDT has been reported to be effective, but a relatively pain option, in the treatment of cutaneous and genital viral warts [9, 20, 52]. A randomized double-blind study has shown that PDT is superior to placebo in the treatment of recalcitrant warts [49].

Several case reports and case series have shown benefits of topical PDT in the treatment of sebaceous hyperplasia [2, 23, 37]. Other diseases that have been described as a potential indication of PDT topical therapy include: recalcitrant hidradenitis suppurativa, linear porokeratosis, recalcitrant skin ulcers, early stage of localized cutaneous T cell lymphoma, and localized morphea [5, 12, 17, 29, 37, 38, 46, 47].

PDT may be an alternative option for several infective and inflammatory dermatological diseases treatment, but further well-designed studies are required.

8.5 Products/Techniques

Topical PDT requires the combination of a photosensitize agent and a specific light source, as shown in Table 8.1.

Currently, a range of light sources, doses, and irradiances continue to be used in ALA-PDT, including lasers, filtered xenon arc and metal halide lamps, fluorescent lamps, and light-emitting diodes (LEDs); whereas in MAL-PDT, the standard procedure now typically involves a LED source.

8.6 Patient Selection

Before undertaking PDT procedure, all patients must be informed about the advantages and disadvantages of this procedure, including possible adverse effects that can occur. Full clinical and dermatological history must be gotten. The preoperative

Table 8.1 Photosensitizer agents and light sources for PDT

Photosensitizer agents:
ALA – Levulan (DUSA Pharmaceuticals, Wilmington, MA, USA)
MAL – Metvix (PhotoCure ASA, Oslo, Norway and Galderma, Paris, France)
Light sources:
Lasers
Filtered xenon arc and metal halide lamps
Fluorescent lamps
Light-emitting diodes (LEDs)

Table 8.2 Common photosensitizer medications

Common photosensitizer medications	
Antiarrhythmics: amiodarone	Phenothiazines: chlorpromazine, prochlorperazine
Diuretics: furosemide	Quinolones: ciprofloxacin, nalidixic acid, lomefloxacin
Thiazides: chlorothiazide, hydrochlorothiazides	Retinoids: isotretinoin, acitretin, etretinate
Nonsteroidal anti-inflammatory: piroxicam, naproxen	Tetracyclines: doxycycline, tetracycline

evaluation must look for history of photosensitivity disorders, medicines in use, and documented allergy to the photosensitizer or to similar chemical structures. Patients with recurrent herpes simplex infections over the treatment site should receive prophylactic or active antiviral therapy.

Before PDT procedure, some documents should be obtained: adequate documentation of the lesion by photography and signed informed consent by the patient [19, 27].

As described before in this chapter, PDT is a well-established treatment modality for premalignant and superficial nonmelanoma skin lesions (NMSC). Regarding the treatment of NMSC lesions, the histopathological diagnosis is always recommended, since there is evidence of efficacy for topical PDT for AK, BCC, and Bowen's disease but limited for SCC [37].

Patients should be advised regarding the risk and the duration of local photosensitivity, usually about 48 h. During this period, patients should use broadband sunscreens and avoid light exposure of any source. To avoid cutaneous hypersensitivity, the use of topical retinoid, glycolic acids, or topical acne treatments should be avoided at least 1 week before and after the procedure.

8.7 Contraindications

Contraindications for PDT include history of porphyria, photodermatosis, and allergy or photoallergy to the photosensitizer [37]. Some medications should be discontinued before PDT treatment, since they may be associated with phototoxic reactions (Table 8.2).

Moreover, the retina is at risk from the photochemical hazard of blue light (400–450 nm), potentially causing irreversible damage to the photosensitive neurotransmitters in the macula [36, 37]. Therefore, adequate protective glasses are always mandatory during this procedure.

PDT is not suitable for treatment of morpheiform BCC, pigmented lesions, or spinocellular carcinoma (SCC) [10].

8.8 Procedure Technique

PDT is a noninvasive and outpatient procedure. After topical application of MAL or ALA, sufficient time must be left to allow for production and accumulation of porphyrins before activation with light. There is preferential production of photoactive porphyrins in neoplastic relative to nonneoplastic cells after ALA and MAL application, with evidence of greater selectivity for neoplastic tissue with MAL [3, 15, 18, 41].

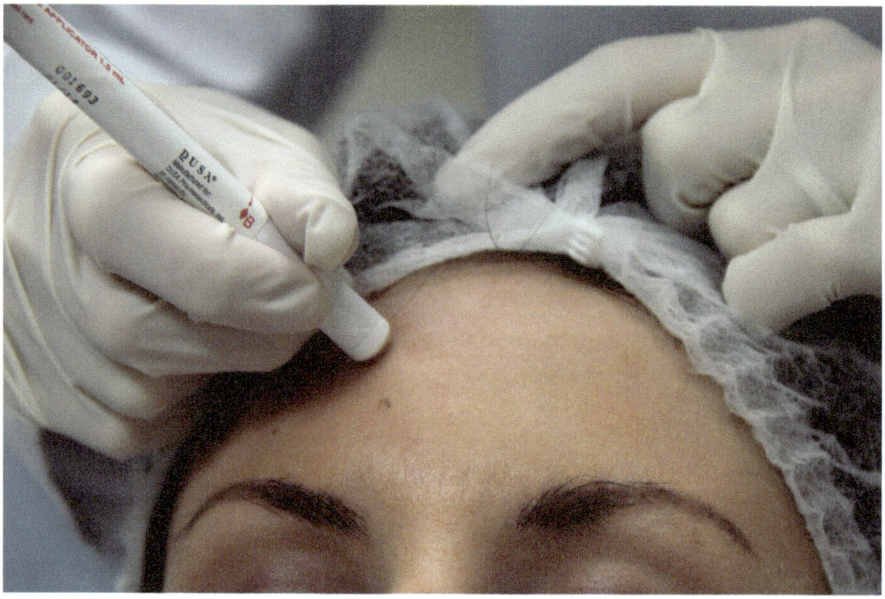

Fig. 8.3 Application of 5-aminolevulinc acid (ALA)

MAL needs to be applied for 3 h under occlusion for the treatment of both AK and BCC. According to US and Canadian monographs, ALA should have an incubation time of 14–18 h, but efficacy of ALA-PDT is reported with the use of shorter the efficacy of this product incubation time (1–3 h) [37].

The use of lesional surface preparation prior to the application of prodrug may enhance tissue penetration of ALA and MAL [37]. Skin preparation can include abrasion, curettage, debulking, and tape stripping [10]. Katz et al. observed that the use of microdermabrasion prior to the application of ALA was associated with consistent superior results than ALA applied alone for 1 h [30].

After the incubation time, the prodrug (ALA or MAL) is removed and the area to be treated should be exposed to a light source. Broadband and narrowband light or lasers may be used for topical PDT [10]. Both patient and therapist should protect their eyes with appropriated glasses.

8.8.1 ALA Procedure

1. To clean the skin with soap and water or alcohol.
2. To remove crust and hyperkeratosis with microdermabrasion procedure or slight curettage.
3. To perform microdermabrasion over the treated area.
4. ALA solution applicator (Levulan®) has a glass capsule containing the alcoholic diluent; it must be crushed and shaken to allow dissolution of ALA into solution.

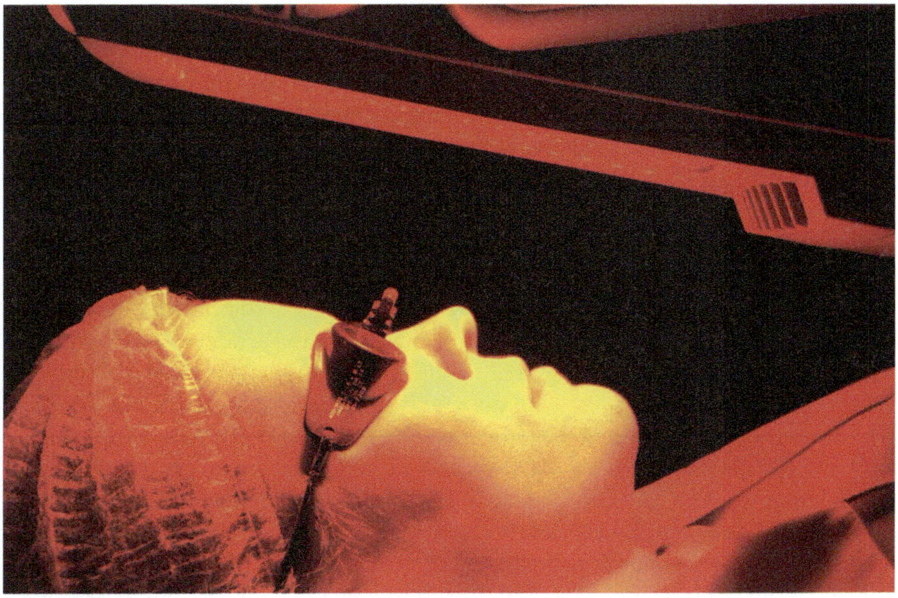

Fig. 8.4 Irradiation with Aktilite® light-emitting diode 37 J/cm^2

Fig. 8.5 Occlusive dressing after methyl aminolevulinate (MAL) cream application

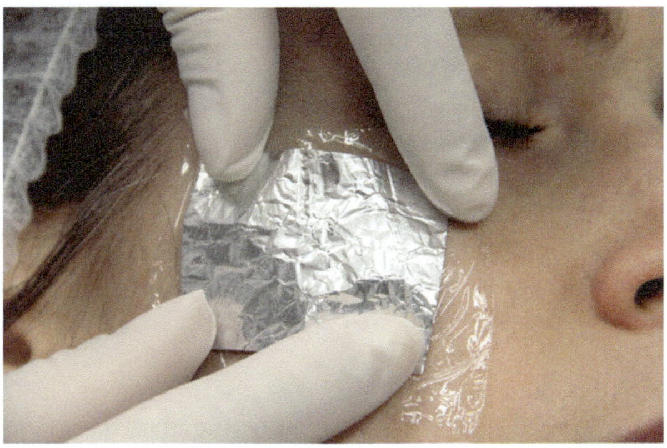

5. To apply the ALA to the desired areas. It does not need to be occluded; time of permanence is 1–3 h (Fig. 8.3).
6. To clean the skin with physiological solution or distilled water.
7. To irradiate the treatment area with LED or IPL [19, 27] (Fig. 8.4).

8.8.2 MAL Procedure

1. To clean the area with alcohol or acetone.
2. To remove any crust and superficial tissue of bulky lesions with gently curettage prior to the application of MAL.

3. If bleeding occurs, carry through homeostasis with compressive measures.
4. To apply MAL 16 % cream at the treated area (1 mm of thickness and 1 cm of edge around the lesion). The site must be occluded with plastic and protected from light with cloudy dressing. The time of permanence is 3 h (Fig. 8.5).
5. To remove the product with gauze and physiological solution.
6. To irradiate the site with LED (Aktilite, PhotoCure ASA): dose 37 J/cm^2, distance of 5–8 cm, duration 5–8 min [19, 27] (Fig. 8.4).

Pain experienced during PDT can be managed using simple steps, like cooling the site of illumination with cold air or cold water. Often, these procedures provide sufficient pain relief, and local anesthesia should be reserved for those who experienced more severe pain [34].

8.9 Advantages

Topical PDT treatment is very safe and associated with good cosmetic outcomes. It is particularly well suited for the treatment of AKs. It is a selective targeted treatment that offers high cure rates with great cosmetic outcome and is generally well tolerated by patients. Furthermore, PDT can be used to over large surface areas, being suitable for the treatment of multiple AK lesions and field of cancerization areas [7]. Cosmetic outcome is an important consideration in the treatment of AKs. Topical PDT offers superior cosmetic outcome over cryotherapy and surgery for the treatment of AKs, SBCC, and BD. Moreover, a study showed that the cost of treatment of NMSC with MAL-PDT is lower than with surgical treatments, even after 2 years of follow-up [1]. And in addition of preventing the development of scars and dyspigmentation that occurs with surgery and cryotherapy, PDT has the added benefit of photorejuvenation.

8.10 Post-procedure Course

It is important to remember that photosensitivity can remain up to 48 h after the procedure [32]. Therefore, patients should use constantly broadband sunscreens and avoid exposure to any light source on the treated area during this period of time [19]. Afterward, patients should maintain the use of broadband sunscreens and avoid sun exposure for 6 weeks after PDT treatment to avoid or limit post-inflammatory hyperpigmentation [1].

PDT is generally well tolerated by patients. The most common complains among patients are pain, irritation, mild exfoliation, edema, and erythema. Occasionally, small areas of crusting may also occur. These findings usually fade away in 1–2 weeks [7, 26, 43].

8.11 Side Effects

The principal and most common acute adverse effect of topical PDT is pain. It is described by most patients as a burning, stinging, or prickling sensation [36, 37, 55]. The intensity of pain has a large interindividual variation, but studies demonstrated that approximately 20 % of patients experience severe pain. It has probably association with nerve stimulation, tissue damage, and hyperthermia [37]. A study with 26 patients with AK and 34 patients with facial acne vulgaris showed that pain during illumination was associated with the PpIX fluorescence in the treatment area and the fluence rate [55]. Pain also appears more intense in patients with AK, lesions located in the head, large areas, or ulcerated lesions [4, 32, 37]. Pain may last for some hours and usually disappears on the same day [1].

Erythema and edema can occur after irradiation. Sometimes it is followed by erosion and crust formation, healing over 2–6 weeks [36, 37]. Clark et al. studied the characteristics of erythema induced by PDT. They found that maximal erythema occurred within 1–2 h of PDT, and interindividual variation in ALA-induced phototoxicity was seen [11].

Contact allergy to PDT is rarely reported [25, 28, 56]. Contact allergy to Metvix® should be expected in around 0.4 % of treated patients, especially those with multiple PDT treatments [28].

Chronic side effects are uncommon, but hyperpigmentation or hypopigmentation can occasionally occur following PDT. Pigmentation disorders were observed in only 1 % of PDT-treated lesions from a study of 762 patients with nonmelanoma skin cancer [37]. Alopecia is a potential side effect of PDT because of the concomitant sensitization of the pilosebaceous units [4, 37]. Topical PDT has a low risk of carcinogenicity. Studies have shown that PDT has very low mutagenic potential [32, 37].

8.12 Recommendations

8.12.1 Actinic Keratosis

Photodynamic therapy with MAL and ALA is a highly effective treatment for AK offering the advantage of excellent cosmetic outcome and could therefore be considered as a first-line therapy. Rating: AI

MAL-PDT has a superior cosmetic outcome compared with cryotherapy. Rating: AI

Thin or moderately thick AK may be treated with one session of MAL-PDT. If after 3 months the treatment effect is insufficient, a repeat treatment is given, with a later 3 month follow-up [1]. Immunosuppressed patients, thicker, hyperkeratotic lesions, and/or lesions with severe atypia should be treated twice, with an interval of 1 week between the sessions [1].

8.12.2 Bowen's Disease

Topical PDT is effective in BD, achieving good cosmesis, and is at least as effective as cryotherapy or 5-FU but with fewer adverse events. Topical PDT should be considered as a first-line therapy for BD. After repeated treatments, nonresponders should be considered for surgery. Rating: AI

Bowen's disease is treated twice with a treatment interval of 1 week [7, 37].

8.12.3 Superficial BCC

PDT is an effective and reliable treatment option for sBCC that offers excellent or good cosmetic outcomes. Rating: AI

PDT offers an advantage in the treatment of large, extensive, and multiple lesions. Rating: AI

MAL-PDT has demonstrated long-term efficacy in BCC. Rating: AI

8.12.4 Nodular BCC

MAL-PDT is an effective and reliable treatment option for nBCC, possibly preferable for thin lesions with the advantage of good cosmetic outcome. Rating: AI

MAL-PDT has demonstrated long-term efficacy for nBCC, backed up with 5-year data. Rating: AI

Basal cell carcinoma is treated twice with a treatment interval of 1 week [7, 37].

8.12.5 PDT for NMSC Prevention in Immunosuppressed Patients and Patients with Gorlin Syndrome

PDT may be considered as a mean of preventing new AK lesions in immunosuppressed transplant patients. Rating: BI. AKs should be treated with two sessions of PDT, with interval of 1 week between then in patients with immunosuppression [1].

PDT may be considered as a mean of preventing SCC in immunosuppressed patients. Rating: CIII

PDT may be considered as a mean of preventing BCC in immunosuppressed patients. Rating: CII

Conclusions

Topical PDT is highly effective in the treatment of actinic keratoses, Bowen's disease, superficial and thin nodular basal cell carcinomas, with cosmesis typically superior to that achieved with existing standard therapies [7].

References

1. Aguilar M, Troya M, Martin L et al (2010) A cost analysis of photodynamic therapy with methylaminolevulinate and imiquimod compared with conventional surgery for the treatment of superficial basal cell carcinoma and Bowen's disease of the lower extremities. J Eur Acad Dermatol Venereol 24:1431–1436
2. Alster TS, Tanzi EL (2003) Photodynamic therapy with topical aminolevulinic acid and pulsed dye laser irradiation for sebaceous hyperplasia. J Drugs Dermatol 2:501–504
3. Angell-Petersen E, Sørensen R, Warloe T et al (2006) Porphyrin formation in actinic keratosis and basal cell carcinoma after topical application of methyl 5-aminolevulinate. J Invest Dermatol 126:265–271
4. Babilas P, Karrer S, Sidoroff A et al (2005) Photodynamic therapy in dermatology – an update. Photodermatol Photoimmunol Photomed 21:142–149
5. Bakos L, Zoratto G, Mazzotti N et al (2009) Photodynamic therapy: a useful adjunct therapy for recalcitrant ulceration in pemphigus vulgaris. J Eur Acad Dermatol Venereol 23(5): 599–600
6. Batchelor RJ, Stables GI, Stringer MR (2007) Successful treatment of scalp actinic keratoses with photodynamic therapy using ambient light. Br J Dermatol 156:779–781
7. Braathen LR, Szeimies RM, Basset-Seguin N et al (2007) Guidelines on use of photodynamic therapy for nonmelanoma skin cancer: an international consensus International Society for Photodynamic Therapy in Dermatology, 2005. J Am Acad Dermatol 56(1):125–143
8. Calzavara-Pinton PG, Venturini M, Sala R (2007) Photodynamic therapy: update 2006 part 1: photochemistry and photobiology. J Eur Acad Dermatol Venereol 21:293–302
9. Chong WS, Kang GY (2009) Dramatic clearance of recalcitrant acral viral wart using aminolevulinate-red light photodynamic therapy. Photodermatol Photoimmunol Photomed 25(4):225–226
10. Christensen E, Warloe T, Kroon S et al (2010) Guidelines for practical use of MAL-PDT in nonmelanoma skin cancer. J Eur Acad Dermatol Venereol 24:505–512
11. Clark C, Dawe RS, Moseley H et al (2004) The characteristics of erythema induced by topical 5-aminolaevulinic acid photodynamic therapy. Photodermatol Photoimmunol Photomed 20:105–107
12. Coors EA, Von der Driesch P (2004) Topical photodynamic therapy for patients with therapy-resistant lesions of cutaneous T-cell lymphoma. J Am Acad Dermatol 50(3):363–367
13. Dover J, Bhatia AC, Stewart B et al (2005) Topical 5-aminolevulinic acid combined with intense pulsed light in the treatment of photoageing. Arch Dermatol 141:1247–1252
14. Fernandez-Guarino M, Garcia-Morales I, Arto A et al (2007) Photodynamic therapy: news indications. Acta Dermosifiliogr 98:377–95
15. Fritsch C, Homey B, Stahl W et al (1998) Preferential relative porphyrin enrichment in solar keratoses upon topical application of delta-aminolevulinic acid methylester. Photochem Photobiol 68:218–221
16. Gad F, Viau G, Boushira M et al (2001) Photodynamic therapy with 5-aminolevulinic acid induces apoptosis and caspase activation in malignant T cells. J Cutan Med Surg 5:8–13
17. Garcia-Navarro X, Garces JR, Baselga E et al (2009) Linear porokeratosis: excellent response to photodynamic therapy. Arch Dermatol 145(5):526–527
18. Gardlo K, Ruzicka T (2002) Metvix (PhotoCure). Curr Opin Investig Drugs 3:1672–1678
19. Gilaberte Y (2008) Procedimiento Clinico. In: Gilaberte Y (ed) Terapia Fotodinámica. Grupo Aula Medica Ediciones, Madrid, pp 85–95
20. Gold MH (2007) Photodynamic therapy update 2007. J Drugs Dermatol 6(11):1131–1137
21. Gold MH, Goldman MP (2004) 5-Aminolaevulinic acid photodynamic therapy: where we have been and where we are going. Dermatol Surg 30:1077–1084
22. Gold MH, Bradshaw MM et al (2006) Split – face comparison of photodynamic therapy with 5-aminolevulinic acid and intense pulsed light versus intense pulsed light alone for photodamage. Dermatol Surg 32:795–801

23. Gold MH, Bradshaw VL, Boring MM et al (2004) Treatment of sebaceous hyperplasia by photodynamic therapy with 5-aminolevulinic acid and blue light or intense pulsed light source. J Drugs Dermatol 3(Suppl 6):S6–S9
24. Gupta AK, Ryder JE (2003) Photodynamic therapy and topical aminolevulinic acid – an overview. Am J Clin Dermatol 4(10):699–708
25. Harries MJ, Street G, Gilmour E (2007) Allergic contact dermatitis to methyl aminolevulinate (Metvix®) cream used in photodynamic therapy. Photodermatol Photoimmunol Photomed 23:35–36
26. Hongcharu W, Taylor CR, Chang Y et al (2000) Topical ALA-photodynamic therapy for the treatment of acne vulgaris. J Invest Dermatol 115:183–192
27. Inãrrairaegui MM, Irazabal MP, Bellón PR (2007) La Práctica Clínica Diaria. Procedimiento y Seguimiento. In: Bellón PR, Viera MS (eds) Terapia Fotodinámica. EDI Complet, Madrid, pp 153–70
28. Jungersted JM, Dam TM, Bryld LE et al (2008) Allergic reactions to Metvix® (ALA_ME). Contact Dermatitis 58:184–186
29. Karrer S, Abel C, Landthaler M et al (2000) Topical photodynamic therapy for localized scleroderma. Acta Derm Venereol 80(1):26–27
30. Katz BE, Truig S, Maiwald DC, Frew KE et al (2007) Efficacy of microdermabrasion preceding ALA application in reducing the incubation time of ALA in laser PDT. J Drugs Dermatol 6(2):140–142
31. Kawauchi S, Morimoto Y, Sato S et al (2004) Differences between cytotoxicity in photodynamic therapy using a pulsed laser and a continuous wave laser: study of oxygen consumption and photobleaching. Lasers Med Sci 18:179–183
32. Kormeili T, Yamauchi PS, Lowe NJ (2004) Topical photodynamic therapy in clinical dermatology. Br J Dermatol 150:1061–1069
33. Kuzelova K, Grebenova D, Pluskalova M et al (2004) Early apoptotic features of K562 cell death induced by 5-aminolaevulinic acid-based photodynamic therapy. J Photochem Photobiol B 73:67–78
34. Lehmann P (2007) Methyl aminolaevulinate-photodynamic therapy: a review of clinical trials in the treatment of actinic keratoses and nonmelanoma skin cancer. Br J Dermatol 156(5): 793–801
35. Marcus SL, Houlihan A, Lundahl S, Ferdon ME (2007) Does ambient light contribute to the therapeutic effects of topical photodynamic therapy (PDT) using aminolevulinic acid (ALA)? Lasers Surg Med 39:201–202
36. Morton CA, Brown SB, Collins S et al (2002) Guidelines for topical photodynamic therapy: report of a workshop of de British Photodermatology Group. Br J Dermatol 146:552–567
37. Morton CA, McKenna KE, Rhodes LE (2008) Guidelines of topical photodynamic therapy: update. Br J Dermatol 159:1245–1266
38. Motta S, Monti M (2007) Photodynamic therapy – a promising treatment option for autoimmune skin ulcers: a case report. Photochem Photobiol Sci 6(11):1150–1151
39. Noodt BB, Berg K, Stokke T, Peng Q, Nesland JM (1996) Apoptosis and necrosis induced with light and 5-aminolaevulinic acid derived protoporphyrin IX. Br J Cancer 74:22–29
40. Palm MD, Goldman MP (2011) Safety and efficacy comparison of blue versus red light sources for photodynamic therapy using methyl aminolevulinate in photodamaged skin. J Drugs Dermatol 10(1):53–60
41. Peng Q, Soler AM, Warloe T et al (2001) Selective distribution of porphyrins in skin thick basal cell carcinoma after topical application of methyl 5-aminolevulinate. J Photochem Photobiol B 15(62):140–145
42. Ruiz-Rodriguez R, Lopez-Rodriguez L (2006) Non ablative skin resurfacing: the role of PDT. J Drugs Dermatol 5:756–762
43. Ruiz-Rodriguez R, Sanz-Sánchez T, Córdoba S (2002) Photodynamic photorejuvenation. Dermatol Surg 28(8):742–744
44. Sakamoto FH, Lopes JD, Anderson RR (2010) Photodynamic therapy for acne vulgaris: a critical review from basics to clinical practice. Part I: acne vulgaris: when and why consider photodynamic therapy? J Am Acad Dermatol 63(2):183–193

45. Sakamoto FH, Torezan L, Anderson RR (2010) Photodynamic therapy for acne vulgaris: a critical review from basics to clinical practice. Part II: understanding parameters for acne treatment with photodynamic therapy. J Am Acad Dermatol 63(2):195–211
46. Saraceno R, Teoli M, Casciello C et al (2009) Methyl aminolevulinate photodynamic therapy for treatment of hidradenitis suppurativa and pilonidal cysts. Photodermatol Photoimmunol Photomed 25(3):164–165
47. Sotiriou E, Apalla Z, Maliamani F et al (2009) Treatment of recalcitrant hidradenitis suppurativa with photodynamic therapy: report of five cases. Clin Exp Dermatol 34(7):235–236
48. Stebbins WG, Wanke WC (2011) MAL- PDT for difficult to treat nonmelanoma skin cancer. Dermatol Ther 24:82–93
49. Stendler IM, Na R, Fogh H et al (2000) Photodynamic therapy with 5-aminolevulinic acid or placebo for recalcitrant foot and hand warts: randomized double-blind trial. Lancet 355:963–966
50. Strasswimmer J, Grande DJ (2006) Do pulsed lasers produce and effective photodynamic therapy response? Lasers Surg Med 38:22–25
51. Tierney E, Baker A, Ahdout J et al (2009) Photodynamic therapy for the treatment of cutaneous neoplasia, inflammatory disorders and photoaging. Dermatol Surg 35(5):725–746
52. Wang YS, Tay YK, Kwok C et al (2007) Photodynamic therapy with 20 % aminolevulinic acid for the treatment of recalcitrant viral warts in an Asia population. Int J Dermatol 46:1180–1184
53. Wiegell S, Wulf HC (2006) Photodynamic therapy of acne vulgaris using 5-aminolevulinic acid versus methyl aminolevulinate. J Am Acad Dermatol 54:647–651
54. Wiegell SR, Haedersdal M, Philipsen PA et al (2008) Continuous activation of PpIX by daylight is as effective as and less painful than conventional photodynamic therapy for actinic keratoses; a randomized, controlled, single-blinded study. Br J Dermatol 158:740
55. Wiegell SR, Skiveren J, Philipsen PA et al (2008) Pain during photodynamic therapy is associated with protoporphyrin IX fluorescence and fluence rate. Br J Dermatol 158:727–733
56. Wulf HC, Philipsen P (2004) Allergic contact dermatitis to 5-aminolaevulinic acid methylester but not to 5-aminolaevulinic acid after photodynamic therapy. Br J Dermatol 150:143–145

Botulinum Toxins

9

Doris Hexsel and Cristiano Brum

Core Messages

- Botulinum toxin type A injection is a safe and efficacious minimally invasive procedure for rejuvenation.
- Patients observe the effects in 3–7 days after the injections and its action lasts for 3–6 months.
- The different commercial brands of botulinum toxin type A have distinctive features, such as the number of units, chemical properties, biological action, molecular weight and inactive ingredients in the formulation.
- Each patient requires individual evaluation and therapeutic plan. Choosing the correct doses and knowing the anatomy is mandatory to achieve the best results, as well as to avoid potential complications.
- Botulinum toxin type A injections can be combined to other treatment modalities such as fillers, lasers and light sources to optimize cosmetic results.

D. Hexsel, M.D. (✉)
Department of Dermatology, Pontifícia Universidade Catolica do Rio Grande do Sul (PUC-RS), Brazilian Center for Studies in Dermatology, Porto Alegre, RS, Brazil

Brazilian Center for Studies in Dermatology, Porto Alegre, RS, Brazil

782 Dr. Timoteo, St., 90570-040 Porto Alegre, RS, Brazil
e-mail: doris@hexsel.com.br

C. Brum, M.D.
Department of Dermatology, Brazilian Center for Studies in Dermatology, Porto Alegre, RS, Brazil
e-mail: cbbrum@yahoo.com.br

A. Tosti, D. Hexsel (eds.), *Update in Cosmetic Dermatology*,
DOI 10.1007/978-3-642-34029-1_9, © Springer-Verlag Berlin Heidelberg 2013

9.1 Introduction

Treatments with botulinum toxin type A (BT-A) became the most common nonsurgical procedure in cosmetic dermatology. Its great acceptance and popularity are result of its safety and efficacy, among being a minimally invasive procedure. To maximize the cosmetic results, BT-A can be also combined with a series of other procedures, such as fillers and lasers.

9.2 Physiology, Immunology, and Pharmacology

Botulinum toxin type A is recognized as the most lethal toxin to humans, responsible for causing botulism. This neurotoxin is a protein originated from anaerobic gram-positive spore-forming bacilli called *Clostridium botulinum*. Seven antigenically distinct serotypes A, B, C, D, E, F, and G are produced from different strains of this bacteria, but only serotypes A and B are in clinical use [1].

Botulinum neurotoxins are synthesized as an inactive single chain polypeptide with a molecular weight of 300–900 kDa, comprising a 150-kDa neurotoxin protein, plus varying amount of nontoxins protein. Their activation happens when the chain is cleaved into heavy and light chains [15]. The heavy chain of the BT-A binds selectively and irreversibly to glycoprotein structure (target receptor) specially found on cholinergic presynaptic membranes. Then, the disulfide bond is cleaved liberating the light chain. The light chain is an endopeptidase with proteolytic activity. It binds with high specificity to the SNARE protein complex, which is the soluble *N*-ethylmaleimide-sensitive factor attachment protein receptor, an acetylcholine transport protein chain, responsible for releasing acetylcholine (ACH) into the synaptic cleft through exocytosis [1].

Distinct serotypes of BT cleave different proteins of SNARE complex. Botulinum toxin type-A cleaves synaptosomal-associated proteins of 25 kDa (SNAP-25) and BT-B cleaves vesicle-associated membrane protein (VAMP). With this process, the nervous impulse that causes depolarization of the muscle membrane is blocked, preventing muscular contraction when the target is a muscle and blockage of glandular secretion when the target is an eccrine gland [15].

After the injection, the onset of action of BT-A is from 24 to 72 h and its peak of effect is around 2 weeks. Patients observe the effects in 3–7 days after the injections. Its action lasts for 3–6 months [34], when the formation of new neuromuscular junctions (neurogenesis) occurs, permitting muscular function again [27]. The anhydrotic outcome tends to have a longer effect than the muscular effect having a symptom-free interval of 6–9 months after each botulinum toxin injection [14].

Botulinum toxin type A is capable to produce circulating IgG antibodies, which may block the therapeutic effects of the drug. The BT-A doses that cause the stimulation of these antibodies remain unclear [36]. However, a possible relationship of antibody formation with higher dose injections and/or more frequent intervals is suggested as neurological patients using the BT-A are more prone to develop antibodies.

In order to reduce the possibility of antigenicity, it is recommended to use the lowest effective dose and avoiding repeating injections at less than 12-week intervals [6]. Patients that develop an immune response to BT-A will produce neutralizing antibodies to type B, conferring also antigenicity activity after some exposure to this substance [1].

9.3 Commercial Preparations

Although the commercial brands are produced from purified cultures of the bacteria *Clostridium botulinum*, each of them has distinctive features, such as the number of units, chemical properties, biological action, molecular weight, and inactive ingredients in the formulation [29]. The most widely known and authorized BTs-A for trading in several countries around the world are the following four:

- Botox® 100 and Vistabel 50U per vial (Allergan Inc, USA) or onabotulinumtoxinA (ONA)
- Dysport® 300 and 500 Speywood Unit (U)/Azzalure® 125 U per vial (Ipsen, England) or abobotulinumtoxinA (ABO)
- Xeomin®100 U and Bocouture® 50 U per vial (Merz Pharmaceuticals, Frankfurt, Germany) or incobotulinumtoxinA (INCO)
- Prosigne®100 U per vial (Lanzhou Institute of Biological Products, Lanzhou, China)

Botulinum toxin type B, also called rimabotulinumtoxin B, is commercialized as Neuroblock®/Myobloc® (Elan Pharmaceuticals, San Francisco, USA/Elan Pharmaceuticals, Dublin, Ireland).

Other serotypes are being studied and might be available in the future.

9.4 Reconstitution, Dilution, and Handling

The commercially available BT-A come in a lyophilized state, and a number of steps are needed to obtain the most efficacious and longest-lasting results of this drug. They should be reconstituted in 0.9 % sterile saline with or without preservatives, gently introduced into the vial to avoid bubble formation [13]. The manufacturers recommend their use in the first hours after reconstitution. However, studies conducted with ONA and ABO showed that these medications keep safe and effective from 2 to 6 weeks after reconstitution [23, 25, 28].

It is also observed that preservatives do not interfere in the results, but apparently allow less painful injections, a longer storage period after reconstitution and reduced risk of bacterial contamination [27]. One study revealed that BT-A lidocaine-reconstituted has equal effectiveness than that reconstituted with saline for treating axillary hyperhidrosis, being associated with reduced pain [37].

Except for INCO, which may be stored at room temperatures up to 25 °C before reconstitution [19], other BTs-A must be stored at temperatures ranging from 2 to 8 °C, prior to and after reconstitution. Freezing must be avoided after reconstitution for all toxins.

The choice for a specific volume to dilute the products is based on physician's experience. Dilutions from 1 to 10 mL have been used for cosmetic purposes. However, most physicians prefer using smaller volumes for cosmetic treatments.

Botulinum toxin type B comes pre-diluted and ready for use in vials with three different volumes containing the same concentration 2,500U/0.5 ml, 5,000U/1.0 ml, and

10,000U/2 ml. It can be stored for up 36 months at temperatures ranging from 2 to 8 °C and at room temperature for at least 9 months without losing stability or potency. The use of slightly acidic formulation at pH of 5.6 confers to BT-B extended stability. This acid formulation is responsible for greater transient discomfort reported for some patients. To avoid this side effect, the pH could be adjusted with sodium bicarbonate, but the injection should be administered immediately to avoid destabilization of the toxin [18].

9.5 Injection Technique

For an adequate treatment, care should be taken regarding injection technique. For better visualization and comfort, the patient should be in a sitting or semi-reclined position. Areas to be treated should be analyzed in its anatomical, static, and dynamic aspects, taking into account each patient's individual characteristics such as facial asymmetries.

Photographs should be performed before treatment at rest and under muscular contraction [22, 35]. Besides, physicians follow a few steps before injections:

- Remove completely the makeup to visualize small vessels prior to injection to decrease the occurrence of hematomas.
- Define and mark out the injection points with a surgical pen or pencil.

Different types of syringes can be used, depending on the volume of reconstituted product [35]. The 0.3 or 0.5 mL Ultra-Fine II syringes equipped with a 30-gauge needle are usually used for low volumes.

Cooling the target area with ice from 3 to 5 s [26] can diminish pain and prevent bruising. Injections are done into the target area superficial or intramuscular, perpendicularly to the skin (Fig. 9.1). When injecting BT-A, the number of units (U) is one of the most important factors determining efficacy as well as injection technique. Patients should also be oriented to avoid aspirin, nonsteroidal anti-inflammatory agents, and high dose of vitamin E for 10 days before the procedure to prevent bleeding and ecchymosis. It is also helpful applying direct pressure and cold compress on the injection site [33, 38].

Patients are usually instructed to avoid manipulating the injected area, practicing physical exercises, lowering their head, and lying down to 4 h after the procedure [10].

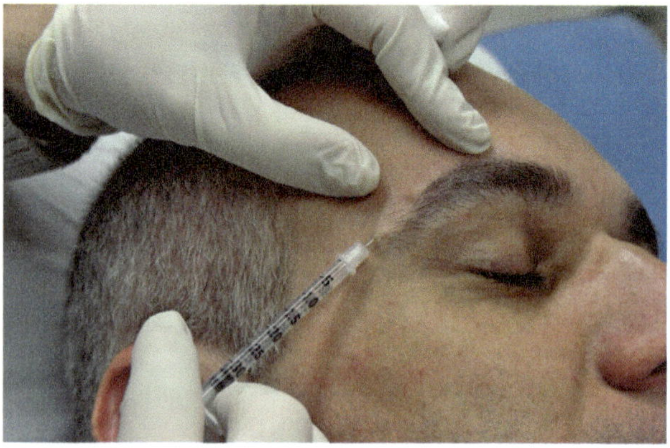

Fig. 9.1 Botulinum toxin injections performed perpendicularly to the skin

Table 9.1 Recommended doses for ONA [12] and ABO [3] in different cosmetic treatments

	ONA	ABO
	Total dose range (U)	Total dose range (s.U)
Upper facial indications		
Glabellar lines	10–40	50
Forehead lines	6–15	20–60
Crow's feet	10–30	30–60
Mid and lower facial indications		
Bunny lines	4–8	10–20
Nasal tip droop/drooping nasal tip	2–4	10
Infraorbital rhytides/lower eyelid wrinkles	2	5
Perioral wrinkles	4–10	4–12
Drooping mouth corner/ marionette lines	4–6	10–20
Dimpled chin	4–10	10–20
Face-lift	2–8	4–20
Gingival smile	4–10	5–15
Extra facial indications		
Platysmal bands	2–12 per band (women)	Maximum dose 50 per side
	3–12 per band (men)	
Décolleté wrinkles	30–100	75–120

Doses are expressed in total number of units per treatment divided in both sides, when applicable

9.6 Cosmetic Use of BT-A

Botulinum toxin type A has become one of the most important nonsurgical tool for facial rejuvenation and acts reducing the motility of the muscles of facial expression, leading to a smoother and more youthful appearance. The usual recommended doses for the most common indications are described in Table 9.1.

9.6.1 Upper Face

The upper third is the most common targeted area for BT-A applications and includes the treatment of forehead, glabellar, and crow's feet lines, and the improvement of brown shape and position.

The dynamic wrinkles on the forehead appear perpendicularly to the direction of the muscle fibers and become static over time. Wrinkles and ptosis of the structures of the frontal region, mainly the eyelids and eyebrows, are striking characteristics of aging, conferring an appearance of fatigue. The same happens in the glabellar area that can express from wrinkles to negative feelings, such as anger, sadness, tension, concern, and disapproval [11, 35].

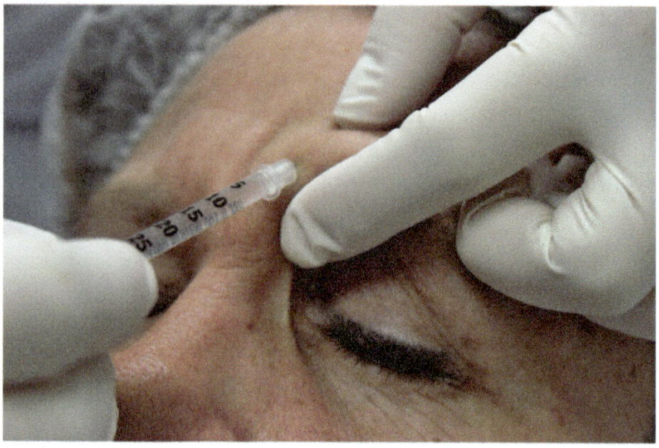

Fig. 9.2 Injection technique for BT-A applications at the glabellar muscles

9.6.1.1 Glabellar Lines

Glabellar frown lines result from the contraction of *procerus* muscle (m.), *corrugator supercilii* m., and *depressor supercilii* m. The BT-A treatment of glabellar lines can also delay physiologic brow ptosis and blepharoplasty. Moreover, it is able to modify the shape and position of the eyebrows, also correcting asymmetries. Because frown muscles are responsible for some facial expressions, a partial paralysis of glabella is desired instead of a complete paralysis [7, 11].

The BT-A is injected slowly into 1–2 points in each *corrugator* m., keeping the needle tip out of the orbital rim. The needle must be placed perpendicularly and pushed slowly upward toward the hair implant line. Two-fingered palpation of these muscles is recommended, since this minimizes the occurrence of side effects (Fig. 9.2).

The BT-A can be applied in 1–2 points of the *procerus* m. to treat the horizontal lines at the root of the nose. A single injection is done along the midline at a point below the line joining the brows and above the crossing point of the "X" formed by joining the medial eyebrow to the contralateral inner canthus, is usually sufficient.

Successive treatments progressively improved appearance at rest [8, 29].

Blepharoptosis is one of the most undesirable adverse events after BT-A injections in glabella, accounting for about 2 % of the injections [38]. This complication occurs when the *levator palpebrae superioris* m. is affected by the action of toxin [7]. It can also occur when injections of nasal bridge are too lateral. Patient with upper eyelid ptosis can be treated with apraclonidine 0.5 % and phenylephrine hydrochloride 2.5 %. These medications stimulate Mueller's muscle, elevating the upper eyelid [38]. Higher volumes and doses of BT-A, besides poor technique, may result in brow or eyelid ptosis. To minimize the risk of ptosis, it is recommended to place the injections no closer than 1 cm above the central eyebrow and inject the minimal dose necessary for efficacy.

Residual nasal lines when the patient smiles, called "botulinum toxin sign," can occur after glabellar Botulinum toxin injection [38].

9.6.1.2 Forehead Lines

The *frontalis* m. is a large but thin muscle with superior insertions in the *galea aponeurotica* and inferior insertion in *procerus* m., *orbicularis oculi* m., *corrugator supercilii* m., *depressor supercilii* m., and in the skin on the brow area. This muscle is responsible for facial expressions of fear and surprise. Raising the eyebrows also results in the horizontal forehead lines [7].

The contraction of *frontalis* m. should be carefully analyzed before the injections because consequent forehead wrinkles vary widely from person to person [20]. Five to ten points are usually injected. These points are generally distributed horizontally or in "V" shape. Sites of injection are established according to the physical exam and patient's needs, also considering the desired brow shape. It is advised to inject 1–2 cm above the orbital rim, in order to avoid eyebrow ptosis, which causes a tired appearance. Another important consideration when treating forehead lines is to avoid a frozen look by using small doses of BT-A and less injection points [2].

Transient brow ptosis involving the lateral brow occurs approximately in 5 % of the cases, and it is associated with over treatment of this area. It is important to maintain some movements of this area, avoiding the freezing aspect [33, 38].

Patients with lateral *frontalis* m. hyperactivity can present unintended quizzical brow lift, with an extreme upward arch of the lateral eyebrows. This undesired event could be corrected by injecting 1–2 U of ONA into the lateral *frontalis* m. fibers, above the outer third of the eyebrow [33].

9.6.1.3 Lateral Canthal Lines (Crow's Feet)

The hyperactivity of *orbicularis oculi* m., a muscle responsible for forceful closure of the eyelids, in association with *levator anguli oris* m., *risorius* m., and *zygomaticus* m. produces radial lines in the lateral canthal area known as "crow's feet." The first point marked to treat this indication is placed at the center of the maximum contraction area, usually located at the lateral canthus, at a minimum distance of 1 cm from the lateral orbital rim. Two or three additional points may be applied, according to patients' needs, 1–1.5 cm above and below the first marked, in a line that follows the orbital curvature. Effects of BT-A last usually less in this area than in other treatable areas due to the frequent contraction during the smile [10, 18].

Attention should be taken to distinguish lines caused by *orbicularis* m. contraction and those produced by *zygomaticus* m. [13].

Some complications involved in the treatment of crow's feet such as ectropion, diplopia, strabismus, and eyelid ptosis can occur. To avoid such effects, caused by effects of the toxins to extraocular muscle and palpebral portion of the *orbicularis oculi* m. [13], the minimum distance from the lateral orbital rim (1 cm) should be respected. Lateral ptosis has been reported in 5 % of patients treated for crow's feet due to denervation of the lateral *frontalis* m. To prevent this complication it is suggested to perform the injections bellow the eyebrow. Lip or cheek ptosis could happen when BT-A is injected bellow the horizontal line between the cheeks. Bell's palsy appears when *zygomaticus* m. is denerved. Lateral rectus palsy is a complication that occurs when the injection is too medial and deep. It is also recommended to use small volumes of 0.1–0.2 mL per injection point, keep the injections 1.5 cm lateral to the lateral canthus, and apply the injections above of the inferior margin of zygomatic arch to reduce the cited complications [33]. Physicians should also be aware of ecchymosis formation in the periorbital region because of the highly vascular and fragile tissue [33].

9.6.1.4 Lateral Eyebrow Lift

A lowered brow and expressions of anger and scowling are results of the over activity of brow depressor. This complex is constituted by medial portion of *corrugator supercilii* m., *procerus* m., and medial and lateral portion of *orbicularis oculi* m. The paralysis of depressor muscles allows for unopposed brow abduction by *frontalis* m. that interdigitates with the three brow depressors in its lower portion [7, 20]. This result can be achieved treating the glabellar complex, producing small degree of brow elevation (1–3 mm). One study reported that injections of 20–40 U of ONA only into the glabella elevate the lateral eyebrow, followed by heighted of medial and central eyebrow portion. Other study showed a significant lateral brow lift after 7–10 U of ONA injected into the lateral *orbicularis* m. lateral to the midpupillary line. According to Ascher et al. [2], it is also indicated to inject one point at each eyebrow tail and the other at the external part of the *frontalis* m. in each side to elevate the lateral portion of the brow [2]. The recommended dose of ABO is 5–10 U per point and the total dose range is 20–40 U [2].

9.6.2 Middle Face

Differently from the upper face, the rejuvenation for middle face requires more volume restoration with fillers than toxins. But BT-A treatments can be combined to fillers to obtain better cosmetic results.

9.6.2.1 Infraorbital Rhytides

Infraorbital folds occur due to hyperfunctional *pretarsal orbicularis* m., and they are present on the lower eyelid.

A snap test can predict good or bad candidates for BT-A in the lower eyelid, usually injected at the midpupillary line, 3 mm bellow the ciliary margin, and if a second point is necessary, it could be placed 1 cm laterally from the first.

This treatment can increase the ocular aperture, which may be desired by some Asian patients. Results are better when associated with treatment of lateral orbital area [17]. Some patients with atopic dermatitis that have Dennie–Morgan folds could also have some benefits with this procedure [16].

Injection of doses higher than the recommended can cause significant side effects such as incomplete function of the eye, lower eyelid edema, and photophobia [16]. Ectropion, fat herniation, and dry eye symptoms can also occur. This indication should not be treated in patients with lower-lid laxity, previous surgery under the eye, and preexisting fat herniation, as those are more prone to have complications.

9.6.2.2 Bunny Lines

The radial lines at the radix of the nose, known as "bunny lines," are created by upper portion of *nasalis* m. contraction. The best point of injection is on the superior lateral aspect of the nasal wall above the nasofacial groove [13]. When the injection is performed in lower sites of the nasal wall, such as the nasofacial groove, an ipsilateral lip ptosis can occur, because the *levator labii superioris alaeque nasi* m. is chemodenerved [10].

9.6.2.3 Cheeks

Many patients, especially when smiling, have furrows and deep wrinkles in the area of the cheeks. These are caused due to the action of *zygomaticus major* m., *zygomaticus minor* m., *buccinator* m., and *risorius* m. [4]. To find these muscles, patient should be asked to smile. Usually cheeks are divided by an imaginary line extending from the oral commissure to the tip of the lobule of the ear. The wrinkles in the upper half are produced by *zygomaticus* muscles, and wrinkles bellow may be produced by either the *buccinator m.* or *risorius* m. or both. These lines are good candidates for fillers, but small doses of 1–2 U ONA or 2.5–5 U of ABO are recommended for *zygomaticus* m., and 1–3 U ONA or 2.5–7.5 U of ABO could be used for *risorius* m. and/or *buccinator* m. Patients should be aware that they can experience and inability to fully smile after treatment [5].

9.6.2.4 Nasal Tip/Repeated Nasal Flare

Botulinum toxin type A injections at the base of columella are used to lift the nasal tip.

Some people dilate or present rhythmic contractions of the nostrils on certain occasions, which may cause embarrassment. Injections of BT-A are indicated on each side in the lower nasal fibers above the lateral nasal ala [9]. The injections are performed intradermically and bilaterally, into the lateral portion of the nasal wings, 0.5 cm from the free edge of the nose.

9.6.3 Lower Face

Aging in this region is characterized by the horizontal lip stretching, downward oral commissures, increase in the distance between the columella and the vermilion border, and loss of lip thickness, perioral wrinkles, marionette lines, and dimpled or *peau d'orange* chin. Although the lower third of the face is the most common area for fillers in facial rejuvenation, BT-A has increased popularity in some indications, such as drooping mouth corner, dimpled chin, perioral wrinkles, and masseter hypertrophy.

9.6.3.1 Drooping Mouth Corner

The corners of the mouth of some people are permanently turned down by the action of the *depressor anguli oris* m. and give an appearance of sadness. Botulinum toxin type A can be used to weaken this muscle to diminish labiomental folds and sad look. It is injected directly above the mandibular angle, along its rim and 1 cm lateral to the oral commissure, bilaterally, [9] in an imaginary line that follows the direction of the nasolabial furrow. Lower lip dysfunction can be caused when the injection is too medial and involve the *depressor labii* m. [33].

9.6.3.2 Dimpled Chin (Peau d' Orange)

An association of *mentalis* m. action and loss of collagen and subcutaneous fat is responsible for dimpled chin appearance. Two techniques of BT-A injections are described to reduce this undesired condition. If the one-point injection is used, it should be placed just below the tip or prominence of the chin located in the midline mass of the muscle [11]. If the BT-A treatment is divided in two points, each one should be injected bilaterally and symmetrically at the most distal point of the *orbicularis oris* m. at the prominence of the chin [30]. Deep injections are recommended because of the reasonable amount of fat that exists in the chin area.

9.6.3.3 Perioral Rhytides

Perioral wrinkles are fine vertical lip rhytides, also called "smokers lines." Botulinum toxin type A can be used to reduce these wrinkles and to produce the appearance of fuller lips, because weakening of this muscle results in slight eversion of the upper lip [10].

The technique consists of injecting in the area of muscle contraction adjacent to the vertical wrinkles superficially at or above the vermilion border. The average number of injections is 5–6 and they should be symmetric.

Injection in mouth corners and midline must be avoided, as they may cause undesirable relaxation of the *depressor anguli oris* m. and lip flattening, respectively [22]. Some complications as failure to drink through a straw or to whistle lip weakening, asymmetry of the mouth, and drooling can occur after BT-A treatment for perioral rhytides, especially if high doses are used. To avoid these complications, lowest effective doses should be used [24].

9.6.3.4 "Face Lift"

Some of the *platysma* m. fibers are located in the malar region and cause lowering of this region. Two to four points along the lateral mandibular border are injected to produce the face lift effect. One study reported high patient satisfaction and a low incidence of adverse effects with this technique [31].

9.6.3.5 Gingival Smile/Gummy Smile

Gingival smile (GS) is characterized by exposure of more than 3 mm of the upper gum when the individual smiles, mainly caused by the contraction of the *levator labii* superioris m. For some patients, GS represents an aesthetic disorder, and the use of BT represents a simple, fast, and effective method for its aesthetic correction [32].

Identifying the type of GS and therefore the main muscles involved is essential to choose the correct injection technique can be used. A new classification of GS into anterior, posterior, mixed, or asymmetric, based on the excessive contraction of specific muscle groups has been described by Mazzuco and Hexsel [32].

Injections of BT-A to treat each type of GS are described as the following [32]:

- Anterior GS: on each side of the nasolabial fold, 1 cm lateral and below the nasal ala, to relax the LLSAN muscle.
- Posterior GS: two points in the malar region – the first point was located in nasolabial fold, at the point of greatest lateral contraction during the smile, and the other point was 2 cm lateral to the first point, at the level of the tragus.

- Mixed GS: at all the points described above.
- Asymmetric GS: two points in the malar region described above, on the side with greater posterior gum exposure. And only at the lowest point on the contralateral side.

9.6.4 Extra Facial Areas

9.6.4.1 Platysmal Muscle (Horizontal Necklace Lines and Platysmal Bands)

Neck wrinkles are more frequently related to photoaging and skin laxity than platysmal bands; however, BT-A can be used in patients with good skin elasticity of platysmal contractions become more prominent, mainly, in some slim patients and when they speak or smile [3].

Platysmal bands are identified by asking patients to contract their necks by clenching their teeth. Bands should be firmly held using the thumb and index, and injections should be performed into various points along the muscle, 1–2 cm apart from each other [9, 21]. Dosage is crucial for good results. In case of horizontal neck lines, deep injections and high dosage should be avoided to prevent dysphagia and neck muscle weakness. Floppy neck may occur if fibers of *sternocleidomastoid* m. are affected by BT-A [38].

9.6.4.2 Chest/Décolleté Wrinkles

Dynamic wrinkles in the upper chest are caused by medial fibers of *pectoralis major* m. and the tail portion of the *platysma* m. movements. The involvement of *pectoralis major* m. can be determined by palpation while having the patient to cross the arms. When properly indicated, the recommended doses can be applied in a V-shape over the wrinkles of this area, divided into 3–6 points on each side [22].

9.7 Combined Treatments with Botulinum Toxins

Botulinum toxin type A injections can be combined to other treatment modalities such as fillers, lasers, and light sources. Treatments that combine the use of fillers and BT-A are capable of correcting the wrinkles by restoring lost volumes and relaxing hyperactive muscles in situations which each treatment alone would provide partial results. Lasers and light sources used in association with BT-A can also optimize cosmetic results as well as to prolong the effects of BT-A, generating greater patients satisfaction [5, 39].

Conclusions

Knowledge of anatomy and choice of the right doses are crucial to achieve best results when using BT for rejuvenation as well as to avoid potential complications. Each patient requires individual evaluation and therapeutic plan that meets doctors' and patients' expectations, with safety, harmony, balance, and naturalness.

References

1. Aoki RK (2003) Pharmacology and immunology of Botulinum toxin type A. Clin Dermatol 21:476–480
2. Ascher B, Talarico S, Cassuto D et al (2010) International consensus recommendations on the aesthetic usage of botulinum toxin type a (Speywood Unit) – part I: upper facial wrinkles. J Eur Acad Dermatol Venereol 24(11):1278–1284
3. Ascher B, Talarico S, Cassuto D et al (2010) International consensus recommendations on the aesthetic usage of botulinum toxin type A (Speywood Unit) – part II: wrinkles on the middle and lower face, neck and chest. J Eur Acad Dermatol Venereol 24(11):1285–1295
4. Atamoros FP (2003) Botulinum toxin in the lower one third of the face. Clin Dermatol 21:505–512
5. Beer K, Waibel J (2007) Botulinum toxin type A enhances the outcome of fractional resurfacing of the cheek. J Drugs Dermatol 6(11):1151–1152
6. Borodic G (2007) Botulinum toxin, immunologic considerations with long-term repeated use, with emphasis on cosmetic applications. Facial Plast Surg Clin North Am 15(1):11–16
7. Carruthers A, Carruthers J (2001) Botulinum toxin type A: history and current cosmetic use in the upper face. Semin Cutan Med Surg 20:71–84
8. Carruthers A, Carruthers J, Lowe NJ et al (2004) One year, randomized, multicenter, two period study of the safety and efficacy of repeated treatments with botulinum toxin type-A in patients with Glabelar lines. J Clin Res 7:1
9. Carruthers J, Carruthers A (2003) Aesthetic botulinum A toxin in the mid and lower face and neck. Dermatol Surg 29(5):468–476
10. Carruthers J, Fagien S, Matarasso SL, Botox Consensus Group (2004) Consensus recommendations on the use of botulinum toxin type A in facial aesthetics. Plast Reconstr Surg 114 (Suppl 6):1–22
11. Carruthers JD, Glogau RG, Blitzer A, Facial Aesthetics Consensus Group Faculty (2008) Advances in facial rejuvenation: botulinum toxin type a, hyaluronic acid dermal fillers, and combination therapies – consensus recommendations. Plast Reconstr Surg 121(Suppl 5):5–30
12. Coleman KR, Carruthers J (2006) Combination therapy with BOTOX and fillers: the new rejuvenation paradigm. Dermatol Ther 19(3):177–188
13. de Sa Earp AP, Marmur ES (2008) The five D´s of botulinum toxin: doses, dilution, diffusion, duration and dogma. J Cosmet Laser Ther 10:93–102
14. Doft MA, Kasten JL, Ascherman JA (2011) Treatment of axillary hyperhidrosis with botulinum toxin: a single surgeon's experience with 53 consecutive patients. Aesthetic Plast Surg 35(6):1079–1086
15. Dressler D, Saberi FA, Barbosa ER (2005) Botulinum toxin: mechanism of action. Arq Neruropsiquiatr 63(1):180–185
16. Flynn TC (2003) Periocular Botulinum toxin. Clin Dermatol 21:498–504
17. Flynn TC, Carruthers J, Carruthers A (2001) Botulinum-A toxin treatment of the lower eyelid improves infraorbital rhytides and widens the eye. Dermatol Surg 27(8):703–708
18. Glogau RG (2002) Review of the use of botulinum toxin for hyperhidrosis and cosmetic purposes. Clin J Pain 18(Suppl 6):191–197
19. Grein S, Mander GJ, Taylor HV (2008) Xeomin® is stable without refrigeration: complexing proteins are not required for stability of botulinum neurotoxin type a preparations. Toxicon 51:10
20. Hexsel D, Dal'Forno T (2003) Type A Botulinum toxin in the upper aspect of the face. Clin Dermatol 21:488–497
21. Hexsel D, Dal'Forno T (2009) The upper trunk: décolleté wrinkles and breast lift. In: Ascher B, Landau M, Rossi B (eds) Injection treatments in cosmetic surgery. Informa Healthcare, London, pp 153–157
22. Hexsel D, Hexsel C (2010) Botulinum toxins. In: Robinson JK, Hanke CW, Siegel DM, Fratila A (eds) Surgery of the skin: procedural dermatology. Mosby Elsevier, Edinburgh, pp 433–446

23. Hexsel DM, Almeida AT, Rutowitsch M et al (2003) Multicenter, double-blind study of the efficacy of injections with botulinum toxin type A reconstituted up to six consecutive weeks before application. Dermatol Surg 29(5):523–529
24. Cohen JL, Dayan SH, Cox SE et al (2012) OnabotulinumtoxinA Dose-Ranging Study for Hyperdynamic Perioral Lines. Dermatol Surg 38(9):1497–1505
25. Hexsel D, Castro IA, Zechmeister D et al (2004) Multicenter, double-blind study of the efficacy of injections with botulinum toxin A reconstituted up to six consecutive weeks before application. Dermatol Surg 30(5):823
26. Hexsel D, DalForno T, Soirefmann M, et al. Effective, low cost, simple, disposable cooling tool for patient comfort in common dermatologic procedures. Dermatol Surg (in press)
27. Hexsel D, Mazzuco R, Dal'Forno T et al (2007) Botulinum toxin for facial wrinkles; history and future. Expert Ver Dermatol 2(4):417–426
28. Hexsel D, Rutowitsch M, Castro LC et al (2009) Blind multicenter study of the efficacy and safety of injections of a commercial preparation of botulinum toxin type A reconstituted up to fifteen weeks prior injection. Dermatol Surg 35(6):933–939; discussion 940
29. Klein AW, Carruthers A, Fagien S, Lowe NJ (2008) Comparisons among botulinum toxins: an evidence-based review. Plast Reconstr Surg 121(6):413–422
30. Kogos L (2002) Mental Wrinkles. In: Hexsel D, de Almeida AT (eds) Cosmetic use of botulinum toxin. AGE, São Paulo, pp 167–170
31. Levy PM (2007) The "Nefertiti lift": a new technique for specific re-contouring of the jawline. J Cosmet Laser Ther 9(4):249–252
32. Mazzuco R, Hexsel D (2010) Gummy smile and botulinum toxin: a new approach based on the gingival exposure area. J Am Acad Dermatol 63(6):1042–1051
33. Pena MA, Alam M, Yoo SS (2007) Complications with the use of botulinum toxin type A for cosmetic applications and hyperhidrosis. Semin Cutan Med Surg 26(1):29–33
34. Rzany B, Ascher B, Monheit G (2010) Treatment of glabellar lines with botulinum toxin type A (Speywood Unit): a clinical overview. J Eur Acad Dermatol Venereol 24(1):1–14
35. Salti G, Ghersetich I (2008) Advanced botulinum toxin techniques against wrinkles in the upper face. Clin Dermatol 26(2):182–191
36. Sposito MM (2004) Toxina botulínica tipo A – propriedades farmacológicas e uso clínico. Acta Fisiatr (Suppl 1):1–44
37. Vadoud-Seyedi J, Simonart T (2007) Treatment of axillary hyperhidrosis with botulinum toxin type A reconstituted in lidocaine or in normal saline: a randomized, side-by-side, double-blind study. Br J Dermatol 156(5):986–989
38. Wollina U, Konrad H (2005) Managing adverse events associated with botulinum toxin type-A: a focus o cosmetic procedures. Am J Clin Dermatol 6(3):141–150
39. Yamauchi PS, Lask G, Lowe NJ (2004) Botulinum toxin type A gives adjunctive benefit to periorbital laser resurfacing. J Cosmet Laser Ther 6(3):145–148

Cryosurgery 10

Cleide Eiko Ishida

Core Messages

- Cryosurgery is a widely used treatment modality in dermatology.
- Knowledge of skin lesion and the differences in the management between benign and malignant lesions and, in some instances, its use combined with other modalities (curettage, shaving, debulking) can produce better cosmetic results.
- New models of accessories such as tips and tip adapters improve the procedure accuracy on benign lesions with short dimensions.
- In the cosmetic cryosurgery, it is fundamental to respect the basic concept of Zacarian SA for cryosurgery in benign lesions: "it is always better to hypofreeze than to hyperfreeze, because the first can be retreated, avoiding definite inaesthetical scars" [32].

10.1 Introduction

Cryosurgery is a consecrate surgical method that uses freezing temperatures to achieve inflammatory and/or destructive response on tissues. It is a widely used treatment modality in dermatology, and its place in the treatment of malignant and premalignant skin diseases is well established. Cryosurgery also has great utility in dermatological benign disease, and some unaesthetic skin diseases are responsive to freezing with excellent cosmetic results. The word cryotherapy is often used for nondestructive treatment of benign condition of dermatological disease.

C.E. Ishida, M.D.
Department of Dermatology,
University Hospital and School of Medicine, Federal University of Rio de Janeiro,
178 Marquês de Abrantes, St. - Apto 704, 22230-061 Rio de Janeiro, RJ, Brazil
e-mail: cleide-ishida@uol.com.br

A. Tosti, D. Hexsel (eds.), *Update in Cosmetic Dermatology*,
DOI 10.1007/978-3-642-34029-1_10, © Springer-Verlag Berlin Heidelberg 2013

Liquid nitrogen (LN) is not the only refrigerant therapy available, but it is the cryogen of choice because it is the coldest (−195. 8°C) and most versatile cryogenic agent, with usefulness for the treatment of benign, premalignant, or malignant conditions. It is nowadays the ideal cryogen due to its availability, manipulating safety, usefulness, and low cost.

10.2 Mechanism of Action

The biologic alterations that occur in cryosurgery are caused by reducing the temperature of the skin. There are two methods of heat transfer. Boiled heat transfer occurs when liquid nitrogen touches the skin when dipstick and spray techniques are used, and conduction heat transfer occurs when a cold metal probe is applied to the skin [18].

The mechanisms of injury from the freezing of tissue include direct effects on the cells and the vascular stasis on tissue after thawing [18]. Slow cooling produces extracellular ice, allowing less overall tissue destruction. Nevertheless, intracellular ice is formed when a lesion is cooled quickly, resulting in a greater degree of cellular damage. The rate of thawing also influences the degree of damage. Slow thawing promotes an increased concentration of electrolytes and recrystallization that is also damaging to cells [18, 26]. The vascular stasis develops in the tissue after thawing, and failure of the microcirculation assures cell destruction [18]. Repeated freeze-thaw cycles (FTC) produce maximum destructive effects in the tissue [18]. Inflammation develops in response to cell death and further contributes to the destruction of the lesion [9, 26].

The cryosurgery produces a selective destruction of cells or tissue, which depends on the minimum temperature reached during the cryogenic injury, because there is an individual variation of the cell types on the minimum temperature for their destruction. In a rising order in relation to the most sensitive to cold-induced damage cell types, the melanocytes are the most sensitive cells, followed by basal cells, keratinocytes, bacteria, connective tissue, nerve connective tissue sheath, blood vessel endothelium, and viruses [5]. The melanocytes are sensitive to a minimum temperature of −4 to−7 °C, the keratinocytes need a minimum temperature of −30 to −40 °C for their destruction, and viruses are resistant to −195.8 °C [26].

Tissue response depends on the gravity of cryogenic injury. On light injury caused by exposure to freezing for seconds and tissue temperature close to −10 °C, the response is an inflammatory reaction, and it is common the formation of vesicle in the dermis-epidermis junction. On severe injury, the freezing occurs for a longer time, reaching −20 °C, and it generates necrosis. Complete freezing of the skin happens when tissue temperature reaches −50 °C; temperature required for the treatment of malignant tumors and necrosis is clearly circumscriptive [18].

10.3 History of Use

Cold use has an extensive history, and the benefits from its use as therapy have been known for several thousand years. There is well-documented use of cold water and ice applications for diverse illnesses and injuries in ancient times. Anesthesia by cooling was also known, and tissue cooling by surface application of snow and ice was used to facilitate amputation in soldiers in Napoleon's Grand Army [9, 19].

In the seventeenth century, scientists observed that atmospheric gases warm when compressed and cool when expanded. Using this principle, all of the permanent gases (oxygen, nitrogen, hydrogen) were liquefied. In 1898, James Dewar developed a vacuum flask to store fluids. These developments permitted the use of cold agents in therapy to enter in a new phase because freezing of some benign skin lesions and early epitheliomas became practical [19].

In 1899, White, a dermatologist from New York, became the first cryosurgeon, when he used a swab dipped in a liquid air to treat successfully benign, premalignant, and some malignant dermatological lesions [9, 19]. Pusey, in 1907, used carbon dioxide snow in the treatment of benign skin lesions. The use of the term cryotherapy was credited to Professor Bordos, in 1912, in relation to his freezing device [19]. Karp et al., in 1939, also used the term cryotherapy in the treatment of acne, using a paste made from ground solid carbon dioxide, acetone, and precipitated sulfur, which was applied directly to the face to obtain superficial exfoliation of the epidermis, in a technique known as "carbon snow" application [16, 17].

Carbon dioxide remained as the main cryogenic agent until the 1940s. Following World War II, cryogenic fluids, oxygen and nitrogen, became readily commercially available. In 1950, Allington introduced the use of liquid nitrogen into clinical practice. He described the technique of using cotton swabs dipped in liquid nitrogen for the treatment of skin diseases [19]. In 1960, cryosurgery was not an important therapeutic modality because the use of cryogenic agents applied topically was limited.

The modern cryosurgery equipments were introduced, in 1961, by Cooper and Lee, neurosurgeons who developed a device that worked with a liquid nitrogen closed system, enabling fast and continuous heat extraction from the tissue [18, 19].

Torre, in 1965, developed a device that allowed the use of spray and probe tips. Later, Zacarian developed a handheld unit to apply liquid nitrogen. Zacarian and Torre, who started instrumental application of liquid nitrogen, helped in the development of new equipments, giving an impulse to dermatologic cryosurgery [18, 19]. Michael Bryne, in 1968, developed the first commercially available handheld cryosurgery device [2].

10.4 Indications

The cryosurgery is indicated for several benign, premalignant, and malignant dermatological lesions. The use of cryosurgery for the treatment of disease and cosmetic use is sometimes difficult to distinguish. Cosmetic cryosurgery has been used in several unaesthetic dermatological diseases with excellent results. It is indicated for benign lesions, where the necessity of tissue destruction is minimum, and the light freezing causes the separation of the epidermis from the dermis, with fast healing of the wound; in some benign vascular tumor lesions, as well as in acne and premalignant lesions, good results are presented because the cell components are more sensitive than stroma, making the cicatrization easier.

The main indications of the cosmetic cryosurgery are [3–6, 8, 9, 12–14, 17, 21, 23, 26, 29]:

- Pigmentation alteration and melanocytic lesions: idiopathic guttate hypomelanosis, solar lentigo, and labial lentiginous macules
- Vascular lesions: venous lake, hemangioma/hemolymphangioma
- Cyst, benign tumors, and other conditions: inflammatory acne, acne cyst, seborrheic keratoses, rhinophyma, and keloid
- Sun-damaged skin: actinic keratoses, solar lentigo, solar elastosis, sebaceous hyperplasia, and fine wrinkles of solar aging

10.5 Relevant Anatomy

Any area of the body can be treated by cryosurgery; however, this method is particularly indicated for lesions located on the nose, ear, and sternum area, because cartilage and bone are resistant to freezing injury and the architecture of the organ is preserved. Cartilage necrosis typically occurs when deep treatments with long freeze times are necessary for malignant tumor treatment [9]. Caution should be taken for tumors located at the inner canthi, free margin of the ala nasi, and auditory canal. Notching and perforation are sometimes the result of cartilage necrosis [5, 9, 18]. It is also indicated for chest and back region because it leaves a minimum hypertrophic scar and it does not require grafting.

Cryosurgery rarely damages nerves because of the resistant nature of the neural sheath, but sometimes superficial nerves are affected by freezing [9]. The freezing often causes hyperesthesia. Permanent loss of neural function is rare because most paresthesias or anesthesias resolve, although it may take up to a year after the treatment. Sensation of pain and cold are slower to return than are sensations of touch. Caution should be taken for lesions that overlie superficial nerves such as lesions on the preauricular or postauricular regions, lateral aspects of the fingers, ulnar fossa, and lateral aspect of the tongue [9].

10.6 Products/Techniques List/Choice

Although some clinicians use nitrous oxide, helium, Freons, fluorocarbonated sprays, and solid carbon dioxide as a cryogen, liquid nitrogen has been widely accepted as an ideal cryogen because it has low temperature (−195.8 °C) and a certificated efficiency in treatment of cutaneous malignant disease, and nowadays it is used for both superficial freezing and deep freezing.

To undertake cosmetic cryosurgery, a vacuuminsulated Dewar tank for the storage of liquid nitrogen, a withdrawal device (Fig. 10.1a), a handheld liquid nitrogen device (Fig. 10.1b), and accessories such as various-sized spray tips, tip adapters, cones, probes, and protective devices (Fig. 10.1c–e) is required.

Among the accessories, having as a reference the ones produced by Brymill, we can highlight the spray tips with different diameters (Fig. 10.1c): A = 1.02 mm,

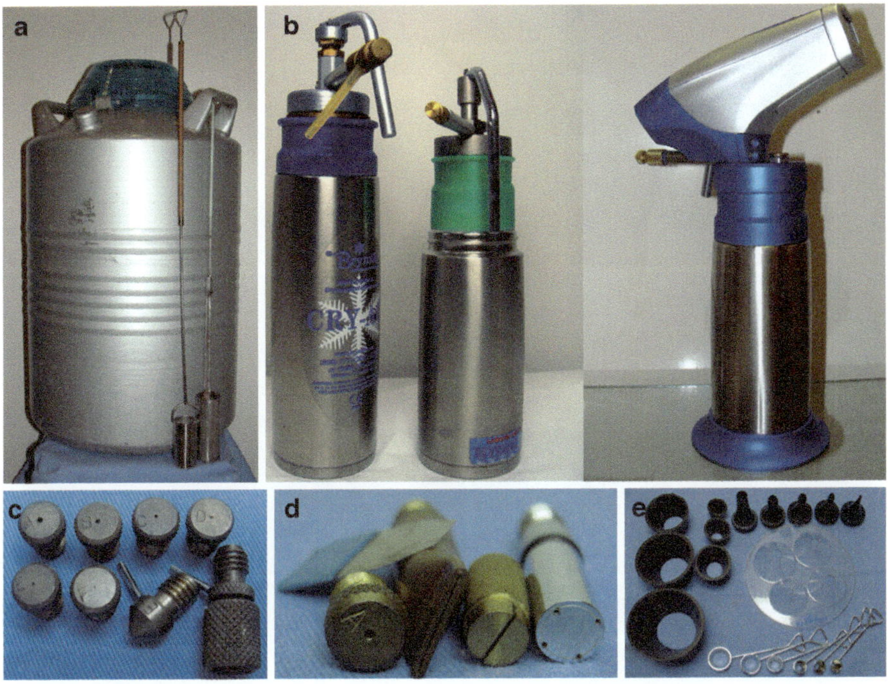

Fig. 10.1 Equipments and accessories: (**a**) vacuum-insulated Dewar tank and withdrawal device, (**b**) handheld device, (**c**) tips and tip adapters for open-spray technique, (**d**) tips for cryopeeling, (**e**) cones and protective device

B=0.80 mm, C=0.57 mm, D=0.40 mm, E=0.34 mm, and F=0.29 mm. The tips with diameters A and B are used on malignant lesions of small and medium dimensions, tips C and D for benign lesions of small dimensions, and tips E and F are useful for small benign lesions and cosmetic means. The back vent adapter eliminates the intermittent vaporization, improving the liquid nitrogen flow, and prevents blockage when used with small diameter open tips, such as the openings D, E, and F (Fig. 10.1c). Spray tips for the treatment of acne and for cryopeeling allow a smooth application that permits a superficial desquamation of the treated area (Fig. 10.1d). In the last few years, a decrease in the size of handheld devices has made using them easier, and new models of accessories such as tips and tip adapters have been developed, improving the procedure accuracy on benign lesions with short dimensions.

The three basic techniques for cryosurgery are dipstick, spray, and probe. Intralesional technique for the treatment of deeper lesions that uses a needle has also been developed [31]. This method involves running a needle through the deep tissue of a tumor, with cryogen passing through the needle and venting to the surface on the opposite end (Fig. 10.2f) [9, 31].

The dipstick technique involves dipping a cotton swab into a cup containing liquid nitrogen and firmly applying the cotton swab to the lesion until a narrow

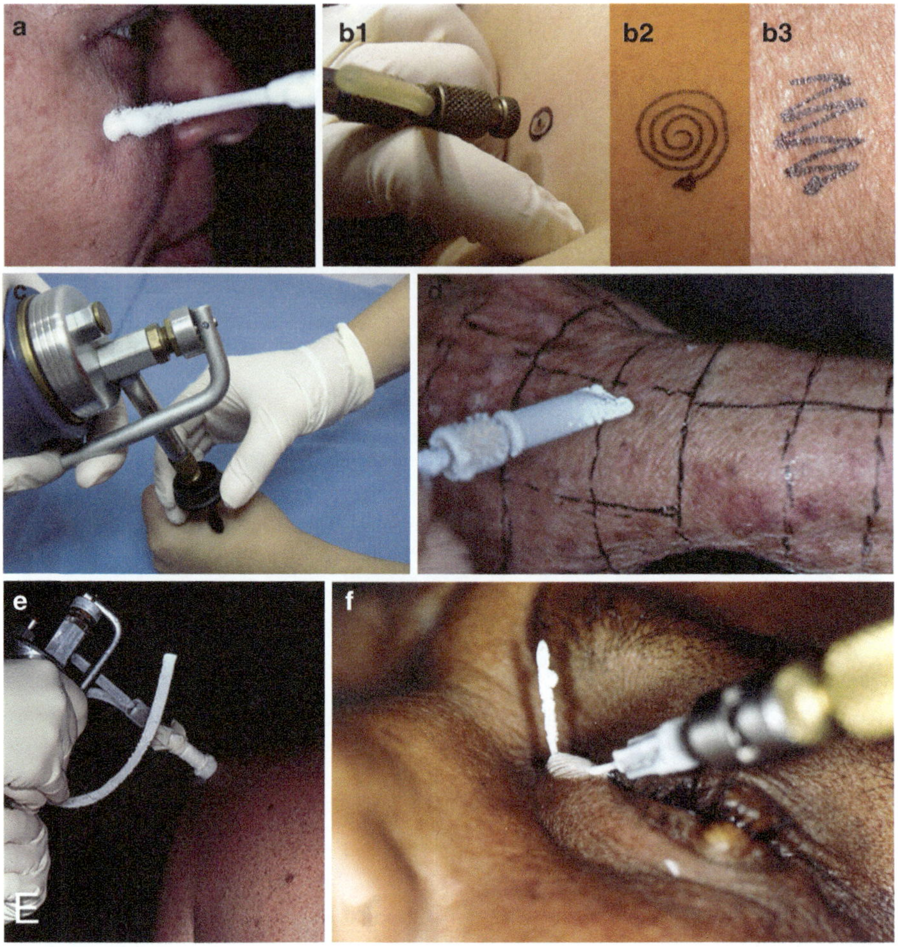

Fig. 10.2 Cryosurgery techniques: (**a**) dipstick; (**b**1) open spray, solid central pattern; (**b**2) open spray, spiral pattern; (**b**3) open spray, paint brush pattern; (**c**) cone-spray technique; (**d**) cryopeeling, area specification for stage application; (**e**) cryoprobe technique; (**f**) intralesional technique

halo of ice forms around the lesion (Fig. 10.2a). The maximum freezing depth is of 2 or 3 mm with this technique, and it is only suitable for treating benign, relatively small, superficial lesions. This method has a disadvantage of necessitating separate allotments of cryogen for each patient because viruses are capable of surviving within liquid nitrogen and cross contaminating the storage of nitrogen [9, 15]. In routine clinical practice, the handheld liquid nitrogen spray/probe equipment is the most used. The open-spray technique is versatile, and commonly used methods are: a solid central spray that may be used on lesions smaller than 0.5 cm (Fig. 10.2b1); a spiral pattern that starts the treatment at the center of the lesion and moves spiraling outward and can be used for slightly larger lesions of 1–2 cm (Fig. 10.2b2); and a paint brush pattern that involves spraying starting from one side of the lesion and moving up and down across the lesion and is used for lesions greater than 2 cm (Fig. 10.2b3). A cone-spray technique involves the use of neoprene, polystyrene or metal cones, or metal cryochambers that are placed directly on the lesion, confining the spray of cryogen to a discrete area, and provides a deeper and faster freezing than the use of spray alone (Fig. 10.2c). They are useful for round, discrete lesions or for lesions close to vital structures that require protection. Cryopeeling uses open-spray technique with paint brush pattern of application, and the area to be treated is marked with multiple 3 × 5 cm rectangles, to avoid skipping or overlaying LN application, which is done by stages, with 1-min intervals, to avoid the freezing of the tip used and also to decrease the pain caused by the application (Fig. 10.2d) [3, 4]. Cryoprobes use a probe tip that is cooled by circulating cryogen and applied directly to the lesion (Fig. 10.2e). Various types of cryoprobes are available in a variety of sizes and shapes, and the choice of probe depends on the type and site of the lesion [9, 26]. It is useful when pressure on the lesion is required such as vascular lesion and keloid.

10.7 Patient Selection

When selecting the patient and planning the treatment, it is crucial to: evaluate if the treatment objective is aesthetical or to heal a disease; evaluate the patient's expectation; discuss if the goal is improvement or healing and the necessity of multiple sessions; evaluate contraindications, side effects, and complications; evaluate the Fitzpatrick skin type of the patients and their ethnic origin; diagnostic tests should include skin biopsy to confirm the diagnosis and the type of lesion and determine the depth of freezing; evaluate the necessity of preoperative topical treatment; run previous test in the anatomic region of the lesion; treat extensive lesions stage by stage; and in some situations, it is better to submit the patients to multiple sessions to avoid excessive freezing and causing an unaesthetic scar.

10.8 Contraindications

Cryosurgery is contraindicated in patients with intercurrent illnesses such as cold urticaria, cold intolerance, cryofibrinogenemia, cryoglobulinemia, Raynaud's disease, pyoderma gangrenosum, collagen and autoimmune disease, agammaglobulinemia, and poorly controlled diabetes [5, 18, 28].

Deep freezing is not recommended for lesions at the corner of the mouth and the vermilion border, because occasional permanent cryosurgical complications like retraction and hypopigmentation can be expected [2].

Caution is advised in the choice of the surgical method for dark-skinned patients, for lesions that overlie nerves, and for lesion in the pretibial region where wound healing may be slow.

10.9 Patient Education

The cryosurgeon should explain to the patient, before the procedure to be undertaken, the risk involved and what to expect during cryosurgery and the postoperative period. An advice sheet on cryosurgery that outlines expected problems and their symptomatic treatment must be given to the patient.

Patient should be informed that cryosurgery does produce discomfort that will persist for several minutes and sometimes up to 20 min after the procedure, and the physicians should be aware that in some cases the discomfort can cause vasovagal reactions.

Before choosing cryosurgery as the method of choice, some factors should be considered, such as the lesion depth, location, quantity of lesions, Fitzpatrick skin type, ethnic origin, cosmetic and functional results, and explaining to the patients the uncomfortable situations that may occur in some locations [9].

10.10 Procedure Technique

In the cosmetic cryosurgery, it is fundamental to respect the basic concept of Zacarian SA for cryosurgery in benign lesions: "it is always better to hypofreeze than to hyperfreeze, because the first can be retreated, avoiding definite inaesthetical scars" [32]. For the treatment of benign lesions, freezing is more superficial than that of malignant lesions, not requiring previous biopsy and freezing depth monitoring. The previous application of local anesthetic depends on the size of the lesion, its location, and the patient's sensitivity to pain.

The freezing time varies, according to the characteristics of the lesion and the applying technique used. The open-spray technique is the most used. The cone-spray and solid contact (probe) are indicated when deeper freezing is necessary. In general, the freezing side margin ranges from 1 to 2 mm, except for keloids, which should not exceed the lesion limit.

The extensive lesions should be treated stage by stage, such as keloid and hemangioma. It is better to treat stage by stage to avoid excessive freezing and cause an unaesthetic definite scar (Table 10.1).

10.10.1 Idiopathic Guttate Hypomelanosis (IGH)

It is a common, unaesthetic, acquired leukodermic dermatosis of unknown cause, consisting of small 2- to 8-mm achromic or hypopigmented macules, without scale or atrophy, mainly affecting the exposed areas of the upper and lower extremities. The condition is observed in persons of both sexes, and the number of lesions tends to increase with age and after excessive sun exposure. Aging, actinic damage, and genetic factors have been proposed as possible etiologic agents [21]. Studies have shown that significantly fewer dopa-positive melanocytes are present in the white macules of IGH than in normal skin, and by electron microscopy, the melanocytes

Table 10.1 Suggested treatment regime for principal unaesthetic dermatological lesion

Lesion	Technique, tip	Time, no. FTC	Margin	Session, intervals	Response
Idiopathic guttate hypomelanosis	OS, D, or E	2–5 s, ×1	1 mm	4–6 weekly intervals According to response	Good
Solar lentigo	OS, C, D, or E	5–10 s, ×1	1 mm	Usually single	Good
Labial lentiginous macules	OS, C, or D	2–3 s, ×2	1 mm	Usually single	Good to excellent
Venous lake	P, probe	10 s, ×2	1–2 mm	Usually single	Good
Hemangioma/ hemolymphangioma	P, probe	5–30 s, ×2	1–2 mm	2–4 at 8 weekly intervals	Good to excellent
Acne cyst	OS Adjunct	5–15 s, ×1	1–2 mm	Usually single	Good
Inflammatory acne	OS, C, or D Adjunct	2–5 s, ×1	1 mm	Usually single	Good
Seborrheic keratosis	OS, C Alone Adjunct with curettage	10–15 s, ×1	1 mm	Usually single	Good to excellent
Keloid	P, OS, cone-S, B, or A	15–30 s, ×2	0 mm	1-month intervals, usually multiple	Variable
Actinic keratoses	OS, B	5–30 s, ×1–2	2–4 mm	Usually single	Good to excellent
Sun-damaged skin[a]	OS, A, acne tip, cryopeeling tips, alone, and adjunct with cryopeeling	×1	Adjoining sun-damaged areas	Usually single	Good

P cryoprobe technique, *OS* open-spray technique, *cone-S* cone-spray technique, *FTC* freeze-thaw cycle
[a]Sun-damaged skin: actinic keratoses, solar lentigo, solar elastosis, fine wrinkles of solar aging

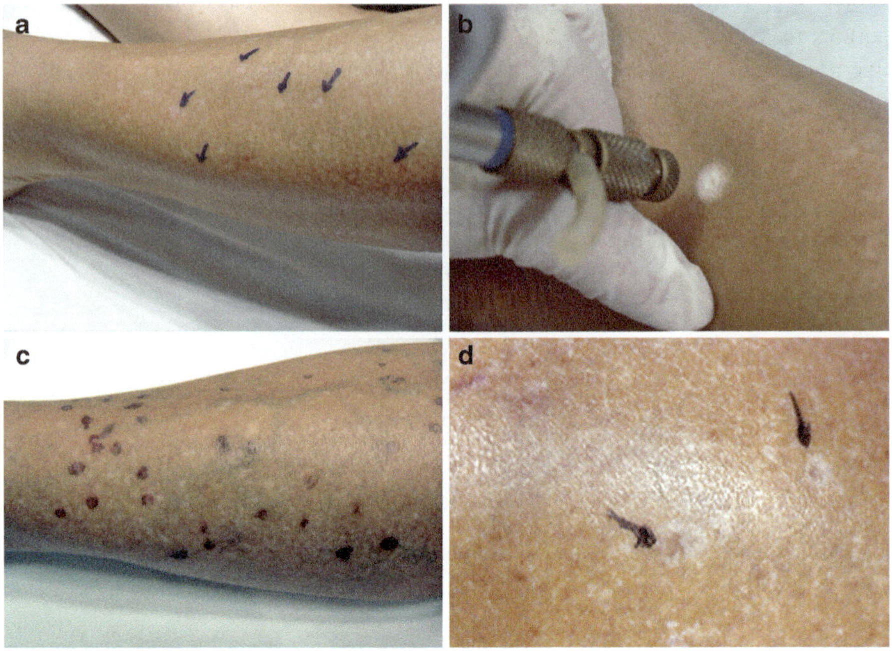

Fig. 10.3 Idiopathic guttate hypomelanosis: (**a**) IGH in lower extremity; (**b**) open-spray technique, back vent adapter with open tip E, 1-mm margin; (**c**) crusting and desquamation of lesion after 10–14 days; (**d**) repigmentation within the lesions 4 weeks after the cryosurgery

in the lesional skin were round and less dendritic with fewer melanosomes than in normal pigment cells [21].

Modality of treatments with a desirable result is limited [21]. The treatment of IGH by localized superficial dermabrasion with good results is reported [10]. This method is recommended in lesions up to 5 mm diameter, because larger lesions prevent melanocyte migration. Cryosurgery is the most used therapeutic option and most successful in repigmenting the IGH, but some patients may not respond to the treatment (Fig. 10.3a). In lesions treated by cryosurgery, the number of dopa-positive melanocytes was significantly greater in repigmented areas than in untreated lesions, but less than in normal skin [21]. Liquid nitrogen is applied with open-spray method, small open tips d, e, and f connected to back vent adapter, a single freeze-thaw cycle, for 2–5 s, with 1-mm margin. Topical or infiltrative anesthesia is not necessary. Liquid nitrogen gives the lesion a snow-white color (Fig. 10.3b). Erythema and discrete edema without vesicle formation occur immediately and evolve with crusting, and the lesion starts to desquamate in 10–14 days (Fig. 10.3c). In this moment, the sun exposure helps the melanocytes' migration to the healing area, favoring repigmentation. Repigmentation was first noted about 4 weeks after cryosurgery and became complete 6 to 8 weeks after treatment (Fig. 10.3d).

As the treatment results may be partial, the application of the cryosurgery in few lesions to evaluate the patient's response is recommended. In some cases, hyperpigmentation of the lesions is observed after sun exposure, or in patients with IV or higher Fitzpatrick skin type, sun filters and topical treatment are used.

10.10.2 Solar Lentigo

Solar lentigines are pigmented macules that appear on sun-exposed skin and are common on the dorsa of the hands, the forearms, and the face. Chronic sun exposure is important in the pathogenesis of the solar lentigo. Histopathologically, they are characterized by numbers of melanocytes, and their melanin contents in dermoepidermal junction increased. Neither pigment incontinence nor cellular abnormalities are found [22]. On the lentiginous lesions, the topical pretreatment with tretinoin, mequinol, hydroquinone, and glycolic acid improves the final cosmetic result [7].

Cryosurgery is a widely used technique to remove solar lentigo, either applied with dipstick method or more commonly with a small handheld spray unit. The aesthetic results are evaluated with a previous test in some lesions [27]. A single freeze-thaw cycle, for 5–10 s, and 1-mm margin are usually sufficient. Topical or infiltrative anesthesia is not necessary. The principle of the treatment is tissue injury by freezing, and melanocytes are especially vulnerable to cold injury. Temporary adverse effects that are commonly observed include local pain during the treatment or shortly after treatment, bulla, and local edema. More permanent side effects are lesional hypopigmentation and/or peripheral hyperpigmentation.

One study reported a recurrence rate of 55 % at 6 months, and topical therapy can also be considered as maintenance therapy to diminish the risk of relapse [20]. Cryosurgery shows better results than TCA 33 % solution in the treatment of solar lentigo particularly in lower Fitzpatrick skin types, and post-inflammatory hyperpigmentation is the major complication of each type of treatment in darker Fitzpatrick skin types [22]. Localized dermabrasion is an efficacious therapeutic alternative for solar lentigo at the back of the hands. Its result is comparable to cryotherapy, and the recurrence rate was the same with both treatments (55 %) [11]. A novel and effective procedure for treatment of light-colored solar lentigo was reported: a combination of cryosurgery plus alexandrite laser, which produced substantial lightening of the whole lentigo after a period between 3 months and 10 months. No adverse effects were detected during the treatment and after 1 year of follow-up [30].

10.10.3 Oral Lesions (Labial Lentiginous Macules and Venous Lake)

Cryosurgery is a very useful technique for treatment of oral lesions because of the characteristics of the oral mucosa. This area is humid and smooth, and it is an ideal site for freezing [13, 14, 25]. It shows a very good aesthetic result and it may be either the first choice or an alternative option to conventional surgery, mainly for benign and premalignant lesions of the oral mucosa [13, 14]. For this procedure, we require good illumination with a fluorescent lamp, so that heat is not created and thaw time is not accelerated, not allowing an adequate cryosurgery. A powerful vacuum cleaner is also required to dissipate the vapors that are formed during the freezing and which cover a clear view of the surgery area when de open-spray or cone-spray techniques are used [29].

The main indications of cryosurgery of benign lesions in the oral mucosa are labial lentiginous macules, venous, angioma, lymphangioma, pyogenic granuloma, mucous cyst, fibroma, and HPV lesions in human immunodeficiency virus (HIV) and non-HIV patients [14, 27, 29]. For precancerous lesions, it can be used in actinic cheilitis, leukoplakia, lichen planus, nicotinic stomatitis, and prostatic hyperplasia [14, 29].

Association of other techniques, such as shaving or eletrosection, can reduce the size of lesion before cryosurgery allowing greater efficacy and can obtain a specimen for histopathologic examination. Cryosurgery can be performed on the lips and on the anterior region of the mouth with or without local anesthesia. The number of freeze-thaw cycle needed depends on the size and nature of the lesion. Open spray and cone-spray are useful for lips and the anterior region of the mouth, while cryoprobes are preferred for deeper lesions and for those with liquid content. There is a risk of ventilatory impairment when performed on the base of the tongue, posterior wall of the larynx, and tonsils. It is necessary to protect the openings of the salivary glands, and the Wharton and Stensen ducts [29].

10.10.3.1 Labial Lentiginous Macules (LLM)

Clinically, it is usually situated on the lower lip and it appears as a roundish, well-circumscribed, light-brown macule. Labial lentiginous macule is frequent in young women, and it presents in histology an increase of melanin in the basal layer, such as freckles. The dermoscopic features of the LLM are rather characteristic, revealing diffuse pigmentation with a peculiar parallel pattern of partially linear and partially curvilinear light-brown to dark-brown streaks, and melanoma-specific criteria have not been found in this benign lesion. The liquid nitrogen spray with C, D, or E open tips, double freeze-thaw cycle with 1-mm margin, and usually a single session is applied with good to excellent result [6].

10.10.3.2 Venous Lake

Some physicians do not consider venous lakes to be true hemangioma but rather simple venous dilatations, and clinically it is a red-blue to black cystic dilatations situated on the lower lip and on the ears. It is usual in the elderly, and it is probably triggered by minimum repetitive trauma. The cryosurgery offers good cosmetic result for its treatment, and a cryoprobe technique is used, and usually no anesthesia is required [26]. A flat or round probe is selected with a diameter either of the same size or slightly smaller than the lesion to be treated. The probe is prechilled and is applied with firm pressure to the center of the lesion to squeeze out the blood content. Freezing is continued until a 1- to 2-mm margin is seen to the outside of the lesion, and at that time the probe is removed. After 3–4 min of total thawing of the lesion, a second freeze-thaw cycle is effectuated. When the venous lake is located on the lips, the ice front should not be allowed to extend beyond the vermilion border as this can result in scar distortion of the site. Venous lake has small size and heals without undue complication or morbidity and it may require 3 to 4 weeks, and sometimes a second session is necessary. When working around the mouth, edema and salivation can occur for several days.

10.10.4 Hemangioma/Hemolymphangioma

The vascular tissue is very sensitive to the cold. Cryosurgery is effective in the hypertrophic vascular lesions, and it is resistant in the plain hemangioma. In the treatment of superficial hemangiomas, a pressure probe is used to empty the lesion and reduce the vascularization, and one freeze-thaw cycle is enough. In the hemangiomas with superficial and deep components, a combination of steroid intralesional infiltration and local anesthesia in the deep part of the hemangioma and freezing of the superficial part can be used [2]. Depending on the location of the hemangioma and on the suspicion of mixed malformations, the patient must go through a complete evaluation including image exams such as color Doppler, selective arteriography and computed tomography to determine the extension of the lesion and the diameter of the vases to avoid damage in deep vessels [2]. In lymphangioma, the process is identical with similar results to hemangiomas [2].

10.10.5 Acne Cyst/Inflammatory Acne

Cryosurgery is a useful adjunctive modality in the management of acne lesions including papules, pustules, and cysts. In the past decade, full-face cryopeeling was effectuated using dry-ice slush made by mixing carbon dioxide, acetone, and sulfur; it was applied with a gauze ball for superficial exfoliation of the epidermis on inflammatory acne treatment [8, 16]. Advances in other systemic and topical therapies of acne have declined the use of cryotherapy, but freezing can continue to find a place in its treatment [28]. For papules and pustules, a light spray of liquid nitrogen for 2–5 s is used until the lesion is slightly blanched white with 1-mm margin. Some firm cysts are best treated by intralesional steroids, but soft fluctuant cysts or cysts covered by eschar can be treated by spraying liquid nitrogen for 5–10 s, 1- to 2-mm margin, until blanching indicates the end point of treatment. For resistant or recalcitrant cysts, particularly those on the back, a longer freeze, of 10–15 s, is necessary.

Cryosurgery also is useful in treating certain patients taking isotretinoin, with pyogenic granuloma-type lesion.

10.10.6 Seborrheic Keratoses

This benign tumor is often accepted as normal change of aging. It is more common after 50 years of age, and single lesions occur but they may be multiple and sometimes familial. The lesions usually are numerous and located on face, neck, trunk, and upper limb; its colors are gray, yellow, brown, or black, but it may be varied and the size varies from 1 mm to many centimeters. The surface of the lesions is usually rough or crumbly and occasionally may have a shiny surface. All seborrheic keratoses begin as flat lesions but most become raised at an early stage. The diagnosis is clinical but they can be confused with other flat pigmented lesions, and when there is doubt with cutaneous melanoma or dysplastic nevus, the histopathologic exam is absolutely indispensable. The dermoscopy is useful in the differentiation of other pigmented lesions by the presence of horn pseudocysts and comedo-like openings. The horn pseudocysts correspond to intraepidermal horn globules and represent a common histopathologic finding in acanthotic seborrheic keratoses, but sometimes it is present also in papillomatous dermal nevi (Unna nevi), and very rarely a few of its structures are observed in melanomas [1]. The thickness and number of lesions help determine the techniques used. Flat and multiple lesions can be treated by application of open spray of short duration, with C open tip, for 5 s, with a frost halo of 1–2 mm. For thicker lesions, an alternative technique is frequently used because when treated by a spray alone, prolonged spraying time is necessary, with B open tip, for 5–30 s, which demands more experience to assess proper depth of freeze and also causes more surrounding hyperpigmentation on healing [28]. The thicker lesion is sprayed superficially just enough to make the raised portion firm but not solidly frozen; then, a lesion is curetted and a hemostatic solution is applied to the surface [28]. Topical or infiltrative anesthesia is not necessary. The cryosurgery on seborrheic keratoses can be treated in a single visit, and good to excellent cosmetic results are usually obtained.

10.10.7 Keloid

Keloids are fibrotic tumors characterized by a collection of atypical fibroblasts with excessive deposition of extracellular matrix components, especially collagen, fibronectin, elastin, and proteoglycans. It responds variably to cryosurgery, and the resistance to cold of fibroblasts and collagen has been blamed for the difficulty in its treatment. Keloidal scars are abnormal healing responses to injury, and there are several modalities to treat these lesions, but there is not a definite treatment yet. Combination therapies tend to give better results. It can be done with cryosurgery, lasers, shaving, excision surgery, or intralesional steroid injections. The rationale for cryosurgery is that the ischemic damage induced by this intervention will lead to necrosis and a reduction in tumor bulk and pigmentary disturbance occur after the healing (Fig. 10.4a–d) [13, 24]. This treatment modality has been used both as monotherapy and in combination with intralesional steroid or preliminary surgical excision. The cryosurgery is an excellent adjunctive therapy for the treatment of hypertrophic scars and keloids when used before intralesional steroid injection increasing favorable results. Usually, a small lesion can be frozen solid and most young keloids respond well; however, multiple treatments are required. Preliminary excision of the bulk of the keloid on the large lesion reduces its size and improves the efficiency of the cryosurgery [12, 13]. Two freeze-thaw cycles are recommended for

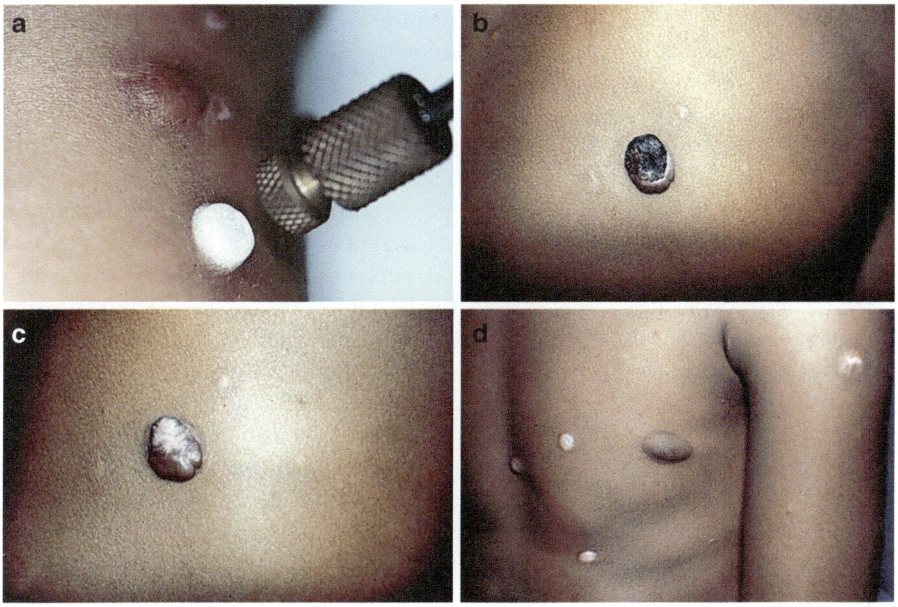

Fig. 10.4 Keloid after chickenpox: (**a**) open-spray technique – side freezing margin should not pass the lesion limit, (**b**) circumscribed necrosis 2 weeks after cryosurgery, (**c**) keloid healed after 4 weeks, (**d**) pigmentary disturbance after the healing

cellular destruction, and the application technique used depends on the format of the lesion. It may be done with a spray, cone-spray, or probes. One freeze-thaw cycle is used to cause the edema and to facilitate the steroid intralesional infiltration [12]. The interval between the cryosurgery sessions is usually 30 days, when the lesion cicatrization occurs. Cryosurgery may produce flattening, but the recurrence rate is not known and there is a high risk of side effects, especially hypopigmentation.

10.10.8 Actinic Keratoses, Sun-Damaged Skin: Cryopeeling

Cryosurgery is an excellent modality for the treatment of actinic keratoses because multiple lesions in any area can be treated and it is rapid and relatively free of complication [9, 18]. The open-spray technique is effective, and the freeze time varies with the type and thickness of the specific lesion. A 2- to 4-mm margin of freeze around the keratoses is adequate, and usually one treatment session is sufficient and various spray patterns are effective [9, 18]. An intermittent spray of 5–7 s is used for small, flat lesions, while hypertrophic keratoses may need freeze times of 20–30 s. Pretreatment with emollients may shorten the freeze time by thinning the keratoses [9]. For a larger lesion, a paintbrush pattern is used, while smaller lesions are treated using the intermittent technique that avoids excessive lateral spreading of the freeze [9].

Cryopeeling is an effective method of treating large areas of actinic keratoses and sun-damaged skin (actinic keratoses, solar lentigo, solar elastosis, sebaceous hyperplasia, fine wrinkles of solar aging), because it not only resolves visible actinic keratoses but also destroys smaller keratoses and lentigines. Sebaceous hyperplasia has a good result and requires a single 5-s freeze time for this lesion to disappear. In cryopeeling, liquid nitrogen is applied directly over the skin, causing exfoliation. It accelerates the epidermis change and eliminates the superficial lesions, stimulating its renewal and making it soft and strong. The skin of the face, hands, arms or bald head is cleaned with chemical antibacterial, applying topical anesthesia in the area to be treated or local anesthesia on the actinic keratoses that are treated individually. The spray technique is used in a paint brush pattern and with specific tips described on the accessories topic. The area to be treated is marked with multiple 3 cm × 5 cm rectangles to avoid skipping or overlaying LN application, which is done stage by stage, with 1-min intervals to avoid freezing the tip used and to decrease the pain caused by the application [3, 4]. Healing is usually completed within 10–14 days. The skin is left smoother, pinker, and tighter [26]. The compared results of recurrence after 1 and 3 years between cryopeeling, 5-fluorouracil, and trichloroacetic acid in discrete or advanced actinic keratoses, with melanosis and wrinkles, showed that cryopeeling had less recurrence [4].

10.11 Advantages/Disadvantages

Among different surgical options, the cryosurgery is extremely competitive with other techniques because it is suitable for office, home nursing, or outpatient facility; it has low cost, efficacy, and no restriction of work or sports; it is useful in pregnancy; and it has excellent aesthetic results [2, 18]. Other advantages of this method are less preoperative and operative time than other techniques, safe and relatively simple procedure, and many lesions can be treated at one time. For the patient, local anesthesia is optional, pain is tolerable (except for children), there is no suture to remove, and wound care is simple.

For the physician, the disadvantages of cryosurgery are minimal because with proper training, its easy delivery allows treatment of common skin diseases, the equipment cost is not expensive, and arranging for delivery and storage of liquid nitrogen is not difficult.

10.12 Postprocedure Course

Patients should be aware, before procedure, of all possible secondary effects of the cryosurgery, and time should be taken to explain the postoperative care, and printed postoperative instruction should be given to patients [2]. The postoperative care is very important because it is the time when there is an increased risk of secondary bacterial infection.

Postoperative care varies according to the lesion, location, and depth of freeze. After freezing, the tissue responds in a predictable manner that leads to healing of the wound by secondary intention [18]. The reaction immediately after freezing includes erythema and urtication, followed by edema which occurs within a few minutes, and the edema may last for several days. This is followed by serous or hemorrhagic exudate and formation of vesicle or bulla after superficial cryosurgery and a gelatinous exudate in the case of deeper treatments, with superficial to deep eschar formation [9].

Most benign lesions require little or no aftercare; care is limited to washing with soap and water with applications of hydrogen peroxide solution. For more complex lesions or malignant lesions, frequent washing of the wound with soap and water and dry gauze dressing are required during the exudative stage. The wound begins to dry between 3 and 10 days after freezing. Then, eschar develops and the patient should keep the area clean and antibiotic ointment is required. The use of systemic antibiotics is reserved for excessive erythema or pus. The cryosurgeon will carry out weekly wound debridement by curettage, and when the wound has been freed of any eschar and as appropriate granulation tissue, the use of hydrophilic pads will accelerate healing [2]. It is related, as an exception, that it is not recommended to remove those eschar formed in neovascularized tumors where removal of the crust could result in bleeding and keloids and where removal of crust can stimulate further fibroblast activity and growth of the keloid [2].

Benign and premalignant lesions usually heal between 2 and 4 weeks [18]. For the healing of a superficially sprayed lesion on the face, one could expect 1 week of postoperative time; for a probe-treated area on the face, it can take 3–4 weeks, and for a same lesion treated with the same technique on the legs, healing can take 2–3 months. Malignant lesions on the face, ears, and neck generally heal between 4 and 6 weeks, and large tumors and those on the trunk and extremities take longer to heal, sometimes up to 14 weeks [18].

After healing, the treated area can look erythematous and this redness can last weeks, and the patient should be advised to use sun protection to avoid hyperpigmentation. Once the redness has disappeared, a hypopigmented area may remain. In benign lesions, this hypopigmentation will last a few weeks and then improve, resulting in a normally pigmented skin. In deep freezing, this hypopigmentation can take years to repigment, while others can be left with a permanent hypopigmented area.

The cosmetic results can be evaluated 4–6 months after cryosurgery, and in some locations, it is often equal or superior to those achieved by other modalities.

10.13 Side Effects

The incidence of complications after cryosurgery is low. It is important to distinguish between side effects and normal and expected signs or symptoms of cutaneous cryosurgery because they represent the normal progression of the physiologic process of freezing tissue. The reaction immediately after freezing includes erythema and urtication, followed by edema which occurs within a few minutes, and the edema may last for several days [9]. This is followed by serous or hemorrhagic exudate and formation of vesicle or bulla after superficial cryosurgery and a gelatinous exudate in the case of deeper treatments, with superficial to deep eschar formation [9]. These effects are transient and usually subside within 1–2 weeks after treatment of benign lesions and within 4–6 weeks after treatment of malignant lesions.

The side effects and complications after cutaneous cryosurgery can be divided into acute, short-term and long-term reactions, and permanent effects [9, 28]. Acute reactions include edema, pain, hemorrhage, nitrogen gas insufflation, and syncope. Pain or a burning sensation is more pronounced during and immediately after treatment, and most discomfort diminishes within 30 min to 2 h. Short-term reactions include bulla formation, infection, delayed bleeding, pyogenic granuloma, and systemic reactions. Long-term reactions include pseudoepitheliomatous hyperplasia, nerve damage, and milia. Permanent effects include hypopigmentation, atrophy and depression, hyperpigmentation, hypertrophic scar, tissue defects (notching and perforation), scarring, and alopecia.

References

1. Argenziano G, Soyer HP, Giorgi V, Piccolo D, Carli P, Delfino M et al (2000) Dermoscopy: a tutorial. EDRA Medical Publishing & New Media, Milan
2. Castro-Ron G, Pasquali P (2005) Cryosurgery. In: Robinson JK, Hanke CW, Sengelmann RD, Siegel DM (eds) Surgery of the skin. Procedural dermatology. Elsevier Mosby, Philadelphia, pp 191–202
3. Chiarello SE (1992) Full-face cryo-(liquid nitrogen) peel. J Dermatol Surg Oncol 18: 329–332
4. Chiarello SE (2000) Cryopeeling (extensive cryosurgery) for treatment of actinic keratoses: an update and comparison. Dermatol Surg 26:728–732
5. Dawber R, Colver G, Jackson A (1992) Cutaneous cryosurgery. Principles and clinical practice. Martin Dunitz Ltd, London
6. Falabella R, Escobar C, Giraldo N, Rovetto P, Gil J, Barona MI et al (1987) On the pathogenesis of idiopathic guttate hypomelanosis. J Am Acad Dermatol 16(1):35–44
7. Farris PK (2004) Combination therapy for solar lentigines. J Drugs Dermatol 3(5):S23–S24
8. Graham GF (1982) Cryosurgery for acne. In: Epstein E, Epstein E Jr (eds) Skin surgery, 5th edn. Charles C. Thomas Publisher, Springfield
9. Grahan GF, Barham KL (2003) Cryosurgery. Curr Probl Dermatol 15:225–250
10. Hexel DM (2001) Treatment of idiopathic guttate hypomelanosis by localized superficial dermabrasion. Dermatol Surg 25:917–918
11. Hexsel DM, Mazzuco R, Bohn J, Borges J, Gobbato DO (2000) Clinical comparative study between cryotherapy and local dermabrasion for the treatment of solar lentigo on the back of the hands. Dermatol Surg 26:457–462
12. Ishida CE (2003) Tratamento das Cicatrizes Hipertróficas e Quelóides. In: Kede MPV, Sabatovich O (eds) Dermatologia Estética. Editora Atheneu, São Paulo, pp 601–607
13. Ishida CE (2009) Criocirurgia. In: Ramos-e-Silva M, Castro MCR (eds) Fundamentos de Dermatologia. Editora Atheneu, Rio de Janeiro, pp 2189–2208
14. Ishida CE, Ramos-e-Silva M (1998) Cryosurgery in oral lesions. Int J Dermatol 37:283–285

15. Jones SK, Darville JM (1989) Transmission of virus particles by cryotherapy and multi-use caustic pencils: a problem to dermatologists? Br J Dermatol 121:481–486
16. Karp F, Nieman H, Lerner C (1939) Cryotherapy for acne and its scars. Arch Dermatol 39:995–998
17. Kempiak SJ, Lee PW, Pelle MT (2009) Rhinophyma treated with cryosurgery. Dermatol Surg 35:543–545
18. Kuflik EG (1994) Cryosurgery updated. J Am Acad Dermatol 31:925–944
19. Kuflik EG, Gage AA, Lubritz RR, Graham GF (2000) History of dermatologic cryosurgery. Dermatol Surg 26:715–722
20. Ortonne JP, Pandya AG, Lui H, Hexsel D (2006) Treatment of solar lentigines. J Am Acad Dermatol 54:S262–S271
21. Ploysangam T, Dee-Ananlap S, Suvanprakorn P (1990) Treatment of idiopathic guttate hypomelanosis with liquid nitrogen: light and electron microscopic studies. J Am Acad Dermatol 23:681–684
22. Razziee M, Balighi K, Shabanzadeh-Dehkordi H, Robati RM (2008) Efficacy and safety of cryotherapy vs. trichloroacetic acid in the treatment of solar lentigo. J Eur Acad Dermatol Venereol 22:316–319
23. Reis CMS, Ishida CE (2002) Criocirurgia: Outras Indicações e Condições Especiais. In: Gadelha AR, Costa IMC (eds) Cirurgia Dermatológica em Consultório. Editora Atheneu, São Paulo, pp 495–517
24. Shaffer JJ, Taylor SC, Cook-Bolden F (2002) Keloidal scars: a review with a critical look at therapeutic options. J Am Acad Dermatol 46:S63–S97
25. Shepherd J, Dawber RPR (1982) The historical and scientific basis of cryosurgery. Clin Exp Dermatol 7:321–328
26. Sinclair RD, Tzermias C, Dawber R (1994) Cosmetic cryosurgery. In: Baran R, Maibach HI (eds) Cosmetic dermatology. Martin Dunitz Limited, London, pp 541–550
27. Thai KE, Sinclair RD (1999) Cryosurgery of benign skin lesions. Australas J Dermatol 40: 175–186
28. Torre D, Lubritz R, Kuflik E (1988) Practical cutaneous cryosurgery. Appleton & Lange, Connecticut
29. Turjansky E, Stolar E (1995) Lesiones de Piel y Mucosas. Técnicas Terapeúticas. Edama – Editorial Asociación Médica Argentina, Buenos Aires
30. Vano-Galvan S, Matarredona J, Harto A, Escudero A, Pascual JC, Jaén P (2009) Treatment of light-coloured solar lentigines with cryosurgery plus alexandrite laser. J Eur Acad Dermatol Venereol 23:850–852
31. Weshahy AH (1993) Intralesional cryosurgery. A new technique using cryoneedles. J Dermatol Surg Oncol 19:123–126
32. Zacarian SA (1985) Cryosurgery for skin cancer and cutaneous disorders. CV Mosby, St Louis

Electrosurgery

11

Sarita Martins de Carvalho Bezerra
and Marcio Martins Lobo Jardim

Core Messages

- Never use flammable antiseptic solution.
- Prefer infiltrative instead topical anesthesia.
- Always clean the electrode tip during the procedure.
- Always plan what to do before start the procedure.
- Mask should be used always by all staff.

11.1 Introduction

ELECTROSURGERY is a general term used to encompass all surgical methods that use electricity [5]. It is a procedure by which tissue is removed or destroyed by the use of an electrical energy current. These currents may be generated by spark gap, radio tube, transistorized or battery-operated electrosurgical equipment [9].

Electrosurgery has been used by dermatologists for well over 80 years. The advantages of this technique, although well known to dermatologists, are less appreciated by other physicians. Electrosurgery is not time-consuming and is ideally suited to outpatient clinical practices of dermatology. It requires few instruments, and patient acceptance of the procedure is high. When used in properly selected cases, it yields acceptable to excellent cosmetic results for both benign and malignant lesions. Over the years, devices for electrosurgical treatment have become increasingly sophisticated [4, 9].

S. Martins C. Bezerra, M.D., Ph.D.
Associated Professor of Dermatology at CEDER - Centro de Estudos Dermatológicos do Recife, 187, Ernesto de Paula Santos, St. - Room 301, 51011-330 Boa Viagem, Recife, PE, Brazil
e-mail: samacabe@gmail.com

M.M.L. Jardim
Medical Student, Av. Beira Mar, 792/301 Piedade Jaboatão dos Guararapes Pernambuco, 54400-010, Brazil

A. Tosti, D. Hexsel (eds.), *Update in Cosmetic Dermatology*,
DOI 10.1007/978-3-642-34029-1_11, © Springer-Verlag Berlin Heidelberg 2013

11.2 Mechanism of Action

To optimize the use of an electrosurgical device, the clinician should have some understanding of how the equipment functions. The circuitries of all electrosurgical instruments share certain design features necessary for production and require suitable electrical outputs for electrosurgery.

Standard household currents first pass through a transformer, which alters the voltage, thereby providing the levels and characteristics required for the instrument's various circuit functions. The current next travels through an oscillating circuit, which increases its frequency. Finally, it is delivered to the treatment electrode [4].

The current may be applied to the patient either mono- or biterminally. Biterminal electrosurgery methods employ large dispersive electrode grounding means and connect the patient to the electrosurgical apparatus via an active treatment needle electrode. The patient is thus incorporated into and is an integral part of the circuit. In monoterminal electrosurgery, the patient is not a part of the circuit, and there is no ground to the apparatus. The electrons are shed from the patient to the air, table, and floor [2].

11.3 History of Use

Medical practitioners have used heat to destroy tissue for centuries. In ancient times, hot cautery was used by the Egyptians and Greeks to treat tumors and abscesses and to stop bleeding [5]. However, the use of electrically generated heat destruction did not occur until the mid-ninth century when electrical physics advanced to the level of practical application. Claude Paquelin developed the use of electrocautery in 1875. This new modality was similar to the old form of hot cautery (in which a hot tip is brought directly in contact with tissue to burn the tissue without passing any current through it) except that it generated heat electrically [5, 13]. The real beginnings of modern electrosurgery occurred with the recognition and development of high-frequency alternating currents. In 1891, Jacques Arsene d'Arsonval developed the circuitry for generating high-frequency electricity. He found that high-frequency currents above 10,000 cycles per second (10,000 Hz) could pass through the body without pain, muscle contraction, or any other obvious harm to the body [4, 5, 8, 12].

In 1893, Oudin designed a resonated circuit with a balance between capacitive and inductive resistance. This allowed for a maximum amount of current flow by minimizing the amount of circuit resistance. Oudin used the resonated gap generator to destroy various skin lesions. In 1908, Walter de Keating-Hart noted that high-frequency currents could spark from the electrode to the tissue in long sparks resembling lightning (fulgur). He used these long sparks to destroy skin cancers and thereby developed the modality of electrofulguration. In 1911, Clark used very high-voltage and low-amperage devices for monopolar tissue destruction. Currents applied directly to tissue produced marked desiccation in the area surrounding the electrical contact. Clark identified the modality as electrodesiccation [5, 8, 13]. In 1908, Doyen apparently was the first to develop a method for delivering lower-voltage, higher-current electrical energy to patients by placing a large indifferent or dispersive electrode under them. In 1926, William Bovie, a physicist, collaborated with Harvey Cushing, a neurosurgeon, to develop a high-frequency electrosurgical instrument that allowed for a variable amount of "damping" as well as variable voltage and current output. This instrument could coagulate vessels of many sizes with or without cutting tissue and was the direct predecessor of modern electrosurgical devices. The next major event in the development of electrosurgery came in 1923 when Dr. George A. Wyeth, a noted tumor surgeon, used electrosurgery for cutting tissues [8]. In 1932, the Bitcher Corporation introduced its spark gap-based Hyfrecator, which has become popular for office-based monoterminal and biterminal electrofulguration, electrodesiccation, and electrocoagulation. Currently, there are numerous commercially available electrosurgical devices [5].

11.4 Electrosurgical Modalities

Variations in voltage, amperage, frequency, and method of application give each of the electrosurgical modalities its unique qualities. Equally important, however, is the waveform of each current [3].

There are four different types of waveforms in electrosurgery. They include fully filtered (undamped wave), e.g., CUT (electrosection), suitable for cutting waveform with minimal coagulation; fully rectified (slightly damped wave), e.g., CUT AND COAGULATION (electrosection with coagulation), which cuts as well as coagulates simultaneously; partially rectified (moderately damped wave), e.g., COAGULATION, suitable for coagulation of bleeding vessels; and spark gap wave (markedly damped wave), e.g., FULGURATION, suitable for fulguration [4].

11.5 Clinical Applications of Electrosurgery [4]

Specific applications of the various electrosurgical modalities depend on the surgeon's preference and experience (Table 11.1).

11.5.1 Electrodesiccation

This is a very common method, used most often by dermatologists. Electrodesiccation is the process by which a monoterminal (one treatment) high-frequency electrosurgical electrode is held in contact with the tissue, resulting in fine sparks that are

Table 11.1 Indications of electrosurgery [4, 6]

Type of lesions	Examples
Benign lesions	Nevi, sebaceous hyperplasia, rhinophyma, acrochordon (skin tags), angiomas, angiofibroma, dermatofibroma, fibrous papula, keratoacanthoma, seborrheic keratosis, syringoma, venous lake, wart
Premalignant lesions	Actinic keratosis
Malignant lesions	Basal cell carcinoma (well-defined, small, superficial, primary, low-risk area)
Cosmetic lesions	Wrinkles

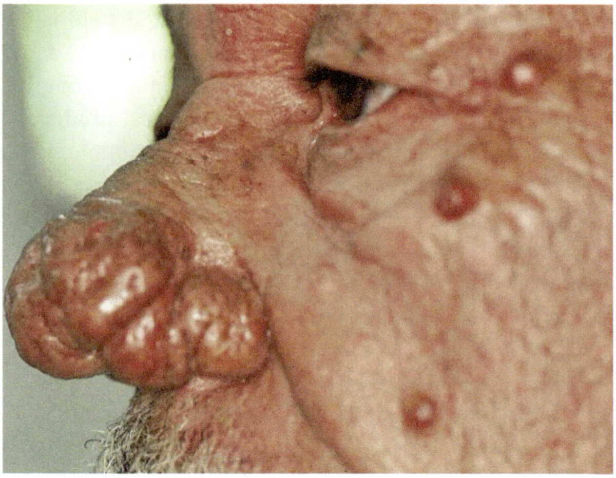

Fig. 11.1 Rhinophima before electrosection

absorbed by the tissue. This procedure causes thermal injury with less carbonization than the amount produced by electrofulguration [4, 5, 13].

Electrodesiccation is used for very superficial lesions, such as those affecting only the epidermis. The treatment electrode makes contacts with the tissue, resulting in dehydration and coagulation [13]. When using minimal power settings with electrodesiccation, most of the damage is epidermal, and there is minimal risk of scarring [3, 4]. However, at high power settings, there is coagulation of the deeper tissues and potential scarring. In practice, there is a combination of electrodesiccation and electrofulguration, because the electrode is not always in complete contact with the tissue, and thus, some degree of arcing occurs [13].

If the electrode is held at a slight distance from the tissue, a spark is formed between the electrode and the tissue. This technique, termed electrofulguration, achieves only very superficial destruction because the surface carbonization it produces insulates the underlying tissue from electrosurgical damage [3, 4]. Electrofulguration is the method of choice when only superficial tissue destruction is desired. For example, it can be used to treat seborrheic and actinic keratoses, spider angiomas, cherry angiomas, angiokeratomas, skin tags (Figs. 11.1 and 11.2), syringomata, warts, condylomata, and small epidermal nevus. Hemostasis of mild capillary bleeding can also be achieved using this type of current. A standard technique for treating keratoses by this method is to move the electrode slowly across the surface of the lesion (for small lesions) or to insert it directly into the lesion (for larger lesions), while applying the current at a low power setting. After a few seconds, the lesion bubbles as the epidermis separates from the underlying dermis. It can then be easily removed with a curette or simply by rubbing a piece of gauze across the treatment site. The clinical endpoint in treating epidermal lesions is punctate bleeding, which is controlled with pressure, by spot electrocoagulation or by topical hemostatic agents such as aluminum chloride. More profuse bleeding indicates probable damage to the dermis, with a greater likelihood of subsequent scarring. Extremely small superficial lesions can be treated by electrofulguration, which causes the least amount of damage to adjacent tissues [4].

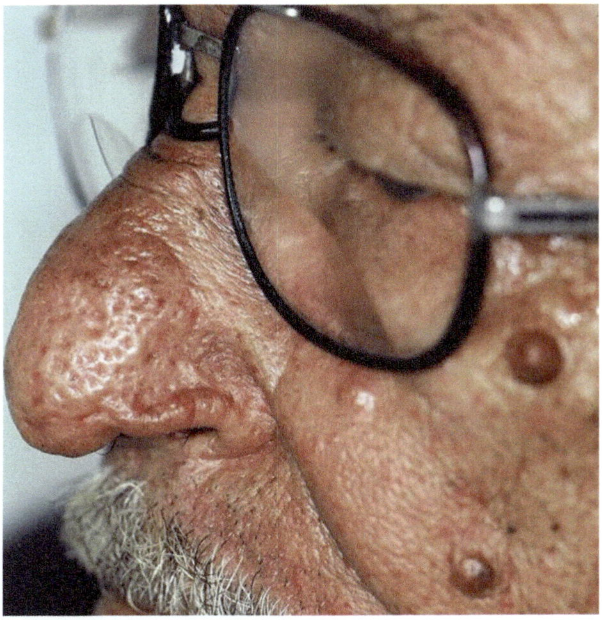

Fig. 11.2 Rhinophima after electrosection

11.5.2 Electrocoagulation

Electrocoagulation is the process by which a biterminal high-frequency, high-current electrosurgical electrode is placed on or near tissue, resulting in significant electrical current passing through the tissue, thereby thermally coagulating it [5].

It is particularly useful for deep and/or wide tissue destruction and surgical hemostasis (clamping of a bleeding point or blood vessel). A moderately damped current is applied in a biterminal manner; that is, both concentrative and dispersive electrodes are used. This current is of higher amperage and lower voltage than that used in electrodesiccation [4, 13].

The electrode is brought into direct contact with the tissue to be treated and is moved slowly across the lesion, which eventually becomes charred. A curette is then used to remove the charred tissue.

The principal use of electrocoagulation is in obtaining hemostasis of larger blood vessels. This method is also indicated to treat warts, superficial telangiectases, unwanted hair, pyogenic granulomas (Figs. 11.3 and 11.4), ingrown toenails, syringomata, xanthelasma, small hemangiomas, mucous cysts, ruby angiomas, sebaceous hyperplasia, seborrheic keratoses, trichoepitheliomas, and small and uncomplicated primary basal cell carcinomas on particular areas. To treat this last condition, the procedure should be repeated multiple times in an attempt to remove any small tumor extensions. During the last curettage, a small curette is often used to remove the final tiny "roots" of the tumor. Scaring is expected with this procedure and should be discussed with the patient [4, 9].

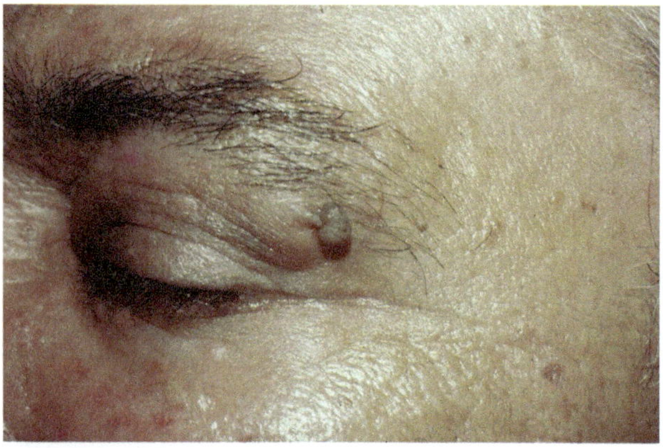

Fig. 11.3 Skin tag before electrocoagulation

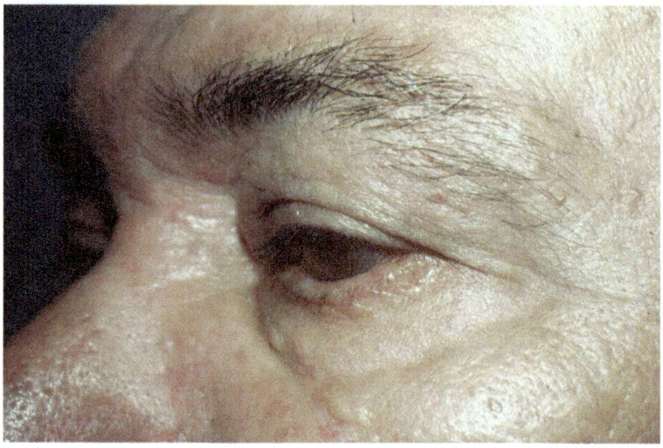

Fig. 11.4 Skin tags after electrocoagulation

While using electrocoagulation for surgical hemostasis, one must perform the procedure in a dry surgical field because if there is a barrier of blood, the electrical current is conducted through the blood and therefore distributed over a wider area of tissue. The coagulation effect is diminished or prevented through dispersion. Avoid high-power outputs whenever possible because there will be a large mass of coagulated and carbonized tissue, which may slough and cause delayed bleeding [13]. An alternative device for electrocoagulation is the biterminal forceps, on which both "poles" of the forceps are alternating active electrodes. The tissue between the two active electrodes receives very concentrated, high-current flow, and coagulation is thorough. Another alternative is the use of a clamp or forceps to hold the blood vessel while contact is made with the active electrode. This technique is not very useful for monoterminal devices, because the current is usually too low and too dispersed to generate sufficient heat for vessel coagulation. However, all too often, because of its deep penetrating, destructive ability, electrocoagulation causes inadvertent damage and necrosis of deeper adjacent tissue, which may affect wound healing and nerve function [5].

11.5.3 Electrofulguration

Electrofulguration is a process by which a monoterminal high-frequency electrosurgical electrode is held at a distance of 4–3 mm from the tissue surface, resulting in a coarse spark that crosses the electrode-skin gap and causes tissue damage and carbonization [1, 5].

The difference between electrofulguration and electrodessication is largely a matter of electrode position. The advantage of electrofulguration is that there is sufficient power to stop bleeding but less damage to the tissue than with direct contact electrodesiccation. It also may produce less scarring than electrodesiccation. High-amperage electrosurgical generators used primarily for coagulation do not produce sufficient voltage to deliver electrofulguration currents. Some units have a secondary coil added to the circuit to boost the current to a voltage level that is sufficient for bridging the air gap. Cutaneous lesions treated by this technique usually heal rapidly because there is a very little thermal damage. The arc need only span a very small distance. A common error in the application of fulguration is to turn the electrosurgical machine to a very high setting so that a large visible spark arcs across a great distance. The large amount of current applied using such a technique can produce excessive tissue damage, charring, and carbonization. Electrofulguration offers no advantage at high power settings [13]. The principal indications for using this current include the treatment of solar melanoses, actinic keratoses, seborrheic keratoses, and peeling.

11.5.4 Electrosection (Cutting)

Electrosection is a process by which a biterminal, high-frequency, high-current electrosurgical electrode is physically passed through tissue, cutting as it moves. It is used to incise, divide, or separate tissue [5].

Electrosection involves the biterminal application of a slightly damped current. The current is of low voltage and high amperage, causes minimal lateral heat spread and tissue damage, and has the additional advantage of simultaneously achieving hemostasis and cutting. "Pure" cutting can be obtained using a true undamped tube current, which provides the least amount of lateral heat spread and causes vaporization of tissue without hemostasis [4]. It can be used to perform rapid and effortless electrosurgical excisions or incisions without bleeding [4, 13, 14]. Virtually no manual pressure by the operator is required. With this method, one can achieve maximum power density with a minimal amount of current. The power density value increases as the radius of the curvature on the electrode decreases. The procedure can be performed with a variety of electrodes, the most common of which are thin wire loops. Blade-shaped electrodes are also available but tend to produce excessive thermal injury because of the greater power required and the greater surface area of the flat electrode. A wire loop electrode also produces greater thermal injury than a straight line wire electrode because of the increased electrical power required to produce cutting power density [5, 13, 14]. The difference between electrosection and scalpel excision is immediately apparent to first-time users of electrosection. At the appropriate power setting, the electrode passes smoothly through the tissue like a "hot knife through butter" [4]. The tissue should be hydrated during the procedure with a wet gauze. If perceptible sparking occurs during incision, the power setting is too high; if the electrode "drags," the power setting is too low [4].

The major advantage of electrosection over scalpel surgery is that hemostasis is achieved immediately as the incision is made. With large blood vessels (greater than 1 mm in diameter), additional spot electrocoagulation is required [4]. However, there can be greater tissue damage and slower healing with cutting current as compared to scalpel use. Wounds that have been created with a cutting current can often be closed initially, but the wound takes longer to achieve satisfactory tensile strength. It is recommended that one use this technique on wounds that are to be closed only if the cutting current is applied judiciously and with considerable skill. Excessive energy levels or a very slow cutting speed can produce overcoagulation, a wider band of tissue damage, and poorer wound healing. Cutting should be at a steady, brisk speed.

The optimal speed will cause clean separation with little or no charring. Charring produces better hemostasis but causes a larger zone of thermal damage. It is important to keep motion at a rate that incises the tissue adequately without resulting in a cooked or charred appearance. An optimal cutting rate is 5–10 mm/s [5, 13, 14]. Because a small amount of charred tissue may adhere to the cutting electrode, thereby interfering with cutting or coagulating action, the electrode should be cleaned regularly during the procedure. If char buildup seems excessive, the power may be too high or the cutting speed too slow [5].

Electrosurgery is extremely useful for achieving relatively bloodless excision on the head and large bulky lesions, using incisional and shave techniques, and to treat rhinophyma (Figs. 11.5 and 11.6), hydrosadenitis, some nevus, benign and malignant

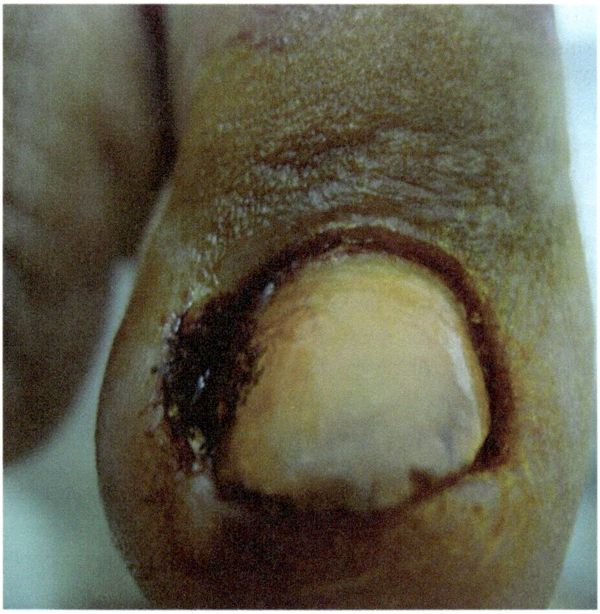

Fig. 11.5 Pyogenic granuloma before electrocoagulation

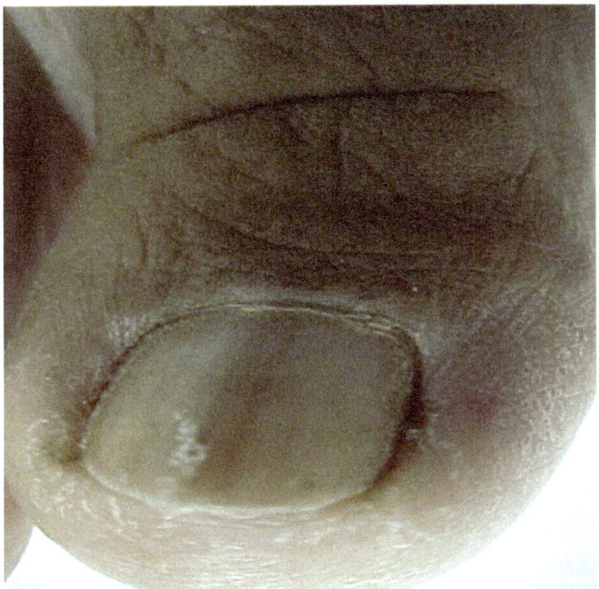

Fig. 11.6 Pyogenic granuloma after electrocoagulation

cutaneous tumor excision, skin biopsies, blepharoplasties, some tumors, scalp reductions, scalp flaps, scalp lifting, and all surgical defects allowed to heal by second intention [4, 5, 9, 11, 14, 16].

11.5.5 Direct-Current Surgical Galvanism

Few dermatologists have the equipment available for the production of a direct galvanic current. Galvanic surgery has very few useful applications in everyday practice. The most common use is in electrolysis. It is a process by which low-flow direct-current electricity is passed through tissue between two electrodes, resulting in tissue damage by a chemical reaction that occurs at the tip of one of the electrodes [5, 10, 13]. It is commonly used to destroy hair follicles (epilation or permanent hair removal). This method is quite effective and is associated with little pain and low risk of scarring. However, it is a time-consuming procedure that has largely been supplanted by the use of laser devices. Therefore, the indications for its use are very restrictive and it is recommended only when one wants to ablate an occasional hair follicle [5].

11.5.6 Electrocautery

Electrocautery is the use of a heat-producing electrode that does not transfer an electrical current. High-frequency equipment has largely replaced cautery today. Electrodesiccation can produce essentially the same results, but electrocautery can cause greater tissue damage and result in slower healing. It may be useful for treating patients who must avoid high-frequency current. One advantage of electrocautery is that it works on non-conductive tissues. High-frequency currents do not conduct to exposed cartilage, bone, or nails, but electrocautery produces its effect in these tissues quite well. Electrocautery can also be effective for use in a bloody surgical field [2, 6, 13].

Overall, this is an old technique that is rarely used anymore [10].

11.5.6.1 Electrodes

There are different types, shapes, and sizes of electrodes on the market. They are available sterile or nonsterile. The choice of electrode is dependent on the waveform and nature of the lesion. Tissue response varies greatly depending on the type of the electrode used. The larger electrodes produce more lateral heat and require higher power settings to operate.

The smaller electrodes produce less lateral heat and require lower power settings to operate [13].

Types

Fine needle electrode
Wire loop electrodes of different sizes
Ball electrode
Scalpel blade electrode
Diamond electrode
Ellipse electrode
Triangle electrode
Epilating needle
Bipolar forceps
Matricectomy electrodes

11.5.6.2 Factors Causing Less Collateral Heat Damage

Smaller electrode diameter
Shorter contact time between the electrode and the lesion
Lower power intensity
Higher frequency of current
Cutting waveform

11.6 Procedural Technique

Most electrosurgical procedures are painful and require the use of anesthesia to reduce or eliminate pain. Anesthesia may be applied topically (2.5 % lidocaine + 2.5 % prilocaine cream), or may be infiltrative or troncular (2 % lidocaine with or without epinephrine), as is used in electrosurgery [10]. We recommend the latter two because the patient should be very comfortable and relaxed during procedures.

Before the anesthesia is administered, the lesion and the surrounding skin should be cleansed with povidone-iodine or chlorhexidine solution (never alcohol due to potential ignition effects).

Electrosurgery should be performed with the patient in a comfortable seated or lying position on the operating table with the lesion exposed and illuminated [16]. The electrode should be kept clean and free of eschar.

Standard postoperative wound management, incorporating semiocclusive dressings, should follow procedures. Patients should be warned of the possibility of delayed bleeding and should be reassured that it can be controlled by 10–30 min of constant direct pressure over the wound. They should also be told that scaring may occur, but that is usually minimal [4]. Cosmetic results are usually excellent [5].

11.7 Risks

There are few risks to the patient from properly applied electrosurgery. However, potential hazards should be understood so they can be minimized. More emphasis is currently being placed on the potential risks to the surgeon and to operating room personnel.

11.8 Burns

Burns may result from the inadvertent contact of the electrode with the skin of the patient or the surgeon; however, the most common burn injury in electrosurgery occurs when there is inadequate contact between the patient and the dispersive electrode plate. Occasionally the patient or the surgeon may inadvertently touch a grounding element such as the metal on the treatment table, resulting in a burn or shock [5, 13].

11.8.1 Channeling

The so-called phenomenon of "channeling" is rarely a problem at the lower power setting used for most office-based cutaneous surgical practices. Channeling is always avoided by use of bipolar forceps or electrosurgery devices [5].

11.8.2 Fire Hazards

It is crucial to be aware of the presence of flammable or explosive liquids or gases in the area. There is a risk of fire or explosion if electrosurgical procedures are conducted in the presence of alcohol, oxygen, or bowel gases (methane). Special attention is necessary in the scalp, where residual alcohol may remain unnoticed [3].

For this reason, nonflammable antiseptic solutions such as povidone-iodine or chlorhexidine should be used. Also, care should always be taken in the perianal region [4, 5].

11.8.3 Other Health Concerns

Much like the smoke from cigarettes, the smoke from electrosurgery has been shown to have mutagenic potential. However, of potentially greater concern is the possible presence of infectious particles on the electrode or in the plume or splatter of electrosurgery cases. Infective hepatitis B virus has been demonstrated to be present on the electrode tips after electrodesiccation. This observation strongly supports the argument against using the same unsterilized electrode on consecutive patients. Electrodesiccation has been shown to produce a fine aerosol and splatter of blood droplets for at least several centimeters around the electrodesiccated site. If inhaled, this aerosol may be infectious. Herpes virus particles have also been shown to be dispersed by these devices. Likewise, transfer of bacteria during electrodesiccation has been demonstrated in a laboratory setting. The presence of human papillomavirus (HPV) particles from carbon dioxide lasers and electrosurgery has also been investigated and found in the plumes of both procedures. A graver implication of these HPV studies is that other viruses such as the human immunodeficiency virus and the hepatitis viruses may also remain intact in the plume and be inhaled by the surgeon or operating room personnel. No laboratory or clinical evidence for this exists as of yet, and additional studies are needed. A smoke evacuator from the operative site and a special mask for the surgeon's face are indicated [4, 5, 12, 15].

11.8.4 Cardiac Pacemaker

Most modern pacemakers operate in a demand mode and require both sensing and output circuits. Either of these circuits may be interfered with by high-frequency electrical currents, which can have adverse effects on pacemaker function. Despite the fact that most modern pacemakers are normally well shielded and filtered to avoid interference from outside electrical currents, high-frequency electrosurgery should be avoided in patients with pacemakers [5, 12, 13]. Although sporadic reports have identified device malfunctions following electrosurgery, the incidence of such events appears to be extremely low, especially with newer generation pacemakers and implantable cardiac defibrillators [7].

Thus, electrosurgery should not be used by anyone who uses a pacemaker without first consulting a physician to insure that the pacemaker is protected and unaffected by high-frequency interference. The surgeon should use appropriate precautions, which include proper grounding and avoiding high-amperage outputs, particularly when using current cutting procedures [12]. The surgeon should also use bipolar forceps with short burst and low voltage and avoid performing electrosurgery within the vicinity of the pacemaker or implantable cardiac defibrillators [7]. However, limited electrodesiccation of small lesions probably poses no risk to the relatively healthy pacemaker patient. Electrocautery is an acceptable substitute, since with this method no electrical current passes into the patient [5].

11.9 Sterilization

Electrodes should be sterilized by autoclave to prevent cross contamination. It has been shown that viral and bacterial infections can be transferred on such electrodes [1, 8, 15]. If one is using a nonsterile electrode tip, the potential for cross contamination and subsequent infection exists either from patient to patient or from patient to physician [1]. Also, disposable electrodes can be used or adapters can be obtained that allow for disposable metal hypodermic needles to be used as electrodes [4, 12]. Another significant contamination potential in the office setting comes from the handling of electrosurgical pencils and cords. Even though the electrode may be changed, the handle itself may be subject to contamination. Therefore, a disposable plastic sheath should be used to envelop the electrosurgical handpiece.

11.10 Advantages

Simple procedure
Rapid healing
Minimal or no bleeding
Aesthetically pleasing scars
Shorter operating time
Histopathological exam of surgical specimens
Fewer surgical risks and complications
Inexpensive
Can be completed outpatient

11.11 Disadvantages

Leads to greater tissue damage.
Creates necrotic tissue within a wound.
Delays wound healing.
Cannot be used near an unshielded pacemaker person.
Smoke and unpleasant odor may be produced.

11.12 Post-procedure Course

After the procedure, the patient is advised to keep the wound clean and dry. The healing process takes at least several weeks or longer, depending on the size of the wound and other factors. Necrotic tissue under the postoperative crust appears as pus and infection to the inexperienced electrosurgeon. Large, loose soggy crusts are best removed, but dry adherent crusts should be left undisturbed. It is desirable that the postoperative site remains dry for healing and should be covered only for protection or cosmetic reasons [2]. These wounds may be cleansed daily and then covered with an antibiotic ointment that provides a moist environment for new tissue growth. The wound may then be covered with common adhesive bandages.

11.13 Adverse Effects

The greatest hazard of electrosurgery involves excessive destruction of tissue and is associated with treatment technique. As a result of excessive tissue destruction, slow healing and tissue necrosis can lead to an unsightly or hypertrophic scar. The surgeon must take special care to avoid causing electrosurgical damage to adjacent areas [13]. Coagulation can cause extreme damage to larger nerves and blood vessels and, at times, delayed hemorrhage from unsuspected injury to blood vessel walls. Delayed postoperative bleeding with the sloughing of the crust can occur, and the patient should be instructed beforehand to apply direct pressure to control any bleeding [2].

11.14 Complications

Complications include occasional hypopigmentation, atrophy of the treated site, hypertrophic scars (especially on the back and chest), and ectropion (e.g., following eyelid electrosurgery). Excessive application of electrodesiccation or electrocoagulation currents can produce tissue destruction extending far beyond the actual treatment site [11, 13].

Destruction of deep lesions may lead to contracture of the upper lip and nasal ala, to depression of the nose tip, and to notching of the rim of the ear [2]. When working near the eyes, special shields should be used to protect corneas [13].

References

1. Bennett RG, Kraffert CA (1990) Bacterial transference during electrodesiccation and electrocoagulation. Arch Dermatol 126:751–755
2. Blankenship ML (1979) Physical modalities: electrosurgery, electrocautery and electrolysis. Int J Dermatol 18(6):443–452
3. Bougthon RS, Spencer SK (1987) Electrosurgical fundamentals. J Am Acad Dermatol 16: 862–867
4. Chiarello SE (2003) Radiovaporization: radiofrequency cutting current to vaporize and sculpt skin lesions. Dermatol Surg 29:755–758
5. Fewkes JL, Cheney ML, Pollack SV (1992) Electrosurgery. In: Illustrated atlas of cutaneous surgery. J.B. Lippincott, Philadelphia, Chapter 9
6. Goodman MM (1994) Principles of electrosurgery. In: Wheeland RG (ed) Cutaneous surgery. W.B. Saunders Company, Philadephia, pp 206–219
7. Hainer BL (2002) Electrosurgery for cutaneous lesions. Am Fam Physician 66(7):1259–1266
8. Matzle TJ, Christenson LJ, Atanashova N et al (2006) Pacemakers and implantable cardiac defibrillators in dermatologic surgery. Dermatol Surg 32:1155–1162; Pollack SV (2000). The history of electrosurgery. Dermatol Surg 26:904–908
9. Popkin GL (1987) Electrosurgery. In: Epstein E, Epstein E Jr (eds) Skin surgery. W.B. Saunders, Philadelphia, pp 164–183

10. Sampaio SAP, Piazza CD (2002) Eletrocirurgia convencional e Eletroncirurgia. In: Gadelha AR, Costa IMC (eds) Cirurgia Dermatológica em Consultório. Atheneu, São Paulo, pp 339–347
11. Sebben JE (1988) Electrosurgery principles: cutting current and cutaneous surgery – part I. J Dermatol Surg Oncol 14(2):147–150
12. Sebben JE (2000) Electrosurgery principles: cutting current and cutaneous surgery – part II. Dermatol Surg 26(2):142–145
13. Sebben JE (1988) The status of electrosurgery in dermatologic practice. J Am Acad Dermatol 19:542–549
14. Sebben JE (1998) Electrosurgery. In: Ratz JL (ed) Textbook of dermatologic surgery. Lippincott-Ravens Publishers, Philadelphia, pp 457–473
15. Shaw DH, Kalkwarf KL, Krejci RF et al (1988) Self-sterilization of the electrosurgery electrode. J Am Acad Dermatol 19(3):542–549
16. Weber PJ, Moody BR, Foster JA (2000) Electrosurgical suspension apparatus. Dermatol Surg 26:142–145

Injectable Treatments for Fat

12

Adam M. Rotunda

Core Messages

- This chapter reviews the history of injectable treatments for small collections of fat, with an emphasis on clarifying terminology and mechanism of action of several medications in development. Guidelines on injection dosing and technique are excluded given the current, experimental nature of these medications.
- Lipodissolve® (an injectable combination of phosphatidylcholine and sodium deoxycholate) and mesotherapy employ unregulated, compounded medications that have been associated with significant adverse events.
- An adipolytic medication based upon purified, non-animal-derived sodium deoxycholate is in FDA registration trials for the reduction of submental fat.
- A lipolytic medication, a combination of a β-agonist (salmeterol xinafoate) and a steroid (fluticasone propionate), is in FDA registration trials for the reduction of abdominal fat and exophthalmos.
- There is currently no data to suggest that injectable medications for cellulite are safe or efficacious.

A.M. Rotunda, M.D., F.A.A.D., F.A.C.M.S.
American Board of Dermatology, Detroit, MI, USA

American College of Mohs Surgery, Milwaukee, WI, USA

Division of Dermatology, David Geffen School of Medicine (UCLA), Los Angeles, CA, USA

Department of Dermatology, University of California, Irvine (UCI), Irvine, CA, USA

1100 Quail Street, Suite 102, Newport Beach, CA 92660, USA
e-mail: arotunda@hotmail.com

A. Tosti, D. Hexsel (eds.), *Update in Cosmetic Dermatology*,
DOI 10.1007/978-3-642-34029-1_12, © Springer-Verlag Berlin Heidelberg 2013

12.1 Introduction

Subcutaneous injections that reduce adipose tissue have been most frequently referred to as injection lipolysis, PC/DC, Lipodissolve®, and mesotherapy [5, 16, 34, 50]. These terms are outdated and associated with controversial, unregulated treatments. Injectable treatments for fat dissolution in development are intended to reduce small pockets of fat, not as a tool for large surface area body contouring. Pharmaceutical-grade, injectable medications that permanently or nonpermanently remove small collections of fat have aptly been referred to as *adipolytic therapy* and *pharmaceutical lipoplasty*, respectively.

If current investigations lead to FDA-approved drugs, the procedure may very well broaden the pool of aesthetic physicians who treat fat as well as open a new market of patients who seek minimally invasive aesthetic treatments. However, the history of fat reducing with injections is marred with controversy. It may therefore be reasonable to view new data about these therapies with a sense of caution and anticipation.

The popularity of colloquially termed "fat-melting" injections can be attributed in part to the Lipodissolve® marketing campaign by Fig. (formerly American Lipodissolve®, St. Louis, MO) commercial treatment centers and the American Society for Aesthetic Lipodissolve (ASAL). As of this writing, however, no commercially available injectable formulations are approved anywhere worldwide for fat removal. The US Food and Drug Administration (FDA) considers injectable fat reduction "unapproved drugs for unapproved uses…," [60] yet interest and even illicit use persists. Notorious reports of cutaneous infections and necrosis, corporate bankruptcies, medical society warning statements, as well as state legislation banning the procedure [2, 8, 10, 11, 13, 26, 54] have contributed to the infamy of this treatment. Despite the alarm, validation of efficacy and an acceptable safety profile by recent well-controlled investigations are evidence for the increasingly exciting prospect of offering patients a nonsurgical, non-device, and minimally invasive remedy to reduce fat.

As none of these medications are current commercial production, this chapter does not fit neatly into the layout used in the rest of this book (Patient Selection, Consultation, Procedure, etc.). Given this constraint, however, the background and research behind an innovative line of medications may be of interest to some readers who wish to be on the "cutting" edge.

12.2 Clarification of Terms and History

12.2.1 Lipolysis, Injection Lipolysis, Pharmaceutical Lipoplasty, Adipolysis, and Adipolytic Therapy

The term *lipolysis* describes the hydrolysis, or degradation, of lipids into their constituent fatty acid and glycerol building blocks [15]. Lipolysis results in the reduction of fat cell volume while preserving the cell viability (Fig. 12.1). Lipolysis occurs within adipocytes and vascular lumen of muscle and fat tissue and is regulated by hormone-sensitive lipase (HSL) and lipoprotein lipase (LPL), respectively [40].

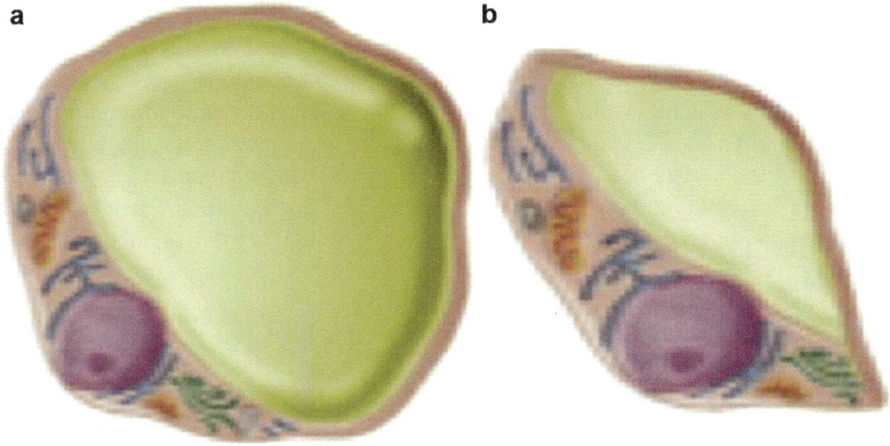

Fig. 12.1 (**a**) Schematic of adipocyte at baseline. (**b**) Schematic of adipocyte lipolysis; adipocyte reduces volume following hormone-sensitive lipase activation and subsequent release of glycerol and free fatty acids (Photographs courtesy of the author)

Hormone-sensitive lipase is expressed in adipose tissue and is activated by cortisone and catecholamines, which are lipolytic, and inhibited by insulin, which is lipogenic. Lipoprotein lipase is located on endothelial walls of capillaries and is responsible for serum chylomicron (from dietary lipids) and very low-density lipoprotein breakdown. Lipolysis may also be induced by medication binding to specific adrenergic receptors (α or β) located on adipocyte membranes [20, 35, 40, 46].

A novel medication currently being developed by Lithera, Inc. (San Diego, CA) is termed "LIPO-102" and its use as an injectable fat reducer is called "pharmaceutical lipoplasty." Understandably, the company prefers this term to "injection lipolysis" although "injection lipolysis" is technically (physiologically) accurate. "Injection lipolysis" has been historically associated with Lipodissolve® or phosphatidylcholine/deoxycholate (PC/DC) injections, which carry a tarnished past. Adding to the confusion, "injection lipolysis" should never have been used to describe treatments that incorporate the detergent, DC. Any detergent-based formulation elicits adipocyte lysis, and so it will not effectively stimulate adipocyte lipolysis, which is a process that requires a fully functioning, or viable, fat cell. Therefore, to more accurately describe injectable methods that employ detergents to diminish fat, the terms "adipolysis" and "adipolytic therapy" are preferred [19].

12.2.2 Brief History of Mesotherapy, Lipostabil®, Lipodissolve®, and the Role of the Compounding Pharmacy

The term *mesotherapy* should not be used interchangeably with PC/DC, DC, Lipodissolve®, injection lipolysis, pharmaceutical lipoplasty, or adipolytic therapy [5, 16, 31, 49]. The repeated, incorrect use of the term in the lay and medical literature has inadvertently confused physicians and patients. Mesotherapy (from the Greek mesos, "middle," and therapeia, "to treat medically") was first introduced in 1952 by French physician Michel Pistor [39] and describes cutaneous injections of minute doses of medication. Mesotherapy has been recognized and traditionally practiced in Europe as a localized treatment in pain medicine, sports medicine, and rheumatology but has been applied over time to cosmetic medicine for conditions like alopecia, cellulite, photoaging, and scarring [34, 38, 39, 49, 50]. The nature of the target condition determines at what depth (epidermal, dermal, or subcutaneous) the injections (often hundreds) of extemporaneously mixed combinations of vasodilators, anti-inflammatory agents, herbs, hormones, antibiotics, enzymes, or coenzymes are placed with a syringe, injection gun, or multineedle device [5, 34, 38, 49]. Several small yet well-designed studies have generated renewed interest in this traditional form of mesotherapy as a treatment for a number of aesthetic and medical conditions [4, 12, 30, 31].

Lipostabil® (Sanofi-Aventis, Paris, France) "fat-melting" injections were introduced onto the worldwide stage by Patricia Rittes [42], a dermatologist in São Paolo, Brazil, who reported reduction of infraorbital fat using direct, transcutaneous injection with Lipostabil®. Lipostabil® is manufactured and marketed for intravenous use in Europe, South America, and South Africa as a treatment for numerous fat-related disorders (i.e., hyperlipidemia, angina pectoris, diabetic angiopathy). Lipostabil® consists of soy-derived PC (5 %), its solvent sodium deoxycholate (2.5 %), dl-α-tocopherol (vitamin E), sodium hydroxide, ethanol, and benzyl alcohol, in sterile water.

Importing Lipostabil® into the USA is illegal, and there are no approved PC/DC or DC medications for which physicians can use "off-label." To meet the demand by physicians and patients, compounding pharmacies have produced formulations similar to Lipostabil®; the most popular was Lipodissolve®. The now defunct company, Fig. (formerly American Lipodissolve®, St. Louis, MO), popularized a chain of treatment centers that used compounded medications of PC and DC based loosely on the original Lipostabil® formulation. Compounded formulations generally consists of 5 % PC combined with 4.2–4.75 % DC [16, 49, 50] or 1–5 % DC alone [16, 36, 49, 51, 56, 61]. At times, collagenase or lipolytic agents (i.e., caffeine, isoproterenol, yohimbine) were added to purportedly [46] augment fat reduction. In the USA, these medications are legally available through compounding [49, 50], although the concentration and purity of medication formulated at a compounding pharmacy can be dubious [19]. As malpractice coverage and standards of care between state and region, physicians may be placing themselves in a precarious position by treating patients with unapproved medication.

Regulations pertaining to compounding vary by state [49, 50]. Traditional compounding involves preparing a specialized, custom drug product to fill an individual patient's prescription when an approved drug cannot meet their needs. With regard to PC/DC, it appears that most, if not all, of the compounded formulations are performed in bulk in anticipation of receiving sales in mass quantities. Interestingly, PC/DC is not being compounded for an individually identified patient, and pharmacies are compounding preestablished and unregulated formulations (i.e., they are not produced within facilities meeting cGMP (Current Good Manufacturing Practice) regulations enforced by the FDA). Local and systemic safety margins of deoxycholate using a cGMP formulation are being used in pivotal clinical studies.

Over the past decade, investigations by Dr. Rittes [27–29] and others [1, 7, 16, 17, 21, 23, 28, 36–38, 51–53, 55, 56, 59, 61] have reported that Lipostabil®, compounded PC/DC, and compounded DC reduce fat on the hips, abdomen, back rolls (known affectionately as "love handles" in men or "bra strap fat" in women), dorsocervical region ("buffalo hump"), neck, jowls, and lipomas (Fig. 12.2). Two relatively recently conducted, IRB-approved prospective, randomized, double-blind clinical trials with compounded PC/DC and DC alone in submental fat [50] (Fig. 12.3) and hips [55] have substantiated the beneficial clinical effects of these medication observed in prior case series and retrospective studies. The indications, technique, safety profile, and so-called standards of practice (a paradox in light of its unregulated use) of PC/DC or Lipodissolve therapy have been reviewed [16, 44, 50]. However, all of these reports utilize non-pharmaceutical-grade (non-cGMP medication) DC derived from bovine sources, using anecdotal, nonstandardized techniques.

12.3 Clarifying the Roles of Deoxycholate and Phosphatidylcholine

12.3.1 The PC Hypothesis

The preponderance of published literature on the subject of injectable fat treatments describes treatment with PC/DC or DC alone. Basic science research, detailed below, has revealed that, invariably, a component of all these formulations was the biologic detergent, DC. It is generally accepted that all published reports describing injectable PC formulations contain DC.

Early publications [22, 26, 41, 46] hypothesized that the lecithin-derived phospholipid, PC, was the active fat-reducing ingredient in Lipostabil®. The premise was that the same mechanism responsible for reducing serum lipids by PC in intravenous Lipostabil® (for which it is approved in Europe) was effective to reduce subcutaneous fat tissue. It was also conjectured [15, 35] that PC induced a cascade of intracellular signals that led to apoptosis or that it directly lysed fat cell membranes, emulsified triglycerides, upregulated LPL, and facilitated transit of triglycerides across cell membranes. None of these theories could be supported experimentally.

12.3.2 Focus on DC

Deoxycholic acid (Fig. 12.4) is a secondary bile acid produced by intestinal bacteria after the release of primary bile acids (i.e., cholic acid) in the liver [49]. Biologically compatible detergents like DC have been conventionally used to improve the solubility of the major constituents of intravenous medications, such as amphotericin B

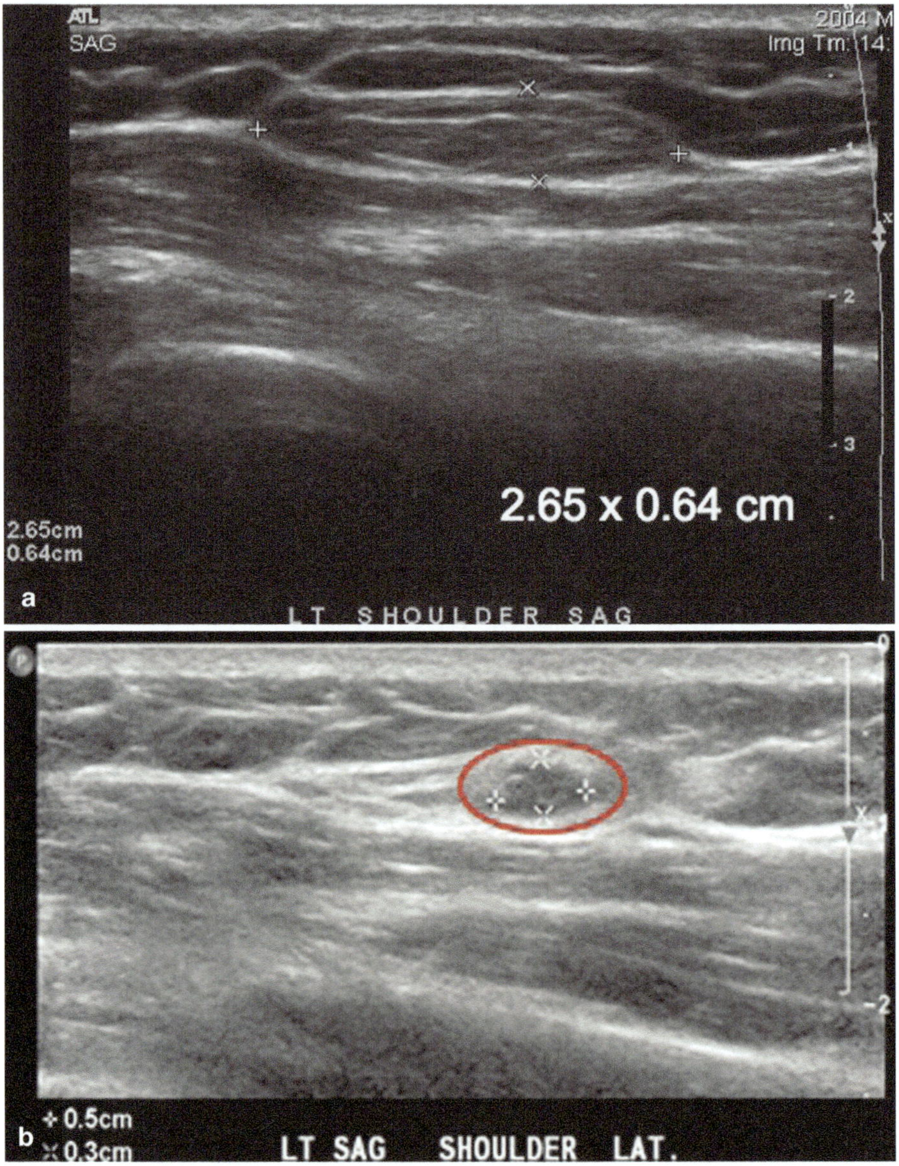

Fig. 12.2 (**a**) Ultrasound of lipoma 7 located on the shoulder measuring 2.65 × 3 × 0.64 cm before sodium deoxycholate (10 mg/mL) treatment. (**b**) Same lipoma measuring 0.5 × 3 × 0.3 cm 4 months after second and last injection (Photographs courtesy of the author)

(Amphocin®, Pfizer) [49]. Sodium deoxycholate is the solvent for PC in Lipostabil®, as phospholipids like PC are essentially water insoluble [49].

An unforeseen discovery [53] revealed that DC alone (without PC) produced cell death and cell lysis in vitro (keratinocytes) and ex vivo (pig adipose tissue) equal to

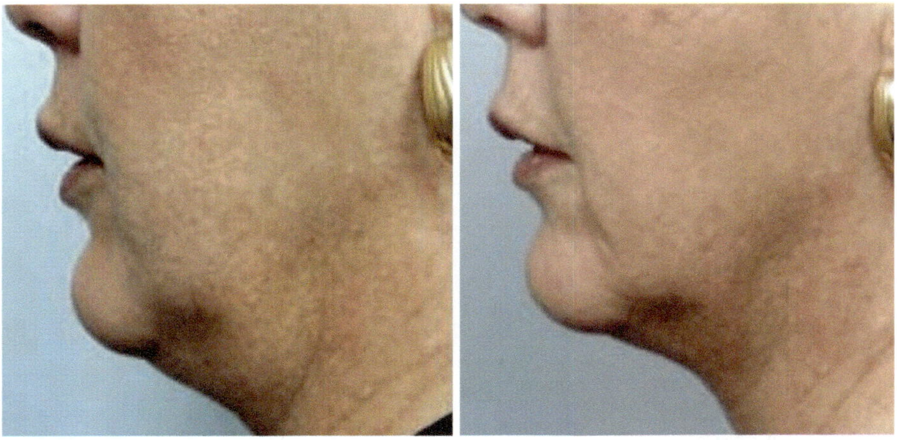

Fig. 12.3 Subject profile before (*left*) and 2 months after (*right*) 5 monthly injections with 1.0 mL of compounded sodium deoxycholate (10 mg/mL) into the submental fat area

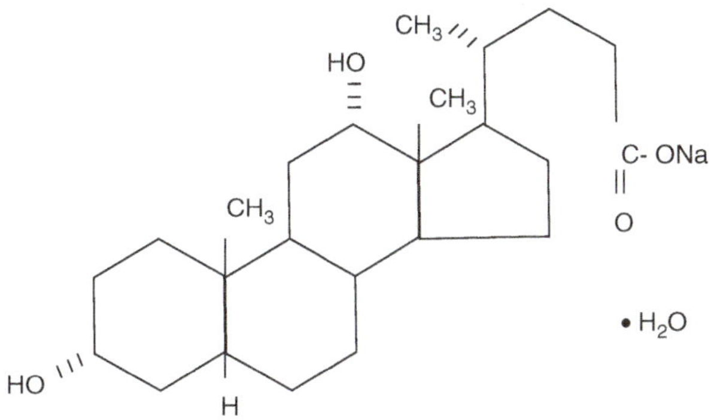

Fig. 12.4 Chemical structure of sodium deoxycholate

the effects produced by the PC/DC combination (Fig. 12.5). These were the first data which called into question the role of PC as the fat-reducing agent by demonstrating that the bile salt, DC, produces nonspecific cell lysis independent of PC.

The strength of the argument that DC acted as the sole active ingredient was based on a mounting evidence from independent sources. Gupta et al. [21] demonstrated that DC alone and PC/DC are comparably cytotoxic on cultured adipocytes, endothelial cells, fibroblasts, and skeletal muscle cells. Schuller-Petrovic et al. [56] extended these laboratory findings into living tissue by performing cell lysis and cell viability studies in vivo (rat adipose tissue) using PC/DC and isolated DC (Fig. 12.6). Additional experiments have corroborated the lytic effects of DC on adipocytes in vivo and in vitro [27, 57]. This laboratory and animal data has been validated through human studies that demonstrate comparable fat-reducing effects when either DC or PC/DC are injected into lipomas [7, 28, 51] and abdominal [15, 17], submental [50], and hip fat [16, 55].

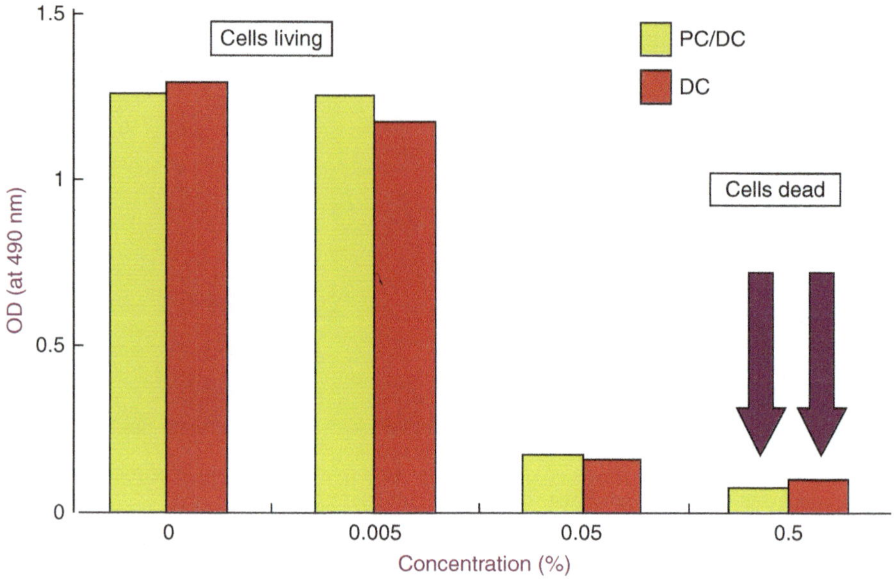

Fig. 12.5 MTS cell viability assay measuring living keratinocytes exposed to phosphatidylcholine/deoxycholate (*PC/DC*) and deoxycholate (*DC*). Absorbance (*OD*) is directly related to cell viability. Increasing concentration of either PC/DC or DC alone produces cell death. DC alone profoundly reduces cell viability, with PC producing minimal effect (Courtesy of the author)

Deoxycholate is an ionic detergent that disrupts the integrity of biological membrane by introducing their polar hydroxyl groups into the cell membrane's phospholipid bilayer hydrophobic core [32]. The process involves first an "attack" of the detergent on the membrane; solubilization of membrane-associated proteins; saturation of the membrane with detergent; and finally, with increasing detergent concentration, membrane integrity breakdown and solubilysis [23, 25, 52, 58] (Fig. 12.7).

While the role of PC as an active participant in localized fat loss had been called into question for years [35, 49], the contention that PC itself could not lyse cells or reduce fat was based only on indirect evidence. Some authors contended that the inclusion of PC was historical artifact [49]. There appeared to be minimal difference in experimental and clinical outcomes when PC was added to DC, and so PC itself was presumed to yield minimal or no fat-reducing effects [6]. Being water soluble, DC's effect on cells and tissue was relatively straightforward to quantify experimentally. On the other hand, it was technically difficult to evaluate PC's direct effect on cells and fat tissue because of its insolubility in the aqueous solutions used in all the prior studies. Conventional laboratory phospholipid solvents like chloroform and ethanol are membrane toxic. This problem was not solved for years.

Duncan and colleagues [16] resolve this quandary by designing a novel method to investigate the effect of PC on adipocytes using mineral oil as its solvent, which could dissolve PC but not affect cell membranes. In this way, the isolated effect of PC on cells could be observed without the confounding lytic effects of PC's solvent.

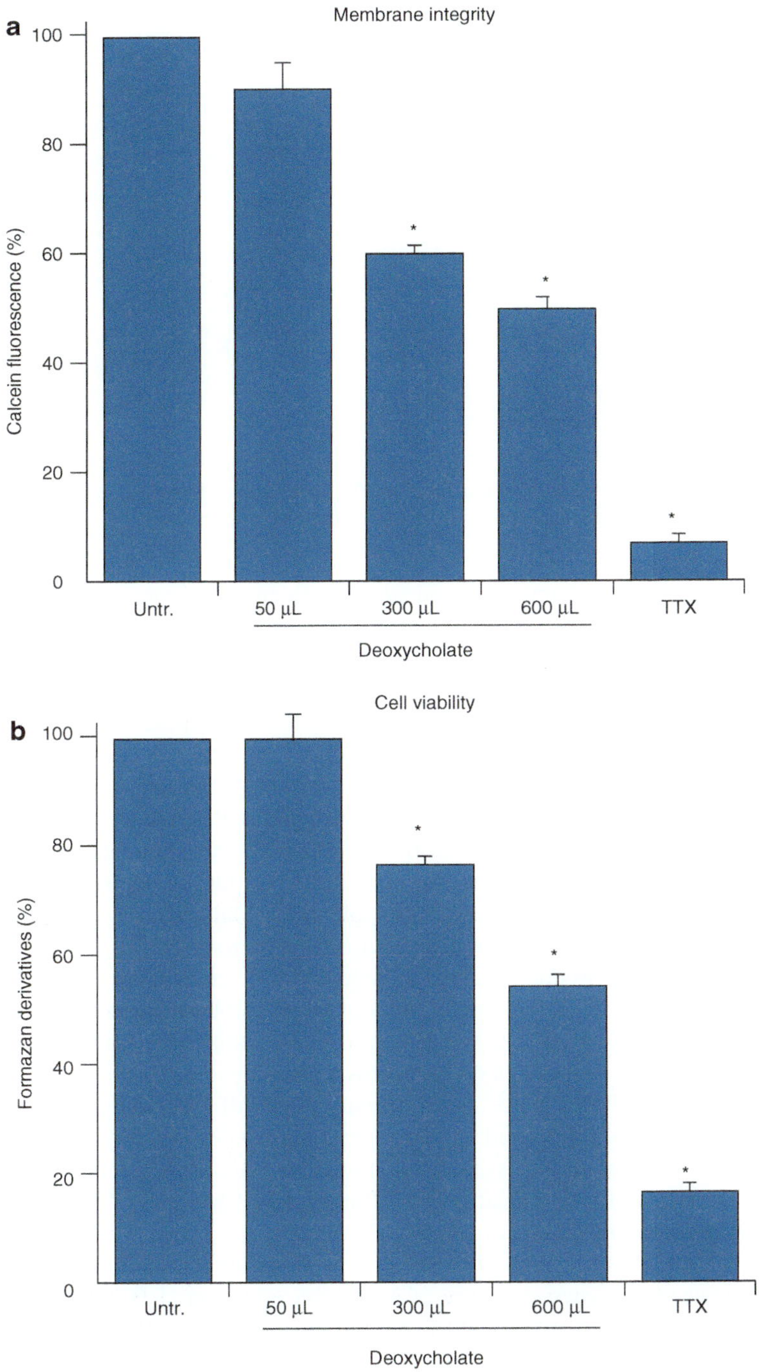

Fig. 12.6 Effects of DC (2.5 %) on (**a**) rat fat cell membrane integrity and (**b**) cell viability after repetitive dosing. The effects were observed after 30 days following application of DC on days 0, 7, and 28. Triton (TTX) 0.5 % served as positive control. These data translate the experimental data summarized in Fig. 12.5 into a living model (Obtained with permission from Medical Insight, Inc.)

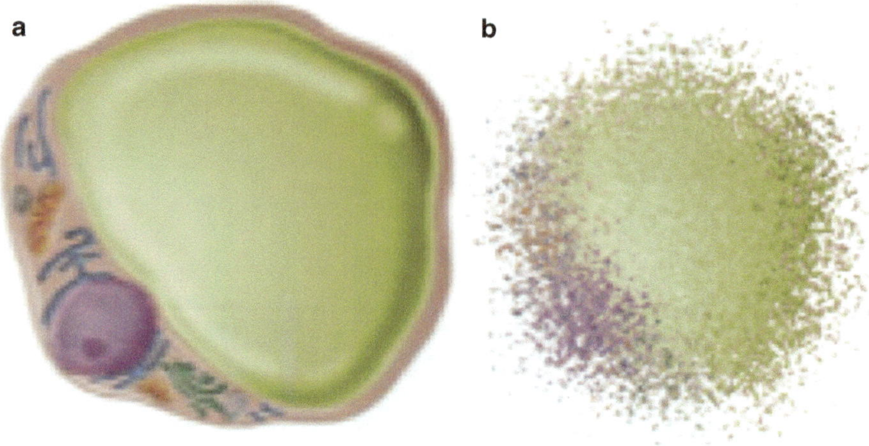

Fig. 12.7 (**a**) Schematic of adipocyte at baseline. (**b**) Schematic of adipolysis; adipocyte becomes nonviable following membrane solubilysis and degradation by detergent

The authors incubated human-derived adipocyte stem cells from abdominal fat and induced them to maturity. Cytotoxicity assays (lactate dehydrogenase and oil red O) and lipolysis assays (glycerol and triglyceride assays) were performed on the cultured adipocytes after exposure to PC (5 %)/mineral oil, DC (1 % and 2.4 %), benzyl alcohol, and isoproterenol (a β-agonist) (Table 12.1). These data are the first to experimentally confirm that PC has no adipolytic (i.e., fat cell lysing) or lipolytic (i.e., triglyceride degrading) effects.

Despite evidence that DC is the sole active ingredient, some clinicians maintain that it is safer for the patient to incorporate PC with DC. To their credit, there is evidence that relatively high concentrations (>1 %) of DC alone produce profound inflammation, prolonged nodularity, and, potentially, skin necrosis [14, 16, 48–51], while PC/DC combinations that use high concentrations of DC (up to 4.75 %) appear less likely to produce these outcomes [16, 55]. In an effort to identify what effects, if any, PC had on the lytic activity of DC [9], found that in the presence of PC, almost ten times more DC was required to lyse adipocytes and that there is a threefold reduction in the area of fat necrosis as compared to when DC was used alone (Fig. 12.8). These results may be a consequence of DC and PC spontaneously forming detergent/phospholipid aggregates called micelles [49, 50]; while unbound DC is capable of lysing fat tissue, it is reasonable to assume that PC/DC micelles have no or minimal lytic capacity [57]. Rather than "protective," PC *inhibits* the desirable fat-reducing effects of DC [9].

A small, double-blind study investigating submental fat reduction demonstrated no differences in efficacy or safety of a low-concentration (1 %) DC formulation compared to a PC (5 %)/DC (4.75 %) formulation. Low-dose DC appears to be an efficacious and safe concentration for subcutaneous injection [50, 51].

Table 12.1 PC in isolation from DC does not cause adipolysis (fat cell lysis) nor lipolysis (triglyceride breakdown)

Test solution	Adipocyte cell lysis obtained with this solution
PC50/DC42	++
Deoxycholate 1 %	+++
Deoxycholate 2.4 %	+++
Phosphatidycholine	0
5 % in mineral oil	
Isuprel 0.08 % injectable	0
Local anesthetic 5 %	0
Saline 0.9 % (control)	0
Benzyl alcohol	0

Used with permission of D. Duncan, M.D.

These data are the first to experimentally confirm prior deductions that PC will not reduce fat without DC

++ *mild effect*, +++ *significant effect*, 0 *no effect*

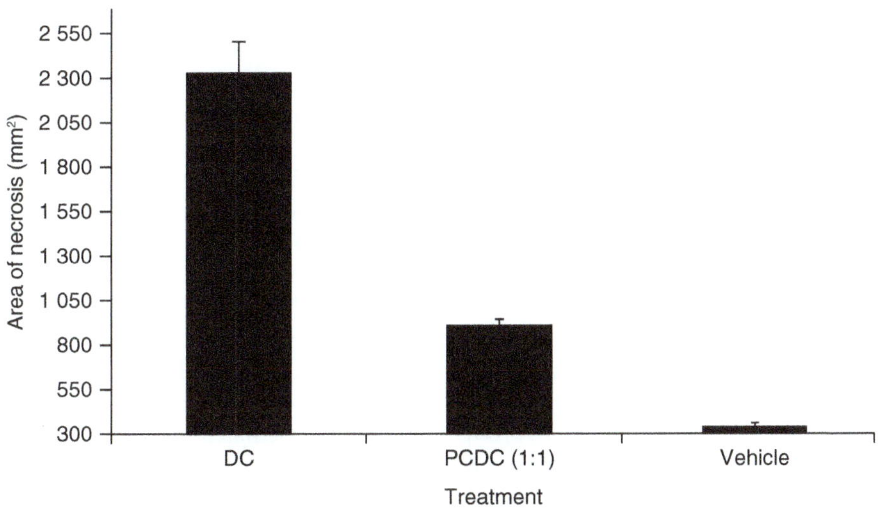

Fig. 12.8 Inclusion of 0.5 % PC with 0.5 % DC produces a threefold reduction in fat cell death (as measured by area of necrosis in vivo) compared to 0.5 % DC. PC inhibits the desirable fat-reducing effect of DC (From Bentow et al. [64])

There are no data from large-scale, rigorous (controlled, randomized, and blinded) trials to conclude any advantage of using PC with DC. As with most drugs, a safe and effective single ingredient medication is more desirable than a multi-ingredient formulation, unless the latter possesses significant advantages.

12.4 Detergents and Tissue Interactions

12.4.1 Mechanism of Fat Reduction and Further Implications on Efficacy and Safety

Fundamentally akin to sclerotherapy [58], subcutaneously injected DC necroses tissue as a result of its cytotoxic effects on the cellular membranes. Isolated DC causes adipocytes to lyse and release their triglyceride contents in the extracellular environment [29, 53]. Almost immediately, inflammation and edema manifest clinically. Living and ex vivo animal human tissue exposed to DC, as well as PC/DC combinations, demonstrates fat cell lysis; erythrocyte extravasation; a mixed infiltrate consisting of polymorphonuclear leukocytes, lymphocytes, macrophages, and multinucleated giant cells; and fibrosis [2, 5, 28, 31, 49–52]. The visible gross and histological progression of events that occurs following detergent injection into a lipoma has been documented [51] (Fig. 12.9). Controlled adipolysis and moderate degrees of postinflammatory fibrosis are desirable for localized subcutaneous volume reduction and for promoting tissue tightening [15, 16, 50].

Under certain conditions, deoxycholate appears to indiscriminately target adipose as well as non-adipose cells and tissue [24]. One study demonstrated that in vitro, high-dose (5 %) DC and PC (5 %)/DC (2.5 %) induce necrosis of porcine fat and muscle [44]. Gupta et al. showed a cytotoxic response to PC/DC of four different cell types' culture [45]. Jancke [59] also found that Lipostabil® had dose-related cytolytic effects on adipose tissue, vascular smooth muscle cells, renal epithelial cells, and myocytes. Schuller-Petrovic [31] found that injection of PC/DC and DC in subcutaneous fat of rats caused fibrosis in adjacent cutaneous muscle.

The proclivity for DC to solubilize adipose as well as non-adipose cell is unsettling and would appear to explain skin ulceration in isolated reports [13, 14, 47]. However, in all reported clinical studies, case series, and FDA registration trials, ulceration with DC is nonexistent. Why the dichotomy? Researchers have recently demonstrated that DC's ability to lyse cells is inversely related to the amount of protein surrounding and within tissue with which it comes into contact, sparing the tissue from necrosis (Fig. 12.10) [60]. This effect is mediated in large part by the presence of albumin (an abundant, ubiquitous physiologic protein), which has a very high affinity to DC and appears to inhibit the lytic activity of DC (Fig. 12.11) [60]. Therefore, albumin's high concentration in vital tissue but relatively low concentration in fat may explain why injections of deoxycholate into fat are relatively safe clinically. In the available data from phase 2a and 2b clinical trials [29], which represents safety reporting on over 350 subjects, skin necrosis and damage to other "bystander" tissue by a DC-based medication was not reported. These results are very encouraging.

However, detergent injections are not without temporary downtime. Injection site erythema, tenderness, paresthesias (primarily numbness), and edema are the primary local adverse reactions to DC-injected fat [3, 40, 42, 43, 57]. These effects are generally mild to moderate and dissipate over days to weeks, with no persistent untoward effects. There does appear to be, however, a dose-dependent response to

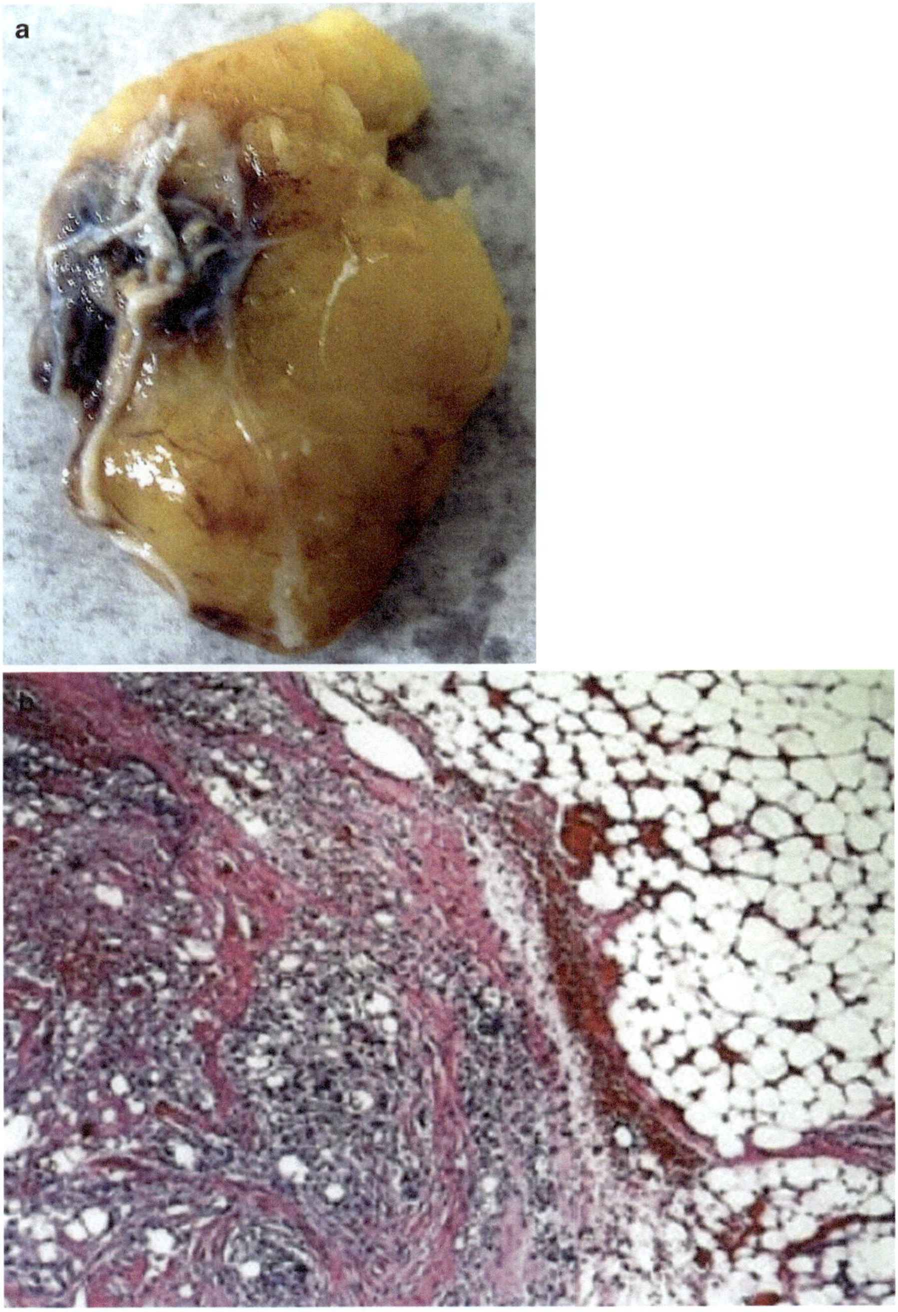

Fig. 12.9 (**a**) Excised lipoma 2 days after injection with sodium deoxycholate (10 mg/mL) revealing a well-demarcated area of necrosis. (**b**) Microscopic findings demonstrating acute inflammation and necrosis (hematoxylin and eosin, original magnification ×10) (Photographs courtesy of the author)

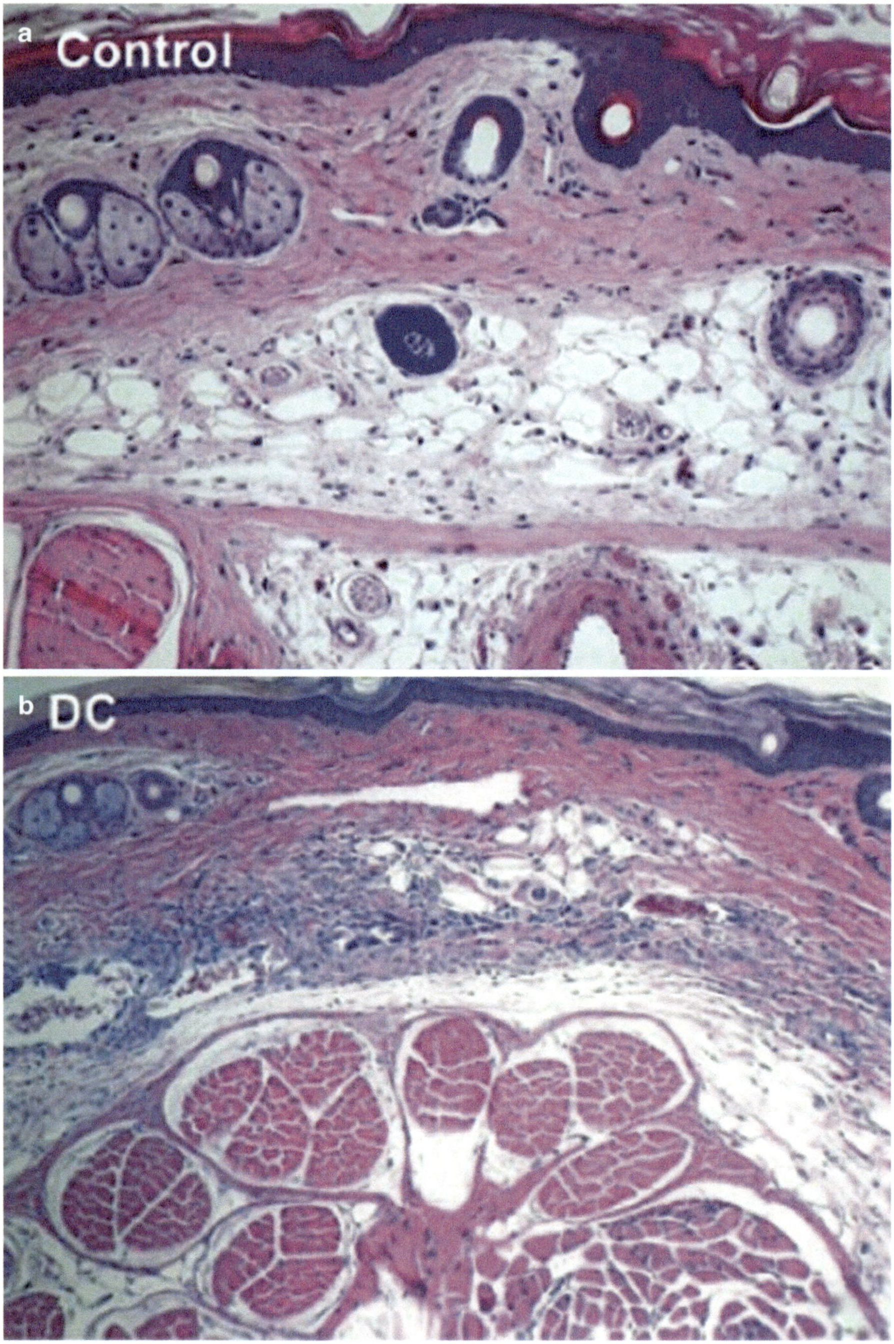

Fig. 12.10 (**a**) Hematoxylin and eosin staining of a mouse tail 20 days postinjection of saline vehicle or (**b**) 0.5 % deoxycholate showing necrosis and inflammatory infiltrate of the subcutaneous fat in the treated tail. (**b**) The tissue architecture of the muscle and skin layers remains preserved in the treated tail, with no signs of necrosis and scant inflammation (Reproduced with permission from John Wiley & Sons)

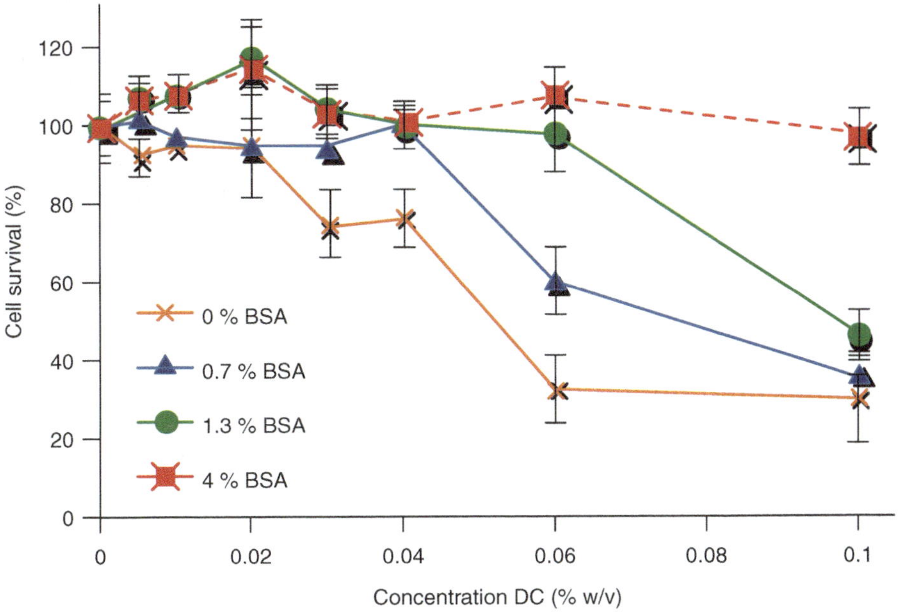

Fig. 12.11 Viability of cultured primary human adipocytes treated with deoxycholate (*DC*) in the presence of increasing concentrations of BSA. Cells were incubated with 0 % BSA (*orange*), 0.7 % BSA (*blue*), 1.3 % BSA (*green*), and 4 % BSA (*red*) and then challenged with increasing concentrations of DC. Cell survival was measured using the 3-(4,5-dimethylthiazol-2-yl)-5-(3-carboxymehtoxyphenyl)-2-(4-sulfophenyl)-2H-tetrazolium colorimetric assay for cell viability. The concentrations of bovine serum albumin used are representative of the concentrations found physiologically in and around the site of injection. Albumin-attenuated DC-mediated cytolysis in a concentration-dependent manner. Error bars represent standard error of the mean (Reproduced with permission from John Wiley & Sons)

DC, whereby increasing DC concentrations produces increasing degrees of cytotoxicity [44, 45] and subcutaneous fat necrosis [2, 36, 42, 64].

These data collectively suggest some safe therapeutic margin, where maximum benefit is achieved with minimal risk, which is currently being defined and exploited [29]. Factors such as injection technique [2, 31, 47], dose (volume and concentration) [2, 15–18, 47], and tissue-detergent interactions [3, 19, 48, 61] most likely influence the extent of this "safety window." Some authors suggest that when DC is used without PC, concentrations of the detergent should be ≤1 % [50] as DC >1 % is associated with pain, profound tissue necrosis, and prolonged nodularity [16, 49, 50]. Correct injection depth of subcutaneous detergent formulations is also critical [16, 47]. Superficial placement may produce cutaneous breakdown and ulceration [16, 47]. Notably, all reports of scarring and ulceration using detergent-based formulations are associated with nonphysician injectors, large injection volumes, unverified dosages of unknown medications, and other unorthodox practices [8, 13, 47, 48]. As with other injectables, injection technique and practitioner skill and experience are paramount to safety.

An additional question – "what happens to the DC after it is injected?" – has been answered with radioisotope-labeled DC injections into fat pads of mice, in an effort to track the body's processing of injected DC [57]. Almost half of the DC injected was transported to the intestinal tract within 24 h of injection into fat tissue. A peak accumulation in the small intestine was noted at 4 h, and at 5 days, the remaining DC was eliminated in the feces. In humans, subcutaneously injected deoxycholate is eliminated from systemic circulation in less than 24 h [57].

12.5 The Fate of Adipolytic Therapy

In contrast to the pathway taken by most novel medical therapies (from discovery to preclinical then clinical testing, regulatory approval then product commercialization), it is apparent that before the acquisition of DC by the pharmaceutical industry, the research and clinical experience with injectable detergents was unconventional and haphazard. A pivotal and "clarifying" moment in the evolution of this treatment came in 2005, when KYTHERA Biopharmaceuticals (Calabasas, CA) acquired the intellectual rights describing the use of sodium deoxycholate as an injectable fat loss medication from the Los Angeles Biomedical Institute and UCLA. Since then, the study of detergent-based medication for localized fat loss has become rigorous and well conceived. Preclinical data and, currently, clinical registration studies performed by KYTHERA have more clearly characterized the safety and clinical potential of DC and distinguished it from Lipostabil®, PC/DC, and Lipodissolve®.

KYTHERA Biopharmaceuticals (Calabasas, CA) is currently seeking approval of a nonanimal source DC fat-reducing formula for submental fat, referred to as ATX-101; as of this writing, they have completed phase 3 (the last phase of clinical drug development before regulatory approval) outside the USA and have initiated phase 3 within the USA and Canada. The strategy of using low-dose DC (i.e., 2 mg/mL) is consistent with prior, non-industry-sponsored investigations and with the experiences of veteran injectors, who recognize that low-dose DC (without PC) is a prudent approach to yield gratifying results while minimizing risks.

A recent phase 2b, randomized, double-blind, placebo-controlled, dose-ranging study showed ATX-101 was well tolerated and demonstrated statistically significant efficacy as compared with placebo [29]. The study enrolled a total of 129 subjects and was conducted across ten dermatology and plastic surgery centers in the USA. Multiple clinician and patient endpoints were assessed as well as MRI to objectively quantify fat reduction. The study tested two drug-dosing regimens (1 and 2 mg/cm^2). In the study, ATX-101 demonstrated statistically significant ($p<0.05$) reductions in submental fat as compared with placebo as assessed by all measures: a validated clinician scale, patient-reported outcome (PRO) scale, and magnetic resonance imaging (MRI) measurement for both fat volume and thickness. Adverse events (i.e., local swelling, tenderness, erythema) were primarily mild to moderate and were transient. In addition, a statistically significant difference versus placebo was also shown on other PRO measures, including instruments measuring subject satisfaction, patient impact, and chin attractiveness.

As of this writing, KYTHERA has completed nine clinical trials and treated more than 1,000 subjects. In two previously conducted ex-US phase 2 studies on 155 patients, ATX-101 was well tolerated and yielded statistically significant reduction of submental fat compared to placebo based on clinician and patient assessments. Results observed from their current phase 2b study confirmed the observations made in previous phase 2 trials. Phase 3 studies of ATX-101 were pursued in Europe in collaboration with Bayer HealthCare, which has licensed rights to ATX-101 outside of the USA and Canada.

12.5.1 LIPO-102 and Related Lipolytic Agents

Using FDA-registered drugs proven safe and effective in other indications (i.e., Advair® Diskus 5/500, marketed for asthma and COPD, GlaxoSmithKline), LIPO-102 targets and stimulates adipocyte (intracellular) lipolysis to produce a non-adipolytic, nonsurgical fat tissue reduction. Like Advair® but in injectable form, LIPO-102 is a combination of salmeterol xinafoate and fluticasone propionate.

Salmeterol xinafoate is a highly selective long-acting β_2-adrenergic receptor agonist. Fluticasone propionate is a synthetic trifluorinated glucocorticoid. Activation of β_2-adrenergic receptors located on human fat cells by salmeterol triggers the breakdown of triglycerides in these cells to free fatty acids and glycerol by lipolysis. Fluticasone propionate has potent anti-inflammatory activity. Glucocorticoids such as fluticasone impart various effects on β-adrenergic receptor function in vivo: They enhance the coupling of β-adrenergic receptors to G proteins and the resulting activation of adenylate cyclase, and they decrease β-adrenergic receptor downregulation (tachyphylaxis) due to chronic receptor stimulation (e.g., by salmeterol) [41], although tachyphylaxis can be still recognized to some degree clinically. In sum, salmeterol stimulates lipolysis through activation of β_2-adrenergic receptors on fat cells and fluticasone upregulates the cellular pathways stimulated by salmeterol.

In clinical testing with sophisticated volumetric imaging technology (Canfield Vectra® analysis), 22 weekly abdominal injections of LIPO-102 (0.5 μg salmeterol and 1 μg fluticasone) in 20 subjects for 4–8 weeks produced rapid (within weeks) and significant reductions in abdominal circumference and volume versus placebo (20 subjects). Prior dose-escalation studies revealed that higher doses of the combination drugs produced tachyphylaxis and minimal efficacy. Plasma levels of fluticasone and salmeterol produced by LIPO-102 injection are a fraction of those produced by the 505(b) (2) reference drug, Advair®500/50. Anticipated weekly dose is ~1/700th of Advair® weekly dose (based on salmeterol).

At 8 weeks, LIPO-102 produced a mean reduction in abdominal circumference >2 cm and a mean reduction in abdominal volume >350 cc in young patients. Interestingly, younger subjects (defined as <40 years of age) also had significantly better responses than older subjects; significant reduction in waist circumference relative to placebo only occurred in young subjects (Fig. 12.12). Overall change in waist circumference was statistically significant at 6 weeks post-dosing, but at the 12-week follow-up, they failed to reach significance. There were no significant hematologic, cardiovascular, or dermatologic adverse effects (i.e., atrophy, pigmentation, nodularity, necrosis). In fact there was minimal difference in swelling, redness, irritation, or any other local injection site reactions between LIPO-102 and placebo.

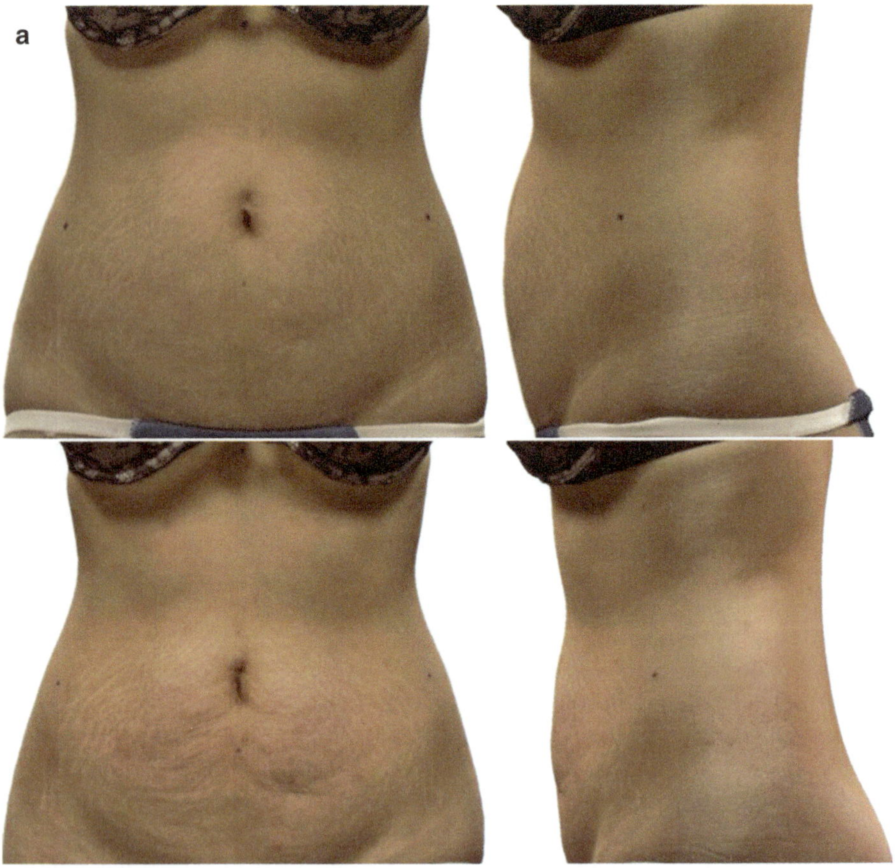

Fig. 12.12 (**a**) Before (*superior*) and after (*inferior*) 1 month of anterior abdomen injections (one injection session weekly) with 1 μg salmeterol xinafoate and 22 μg fluticasone propionate (total weekly dose) at 8-week follow-up. Volumetric reduction (as measured by Canfield Vectra imaging system): waist reduction is 2.85 cm and volume reduction is 355 cc. (**b**) Before (*superior*) and after (*inferior*) 1 month of anterior abdomen injections (one injection session weekly) with 1 μg salmeterol xinafoate and 22 μg fluticasone propionate (total weekly dose) at 8-week follow-up. Volumetric reduction (as measured by Canfield Vectra imaging system): waist reduction is 4.52 cm and volume reduction is 857 cc (Photographs courtesy of Lithera, Inc.)

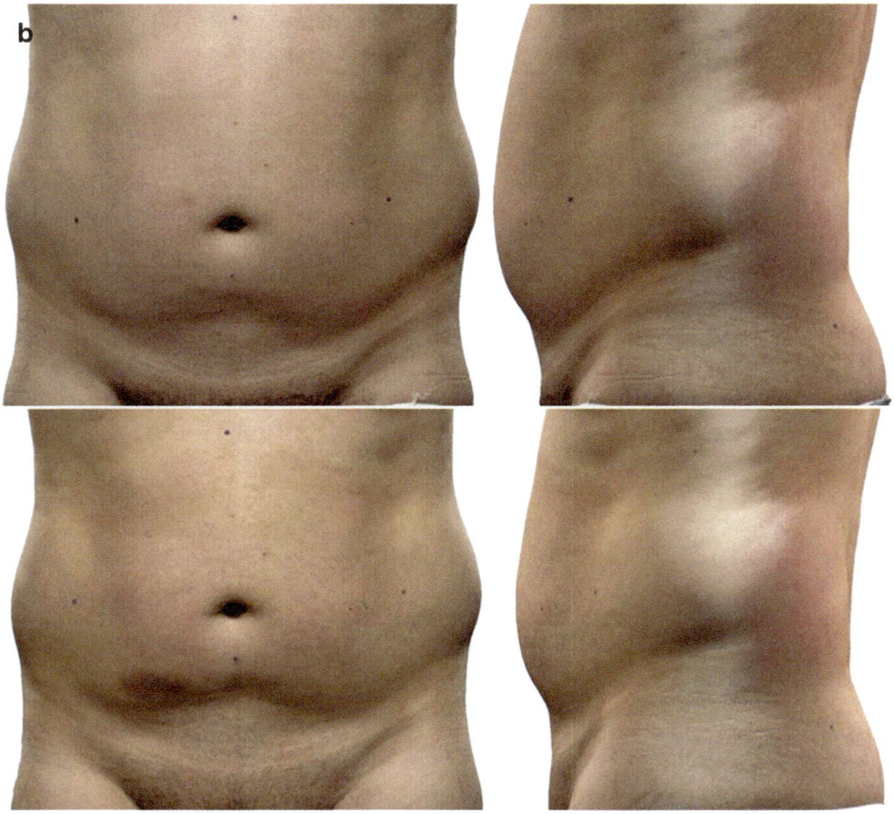

Fig. 12.12 (continued)

Another small but methodologically compelling study provides additional insight into the response of subcutaneous fat to lipolytic compounds [41]. An injected combination of steroid (prednisolone) and a nonselective β-agonist (isoproterenol) produced an average volume decrease of 50 % in ten lipomas injected five times a week for 1 month. There were no acute or chronic adverse effects. All except one of the lipomas, which were measured up to 1 year posttreatment, recurred.

It is perhaps too early to tell whether LIPO-102 or any similarly acting lipolytic compound becomes a very useful minimally invasive (injectable) treatment for fat reduction. Ideal injection technique, dosing, and patient selection are still unknown. The data suggests rapid onset after frequent treatment but some (yet undefined) likelihood of fat re-accumulation several months after treatment. Lithera is seeking approval of its drug for anterior abdominal fat reduction as well as exophthalmos related to retro-orbital fat accumulation. Should the durability of the treatment response be limited to only to several months, pharmaceutical lipoplasty may be a boon to aesthetic medicine (recurrent, nonpermanent treatments like hyaluronic acid tissue fillers and botulinum toxin are the gold standard among injectables). On the other hand, lipolytic agents may fall short if expectations are that any fat treatment, including a simple, "no downtime" injectable, be permanent.

Conclusions

A safe and effective injectable capable of reducing fat may become available in the near future. Injectable fat-reducing therapies are not an alternative to liposuction or other forms of "body sculpting." Rather, they may be best and more appropriate for patients unwilling or unable to have surgical reduction of small collections of fat or for those patients who desire touch-ups for liposuction-induced irregularities. Extensive preclinical safety testing and rigorous clinical trials demonstrating a favorable product profile using a pharmaceutical-grade formulation will be required for regulatory authority approval. Novel lipolytic (LIPO-102) and adipolytic (ATX-101) agents are currently in registration trials. Physicians should avoid compounded, nonregulated medications for the purpose of reducing fat and anticipate the outcome of FDA-registered clinical trials shortly.

Disclosure Dr. Rotunda is the coinventor of several patents that describe methods to reduce subcutaneous fat with deoxycholate. Dr. Rotunda is a consultant to KYTHERA Biopharmaceuticals, Lithera, and Allergan.

References

1. Ablon G, Rotunda AM (2004) Treatment of lower eyelid fat pads using phosphatidylcholine: clinical trial and review. Dermatol Surg 30:422–427
2. American Society for Dermatologic Surgery (2005) Emerging technology report: mesotherapy. Available at: http://www.asds-net.org/Media/PositionStatements/emerging_technology-mesotherapy.html. Accessed 15 June 2009
3. American Society for Aesthetic Plastic Surgery (2007) American Society for Aesthetic Plastic Surgery warns patients to steer clear of injection fat loss treatments. Available at: http://www.surgery.org/press/news-release.php?iid1⁄4475. Accessed 15 June 2009
4. Amin SP, Phelps RG, Goldberg DJ (2006) Mesotherapy for facial skin rejuvenation: a clinical, histologic, and electron microscopic evaluation. Dermatol Surg 32:1467–1472
5. Atiyeh BS, Ibrahim AE, Dibo SA (2008) Cosmetic mesotherapy: between scientific evidence, science fiction, and lucrative business. Aesthetic Plast Surg 32:842–849
6. Bangham JA, Lea EJ (1978) The interaction of detergents with bilayer lipid membranes. Biochim Biophys Acta 511:388–396
7. Bechara FG, Sand M, Hoffmann K et al (2007) Fat tissue after lipolysis of lipomas: a histopathological and immunohistochemical study. J Cutan Pathol 34:552–557
8. Beer K, Waibel J (2009) Disfiguring scarring following mesotherapy associated Mycobacterium cosmeticum infection. J Drugs Dermatol 8:391–393
9. Bentow J, Suzuki H, Nahmood N et al (2009) Phosphatidylcholine inhibits the adipolytic activity of deoxycholate in vitro and in vivo. The 5th Continent Congress. Abstract
10. Boodman SG (2007) Can shots safely 'Melt Away Fat'? Washington Post. Available at: http://www.washingtonpost.com/wp-dyn/content/article/2007/06/22/AR2007062201870.html. Accessed 15 June 2009
11. Carbonne A, Brossier F, Arnaud I et al (2009) Outbreak of nontuberculous Mycobacterial subcutaneous infections related to multiple mesotherapy injections. J Clin Microbiol 47:1961–1964
12. Cacchio A, De Blasis E, Desiati P et al (2009) Effectiveness of treatment of calcific tendinitis of the shoulder by disodium EDTA. Arthritis Rheum 15:84–91

13. Consumer Safety Alert on Fat Dissolving Injections (2007) Available at: http://www.prnewswire.com. Accessed 15 June 2009
14. Davis MD, Wright TI, Shehan JM (2008) A complication of mesotherapy: noninfectious granulomatous panniculitis. Arch Dermatol 144:808–809
15. Duncan DI, Hasengschwandtner F (2005) Lipodissolve for subcutaneous fat reduction and skin retraction. Aesthetic Surg J 25:530–543
16. Duncan D, Rubin JP, Golitz L, Badylak S, Kesel L, Freund J, Duncan D et al (2009) Refinement of technique in injection lipolysis based on scientific studies and clinical evaluation. Clin Plast Surg 36:195–209
17. Duncan D (2005) Lipodissolve for subcutaneous fat reduction and skin retraction. Aesthetic Surg J 25:530–543
18. Durr M, Hager J, Lohr JP (1994) Investigations on mixed micelle and liposome preparations for parenteral use based on soya phosphatidylcholine. Eur J Biopharma 40:147–156
19. Goldman MP (2004) Sodium tetradecyl sulfate for sclerotherapy treatment of veins: is compounding pharmacy solution safe? Dermatol Surg 30:1454–1456
20. Greenway FL, Bray GA (1987) Regional fat loss from the thigh in obese women after adrenergic modulation. Clin Ther 9:663–669
21. Gupta A, Lobocki C, Singh S et al (2009) Actions and comparative efficacy of phosphatidylcholine formulation and isolated sodium deoxycholate for different cell types. Aesthetic Plast Surg 33:346–352
22. Hexsel DM, Serra M, de Oliveira Dal'Forno T et al (2003) Phosphatidylcholine in the treatment of localized fat. J Drugs Dermatol 2:511–518
23. Hexsel DM, Serra M, de Oliveira Dal'Forno T, Zechmeister do Prado D (2005) Cosmetic uses of injectable PC on the face. Otolarngol Clin N Am 38:1119–1129
24. Janke J, Engeli S et al (2009) Compounds used for injection lipolysis destroy adipocytes and other cells found in adipose tissue. Obes Facts 2:36–39
25. Jones MN (1999) Surfactants in membrane solubilisation. Int J Pharm 177:137–159
26. KCTV 5 News (2007) Lipodissolve company to file bankruptcy. Available at: http://www.kctv5.com/news/14822891/detail.html. Accessed 15 June 2009
27. Klein SM, Schreml S, Nerlich M et al (2009) In vitro studies investigating the effect of subcutaneous phosphatidylcholine injections in the 3T3-L1 adipocyte model: lipolysis or lipid dissolution? Plast Reconstr Surg 124:419–427
28. Kopera D, Binder B, Toplak H (2006) Intralesional lipolysis with phosphatidylcholine for the treatment of lipomas: pilot study. Arch Dermatol 142:395–396
29. Kythera Biopharmaceuticals. Available at: http://www.kytherabiopharma.com/newsroom/. Accessed 13 Feb 2011
30. Lacarrubba F, Tedeschi A, Nardone B et al (2008) Mesotherapy for skin rejuvenation: assessment of the subepidermal low-echogenic band by ultrasound evaluation with cross-sectional B-mode scanning. Dermatol Ther 21:S1–S5
31. Lee JH, Park JG, Lim SH et al (2006) Localized intradermal microinjection of tranexamic acid for treatment of melasma in Asian patients: a preliminary clinical trial. Dermatol Surg 32:626–631
32. Lichtenberg D (1985) Characterization of the solubilization of lipid bilayers by surfactants. Biochim Biophys Acta 821:470–478
33. Lichtenberg D, Zilberman Y, Greenzaid P et al (1979) Structural and kinetic studies on the solubilization of lecithin by sodium deoxycholate. Biochemistry 18:3517–3525
34. Matarasso A, Pfeifer TM (2009) Mesotherapy and injection lipolysis. Clin Plast Surg 36:181–192
35. Motolese P (2008) Phospholipids do not have lipolytic activity. A critical review. J Cosmet Laser Ther 10:114–118
36. Myers P (2006) The cosmetic use of phosphatidylcholine in the treatment of localized fat deposits. Cosmet Dermatol 19:4120–4160
37. Palmer M, Curran J, Bowler P (2006) Clinical experience and safety using phosphatidylcholine injections for the localized reduction of subcutaneous fat: a multicentre, retrospective UK study. J Cosmet Dermatol 5:218–226

38. Park SH, Kim DW, Lee MA et al (2008) Effectiveness of mesotherapy on body contouring. Plast Reconstr Surg 121:179e–185e
39. Pistor M (1964) Mesotherapy. Librairie Maloine S.A., Paris
40. Rang HP, Dale MM, Ritter JM et al (2003) Chapter 11: Pharmacology. Elsevier Churchill Livingstone, Philadelphia
41. Redman LM, Moro C, Dobak J et al (2011) Association of beta-2 adrenergic agonist and corticosteroid injection in the treatment of lipomas. Diabetes Obes Metab 13:517–522
42. Rittes PG (2001) The use of phosphatidylcholine for correction of lower lid bulging due to prominent fat pads. Dermatol Surg 27:391–392
43. Rittes PG (2007) Complications of Lipostabil Endova for treating localized fat deposits. Aesthetic Surg J 27:146–149
44. Rittes PG, Rittes JC, Carriel Amary MF (2006) Injection of phosphatidylcholine in fat tissue: experimental study of local action in rabbits. Aesthetic Plast Surg 30:474–478
45. Rittes PG (2009) The lipodissolve technique: clinical experience. Clin Plast Surg 36:215–221
46. Rotunda AM, Avram MM, Avram AS (2005) Cellulite: is there a role for injectables? J Cosmet Laser Ther 7:147–154
47. Rotunda AM, Avram MM (2009) The importance of caution in the use of unregulated anticellulite treatments. Arch Dermatol 145:337
48. Rotunda AM, Commentary to Schuller-Petrovic et al (2008) Tissue-toxic effects of phosphatidylcholine/deoxycholate after subcutaneous injection for fat dissolution in rats and a human volunteer. Dermatol Surg 34:534–535
49. Rotunda AM, Kolodney MS (2006) Mesotherapy and phosphatidylcholine injections: historical clarification and review. Dermatol Surg 32:465–480
50. Rotunda AM, Weiss SR, Rivkin LS (2009) Randomized double-blind clinical trial of subcutaneously injected deoxycholate versus a phosphatidylcholine-deoxycholate combination for the reduction of submental fat. Dermatol Surg 35:792–803
51. Rotunda AM, Ablon G, Kolodney MS (2005) Lipomas treated with subcutaneous deoxycholate injections. J Am Acad Dermatol 53:973–978
52. Rotunda AM, Jones DH (2010) HIV-associated lipohypertrophy (buccal fat-pad lipoma-like lesions) reduced with subcutaneously injected sodium deoxycholate. Dermatol Surg 36:1348–1354
53. Rotunda AM, Suzuki H, Moy RL et al (2004) Detergent effects of sodium deoxycholate are a major feature of an injectable phosphatidylcholine formulation used for localized fat dissolution. Dermatol Surg 30:1001–1008
54. Rundle RL (2007) Popular treatment that aims to melt fat draws scrutiny. *Wall Street Journal.* Available at: http://online.wsj.com/article/SB118160554567831887.html?mod1⁄4home_health_right. Accessed 15 June 2009
55. Salti G, Ghersetich I, Tantussi F et al (2008) Phosphatidylcholine and sodium deoxycholate in the treatment of localized fat: a double-blind, randomized study. Dermatol Surg 34:60–66
56. Schuller-Petrovic S, Wolkart G, Hofler G et al (2008) Tissue-toxic effects of phosphatidylcholine/deoxycholate after subcutaneous injection for fat dissolution in rats and a human volunteer. Dermatol Surg 34:524–529
57. Thuangtong R, Bentow JJ, Knopp K et al (2010) Tissue-selective effects of injected deoxycholate. Dermatol Surg 36:899–908
58. Tisi PV, Beverley C, Rees A (2006) Injection sclerotherapy for varicose veins. Cochrane Database Syst Rev 4:CD001732
59. Treacy P, Goldberg D (2006) Use of phosphatidylcholine for the correction of lower lid bulging due to prominent fat pads. J Cosmet Laser Ther 8:129–132
60. United States Food and Drug Administration (USFDA) (2008) Statement on lipo dissolve. Available at: http://www.fda.gov. Accessed 15 June 2009
61. Yagina Odo YME, Cuce LC, Odo LM et al (2007) Action of sodium deoxycholate on subcutaneous human tissue: local and systemic effects. Dermatol Surg 33:178–188

Cosmetic Procedures in Asian Skin

13

Evangeline B. Handog, Ma. Teresita G. Gabriel, and Jonathan A. Dizon

Core Messages

- Various studies by Asian dermatologists showed that Asian skin types encompassed SPTs II–V.
- Asian skin is less prone to premature aging, wrinkling, and sagging, than their Caucasian counterparts.
- The aging Asian skin is more prone to pigmentary alterations, in contrast to Caucasian skin.
- Cosmetic procedures in Asian patients require more caution and deep understanding of possible complications.
- The less invasive, non-ablative procedures are more suited and favored by Asians because of the low downtime and decreased risk of unwanted reactions.

E.B. Handog, M.D., FPDS (✉)
Department of Dermatology, Room 316, Asian Hospital and Medical Center, 2205 Civic Drive, Filinvest Corporate City, Alabang, Muntinlupa City, Metro Manila 1780, Philippines

Department of Health Philippines, Research Institute for Tropical Medicine, Muntinlupa City, Philippines
e-mail: vangee@handog.net

M.T.G. Gabriel, M.D., FPDS
Department of Dermatology, Research Institute for Tropical Medicine, Alabang, Muntinlupa City, Philippines
e-mail: tcilygab@pldtdsl.net

J.A. Dizon, M.D., FPDS
Cosmetic Dermatology Unit, Ospital ng Maynila Medical Center, Manila, Philippines

A. Tosti, D. Hexsel (eds.), *Update in Cosmetic Dermatology*,
DOI 10.1007/978-3-642-34029-1_13,

St. Luke's Medical Center,
Suite 1410- North Tower Cathedral Heights Building Complex, 279 E.
Rodriguez Sr. Boulevard, Quezon City 1100, Philippines
e-mail: jonathandizonmd@yahoo.com

13.1 Background

Asia is the world's largest and most inhabited continent, covering 8.6 % of the Earth's total surface area (or 29.9 % of its land area), and with over four billion people, it contains more than 60 % of the world's current human population. Given its size and diversity, Asian ethnic features vary. There are the East Asians (Chinese, Japanese, Koreans, Mongolians), the South Asians (Indians, Pakistanis, Sri Lankans, Bangladeshi), and Southeast Asians (Filipinos, Thais, Indonesians, Malaysians, Singaporeans, Vietnamese, Cambodians, and the people from Brunei, Laos, Myanmar, Timor-Leste). The origin of Asians dates back to classical antiquity. Asia now is more of a cultural concept incorporating vast regions and peoples, rather than a homogeneous physical entity [25].

Scholarly attempts at classification of Asians as a group have been berthed by controversies between anthropologists, forensic scientists, sociologists, and biogeneticist, and various terms had been coined to describe Asians based mainly but not exclusively on ethnicities, origin, ancestry, culture, traditions, religious practices, or convenience [20, 24]. This is because Asians belong to a heterogeneous group having divergent features. Those from East Asia are of Mongoloid ethnic origin and tend to have lighter skin color. South Asians are of Caucasian ethnicity but generally have brown skin. Southeast Asians are of Malay and Mongoloid ethnicity and have very light to very dark brown skin color.

Most medical practitioners, notably the dermatologists, rely upon one or more skin classification systems as a valuable tool in diagnostics and therapeutics [3, 6]. The denominating factors are based mainly on skin and hair color and the ability to tan or burn or to produce dyschromias. In the Fitzpatrick skin phototype (SPT) system, modern Asian skin is considered as "skin of color" falling within SPTs IV and V but is expanded to include SPTs II and III [14, 34]. There are many Asian Americans (e.g., Vietnamese and Koreans) and even fair-skinned persons (e.g., Arabs, Pakistanis, Indians) who also would be classified as having types IV and V skin. A segment of each of the previously described ethnic groups could be classified as having SPT III or even SPT II skin. This reflects the variability between the races as well as intermarriage between races [26]. Hence, Asian skin tone may vary from the palest to the darkest shade of brown, while textural variations may range from smooth and fine to rough and thick. Youn and colleagues demonstrated in their study of a Korean population that skin types encompassed SPTs of II, III, IV, and V rather than only V [34].

The exact history of cosmetic dermatology is vague. Man's inherent quest for self-preservation and beauty can be seen recorded in prehistoric wall carvings and ancient manuscripts. Evidences and descriptions of aesthetic concerns and interventions were recorded not only by the Egyptians, Sumerians, Persians, Turks, Arabs, Greeks, or Romans but also by the Aztecs and Incas, the ancient Chinese, and the Indian civilization [1].

The era of cosmetic dermatology, as we know it today, may have started in the 1950s since almost all of the relevant equipment of contemporary aesthetic dermatology were developed after 1950 [31].

In the Philippines, dermatology as a specialty started with the founding of the Philippine Dermatological Society in 1952. Within Asia and elsewhere in the 1970s, the origins of cosmetic dermatology started to be felt with procedures like dermabrasion and chemical peeling. The advent of cosmetic botulinum toxin and ablative laser resurfacing using the CO_2 laser in the early 1980s paved the way for the exodus of emerging technologies, gadgets, and new techniques [31].

The skylines in Asian cities are changing. Similarly, the field of cosmetic and procedural dermatologic research and biotechnological advancements has evolved dramatically over the last several years. The specialists of today, apart from pathologic dermatology, are becoming more adept in aesthetic procedures and are faced with different and newer challenges compared with their counterparts several generations back. Participation in this new environment of modernization is increasing in Asian dermatology clinics across the continents. Due to globalization, recent trends have evolved and will surely spread radially as the demand by more Asians continues to grow. The popularity of cosmetic dermatologic procedures is an all-time high and has become a billion-dollar industry. The challenge now for dermatologists caring for Asian skin is to establish a more solid scientific base for its own techniques and procedures. Contrary to existing trend, the adage "newer is always better" does not hold true for Asian skin.

13.2 Clinical Features

Biological differences and factors like diet and nutrition, the presence of comorbid conditions or sequelae from endemic diseases, and certain social-cultural-religious practices potentially alter the expression of diseases and the physio-pharmaco-pathologic response to treatment [20].

Ethnic variations significantly alter the treatment milieu and preclude clinicians to exercise caution and care when treating Asian skin.

The Philippines is a merry mix of Asian ethnicities. Originally Malay, we were conquered by the Spaniards for more than three centuries and were under the Japanese and the Americans for decades. People with skin of color constitute a wide range of racial and ethnic groups—including Africans, African Americans, African Caribbeans, Chinese and Japanese, Native American Navajo Indians, certain groups of fair-skinned persons (e.g., Indians, Pakistanis, Arabs), and Hispanics. It has been predicted that people with skin of color will constitute a majority of the USA and international populations in the twenty-first century [26]. In the future, because of intermarriages and migration, it may be difficult to find a pure-blooded Filipino, Japanese, or Thai.

Acne and melasma consistently belong to the top ten reasons for consulting at the Research Institute for Tropical Medicine (RITM) Department of Health, Philippines, among 32,312 new general dermatology consults (RITM Census, 2004–2008). At the Dermatology Outpatient Department of the Ospital ng Maynila Medical Center (OMMC), Manila Health Department, Philippines, among 29,991 new consults, acne, post-inflammatory hyperpigmentation, and melasma were among the top ten diseases (OMMC Census, 2004–2008). Most of the patients' acnes were moderate and severe with predominance of inflammatory papules and pustules, and nodules and cysts, respectively. Among those with melasma aged 40–50 years, centrofacial and malar areas were the most common sites affected. Majority of these patients had the mixed type and on the average had melasma for about 5 years (Figs. 13.1 and 13.2).

Photoaging is universal and is a growing concern. Inevitably, people living near the equator will have visible signs of photoaging sooner than those living in other countries. The clinical signs associated with photoaging are dyspigmentation, laxity,

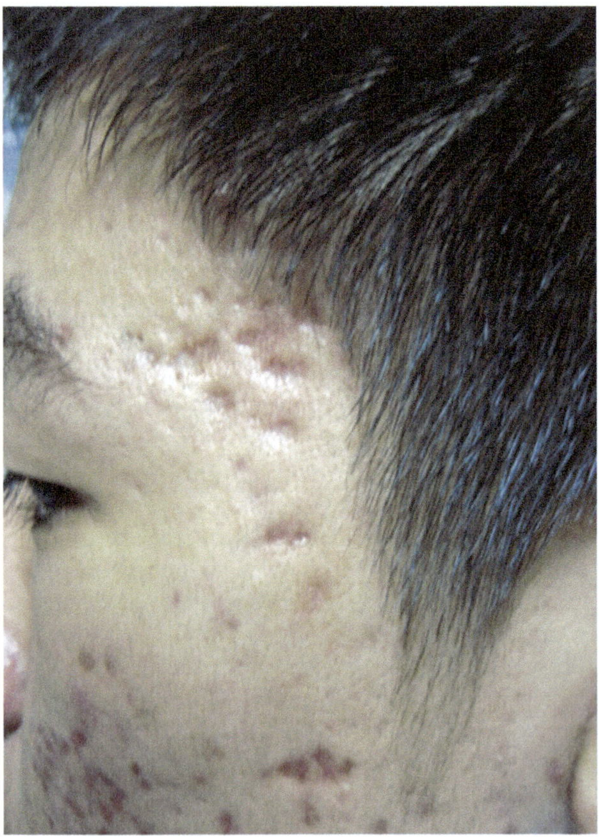

Fig. 13.1 Acne Scarring is a major concern among Filipinos

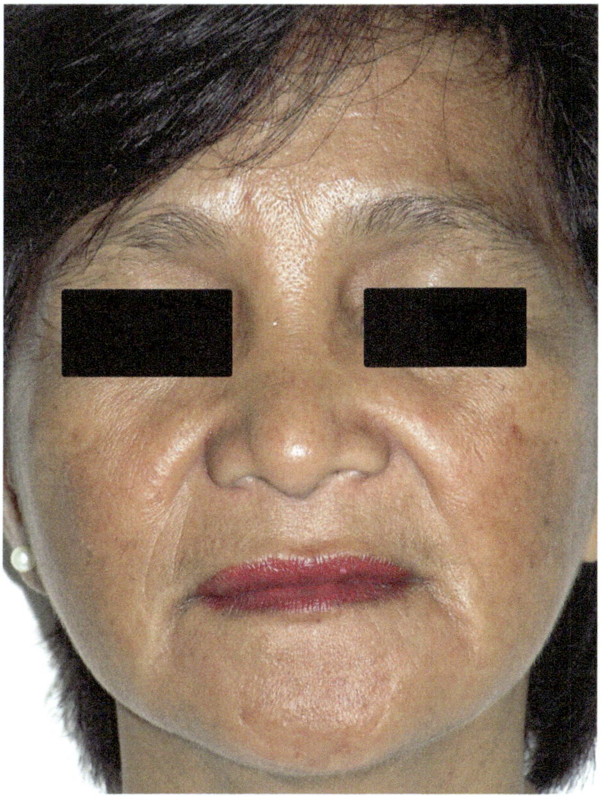

Fig. 13.2 Aging Skin includes melasma, wrinkles and sagging skin

a yellow hue, wrinkles, telangiectasia, a leathery appearance, and cutaneous malignancies [9, 15, 16, 30]. Old, photoprotected skin may have increased laxity and fold accentuation, but it is thin and lacks signs of actinic damage [13]. Seborrheic keratoses are common benign proliferative growths characteristic of aged skin and may be related to sun exposure [32].

An informal survey on the most common consults and dermatologic procedures was conducted last November 2008 by the authors among 450 Filipino board-certified dermatologists who are members of the Philippine Dermatological Society. Results showed that treatments for acne scarring, verruca plana, seborrheic keratoses, photorejuvenation, and hair reduction were among the five main reasons why patients consult in aesthetic dermatology. Patients also consult for dyschromia; telangiectasia; pathologic conditions like warts, small benign tumors, vascular malformations, or genodermatoses; and mesotherapy. Interestingly, more males were found to have seborrheic keratoses, most of which were located on the face. The most common procedures done were acne surgery for acne and subcision for rolling and boxcar scars acne scars; skin resurfacing (microdermabrasion, chemical peeling, and lasers); electrocautery/electrosurgery for warts and benign tumors; various laser therapy procedures for photorejuvenation and hair reduction; and botulinum toxin injections for hyperhidrosis. Also done were contouring procedures for the face and body using

Table 13.1 Ten [10] most common cosmetic procedures

1. Acne surgery and subcision
2. Microdermabrasion
3. Chemical peeling
4. Electrocautery/electrosurgery
5. IPL and lasers
6. Hair removal
7. Botox
8. Fillers
9. Mesotherapy
10. Sclerotherapy

injectable fillers, botulinum toxin injections, fat transfer, and radiofrequency and energy devices (Table 13.1). Important to note were consultations for skin whitening. Filipinos in general have brown complexion and prefer to be fair.

13.3 Pathophysiology

Evolutional adaptation resulted in ethnic biological differences. This diversity in skin coloration is thought to be an evolutional response to the interplay of intrinsic and extrinsic factors exemplified by genetics and environmental effects, mainly from ultraviolet light exposure [4, 7, 11, 23].

Moschella defines aging as a progressive, intrinsic, time-dependent deterioration of an organism's structural or functional integrity and may be reflected in the ability of that organism to interact with and respond to its environment. The aging process encompasses progressive physiological changes that lead to senescence; it refers to the decline of biological functions and the organism's ability to adapt to metabolic stress with time [8]. Aging comes in two forms, intrinsic and extrinsic.

Intrinsic or biological aging is genetically programmed and a continuous non-preventable process that occurs over a certain number of years regardless of ethnicity. In the natural aging process, oxidative stress occurs at a rate at which the skin is no longer able to fully neutralize free radicals. Free radicals damage cellular DNA resulting in an aged appearance. Genes control how quickly the normal aging process manifests. The signs of intrinsic aging are typically not visible till much later in life, usually starting by the second decade of life. As collagen and elastin productions slow, the following physical changes appear: fine wrinkles; thin, dry, and transparent (atrophic) skin; loss of underlying fat leading to hollowed cheeks and eye sockets; and bones shrinking away from the skin due to bone loss, all of which cause the skin to fold and sag. Hair changes are inevitable, such as thinning, graying or loss of hair, or appearance of unwanted hair growth.

Extrinsic or environmental aging results from the cumulative exogenous effects of oxidative stress like prolonged unprotected sun or ultraviolet exposure, pollution, smoking, severe psychological and physical stress, overeating, and physical inactivity.

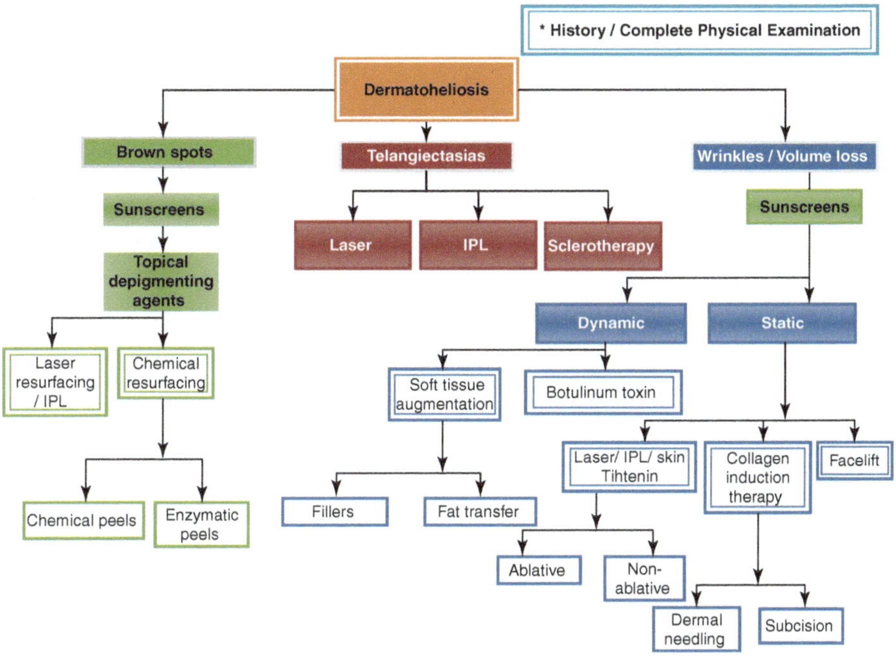

Fig. 13.3 Approach to aging Asian skin

This results to the release of free radicals giving rise to cytokines (e.g., IL-1 and IL-6) responsible for inflammation and increase in metallomyeloproteinases, which then leads to collagen breakdown, all of these directing to premature aging. *Dermatoheliosis or photoaging* is a term to describe the array of clinical and histological findings which characterize chronically sun-exposed skin [12, 13]. Common among Asians, it is characterized by hyperpigmentation or brown spots, telangiectasia, and wrinkling plus volume loss. Together, these represent a spectrum of clinical conditions requiring cosmetic procedures for treatment (Fig. 13.3).

Racial and ethnic differences in skin color are due to variations in the number, size, and aggregation of the melanosomes within the melanocyte and keratinocyte. Clearly demonstrated are racial or ethnic differences in the melanosome size and aggregation within keratinocytes [12, 19, 27]. The color of the skin is determined by the quantity and types of melanin synthesized in melanocytes located on the stratum basalis (epidermal basal cell layer) [21]. Keratinocytes also play a significant role in skin color determination by regulating the distribution pattern of melanosomes in the epidermis and by producing cytokines involved in melanogenesis [33].

All skin types have the same number of melanocytes and common melanogenic mechanisms but differ in melanosome size and melanin pigment content [2, 5]. Ethnic pigmented skin, as seen among Asians, are more melanized and have bigger melanosomes, whereas Caucasian skin is lighter because of the smaller, more lightly pigmented melanosomes. People of African ethnicity have much darker skin due to larger, more melanized melanosomes located not just in the basal cell layer but throughout the epidermis [19]. Larger, more melanized melanosomes scatter and absorb more energy thereby providing greater inherent photoprotection. Furthermore, the melanocytes and mesenchyma in darker skin types seem to be more vulnerable to trauma and inflammatory conditions [26]. An increased mesenchymal reactivity may result in hypertrophic scarring and keloid formation. Although the exact mechanisms are now just being understood, these findings help explain why almost any procedure that produces severe or prolonged inflammation in Asians and other "people of color" have consequential adverse risks of pigmentary alterations, textural changes, prolonged erythema, and keloid formation [18].

Being more pigmented, Asian skin manifests with more dyschromias like brown age spots when compared to white Caucasian skin. Other findings are loose inelastic skin, a blotchy complexion, telangiectasia on the face, rough and leathery skin, and lines, wrinkles, and folds. *Poikiloderma* refers to varied skin conditions with a mottled appearance, characterized by patchy areas of telangiectasia, atrophy, and hyperpigmentation.

Telangiectasias are small dilated blood vessels near the surface of the skin or mucous membranes, measuring between 0.5 and 1 mm in diameter. They can develop anywhere on the body but are commonly seen on the face around the nose, cheeks, and chin. They can also develop on the legs, specifically on the upper thigh, below the knee joint, and around the ankles. Because these are vascular lesions, they blanch when tested with diascopy.

Current concepts view wrinkles to be the result of volume loss secondary to collagen and elastin depletion and to fat and bone atrophy. Wrinkles come in various degrees of severity and are classified either as dynamic (in motion) or static (at rest). The predominant wrinkle form will depend on age, habits, and lifestyle.

13.4 Methods/Products

The reduction of pigment, scars, and other skin lesions from the skin is dependent on a process called "skin remodeling."

Benign pigmentary changes, like hyperpigmentation or brown spots, can be managed with depigmenting agents as first-line therapy. More frequently used by Filipino dermatologists as lightening agents are hydroquinone, arbutin, kojic acid, licorice, azelaic acid, salicylic acid, lactic acid, alpha-hydroxy acids, and tretinoin. These regimens are easily available, cost-effective, and offer minimal side effects. Patient compliance is likewise better. Procedures that are being used for pigment alterations are Q-switched ND-YAG laser or IPL, mechanical resurfacing with microdermabrasion, and chemical resurfacing using various acid peels or fruit enzymes. The Q-switched ND-YAG is the optimal laser for treating melanocytic processes in SPTs III–VI. However, these technologies are skill dependent and more expensive and carry a higher risk of possible complications. Due to prohibitive cost, patients are unable to complete treatment sessions. Standard laser parameters may not necessarily apply to Asian skin since most studies were done on Caucasians.

Aggressive chemical resurfacing among Asian skin is associated with higher incidence of post-inflammatory hyperpigmentation, rarely hypertrophic scarring.

Telangiectasias can be managed with IPL, various vascular lasers like pulsed-dye laser, diode and sclerotherapy.

Strategies for medical treatment and intervention for photoaging can be categorized into a unique paradigm based on disease prevention. Primary prevention refers to the reduction of risk factors before a disease or condition has occurred. The goal of secondary prevention is early detection of the disease, potentially while still asymptomatic; this allows positive interference to prevent, postpone, or attenuate the symptomatic clinical condition. Tertiary prevention is the treatment of an existing symptomatic disease process to ameliorate its effects or delay its progress [17].

Primary prevention entails the use of photoprotection. The single most cost-effective therapy that can be offered to patients is sun protection [10]. Most quality sunscreen would combine ingredients to yield a product with excellent photoprotection. Since filters would have different peak absorption range, it is ideal to have a sunscreen that is broad spectrum with coverage against UVB and UVA.

Secondary treatment options include the use of retinoic acid, antioxidants, estrogens, and growth factors. Retinoids have been the mainstay of topical therapy for the prevention and treatment of photoaging [10]. Tretinoin (all-transretinoic acid), a nonselective agent that activates all retinoic acid receptors (RARs) directly and retinoid X receptor (RXR), has been shown to improve the clinical signs of photoaging in controlled clinical trials [28, 29].

Tertiary therapies have been popularized because they not only target the clinical characteristics of photoaged skin but can also be used in intrinsic aging as well as cosmetic augmentation [22]. Under tertiary management, the following are being utilized: chemical peels, resurfacing techniques like microdermabrasion or microablation, lasers including ablative and non-ablative systems, radiofrequency technologies, botulinum toxins, and soft tissue augmentation.

In the Philippines, wrinkles are being treated using a variety of combination regimen: laser resurfacing; botulinum toxin injections, soft tissue augmentation, and volumization using fillers or autologous fat; skin tightening procedures using lasers, IPL, or radiofrequency devices; and collagen induction treatments using dermal needles and subcision wires or needles.

Laser resurfacing is a technique to remove areas of damaged or wrinkled skin layer by layer. It may be performed in specific regions or on the entire face. The procedure is most commonly used to minimize the appearance of fine lines. In many instances, invasive procedures like thread lifts or even surgical rhytidectomy (facelifts) are other options.

Botulinum toxin injections are being used for dynamic wrinkles. Patient satisfaction is evident in a week's time. This procedure is repeated every 4–6 months. Likewise, there is an increasing number of patients using this modality for contouring of the jawline.

For acne scars, Filipino dermatologists do the following procedures: subcision for rolling and box-type scars, skin resurfacing using microdermabrasion or lasers, and moderately deep chemical peeling.

IPL and diode laser for hair reduction are more popular among the younger age group.

The clinical indications of lasers and light sources among Asians are similar to their Caucasian counterparts and are classified based on the chromophore target of destruction. These include the use of pigment-specific vascular, hair reduction, and ablative and non-ablative laser systems. In our practice of using these systems, we usually follow the preset parameters recommended by the device manufacturers based on the patients' individual skin phototype. But with the knowledge that Asians tend to have an increased risk for dyschromias or textural changes, we lower the parameters by 10–20 % below the recommended preset parameters. Initiating a test spot treatment for each patient, we then adjust the parameters, going higher or lower, based on our results. This is especially true with the use of Q-switched lasers and IPL. To further prevent epidermal damage, we do precooling of the skin using cool air, cold packs, gels, or cryospray devices. We likewise recommend pretreatment medications composed of a depigmenting agent for 2–4 weeks and avoidance of sun and heat exposure.

When treating benign epidermal lesions in Asians, we choose a pulse width (millisecond) that matches the thermal relaxation time of the epidermis (10 ms), so the risk of thermal injury to the dermis is minimized.

With the advent of several types of fillers, soft tissue augmentation has gained popularity mostly for nasolabial folds and Marionette's lines. Volumization is also indicated for lipoatrophy. Disadvantages include bruising, beading, and pain during the procedure. Only a few patients submit to this procedure due to its prohibitive cost.

Skin tightening procedures have been recently introduced, mostly with the use of radiofrequency devices and IPL. Results are not that remarkable unless patients complete several sessions. Lower settings are recommended for Asian skin to prevent complications like burning or hyperpigmentation.

Use of dermal needles or subcision wires/needles for deep wrinkles has been employed by a few dermatologists in the Philippines to date.

Electrocautery/electrosurgery is used with ease, within the clinic setup, to remove warts and benign tumors.

For patients with excessive palmar hyperhidrosis, aside from topical aluminum chloride application, botulinum toxin injections may be used but they have the disadvantage of being very expensive and painful.

For volume loss, fillers and autologous fat transfer are being suggested. Mesotherapy, carboxytherapy, and radiofrequency used for contouring are new technologies being utilized but not very popular. In our setting, these procedures are well tolerated.

All procedures which have been enumerated are skill dependent. The success of the different regimens is dependent on various factors, namely, dermatologist's training, parameters, patient compliance, and lifestyle.

Among the adjunct therapy that may help retard skin aging are music therapy, exercise, dancing, balanced diet, enough sleep, aromatherapy, yoga, power of touch, increased fluid intake, and moisturization. More so, "laughter is still the best medicine."

Acknowledgment The authors wish to thank Dr. Clarisse G. Mendoza for the technical assistance in the preparation of this chapter.

References

1. Akerknecht EH (1982) A short history of medicine, 2nd edn. JHU Press, Baltimore
2. Alaluf S, Atkins D, Barret K, Blount M, Carter N, Heath A (2002) Ethnic variation in melanin content and composition in photoexposed and protected human skin. Pigment Cell Res 15: 112–118
3. Bauman L (2006) New skin typing system. Skin Aging 14:2 http://www.skinandaging.com/article/5334
4. Berardesca E, Maibach HI (1996) Racial differences in skin pathophysiology. J Am Acad Dermatol 34:667–672
5. Boissy RE, Huizing M, Gahl WA (2006) Chapter 7: Biogenesis of melanosomes. In: Nordlund JJ, Boissy RE, Hearing VJ, King RA, Oetting WS, Ortonne J-P (eds) The pigmentary system. Blackwell Publishing, Oxford, pp 155–170
6. Caulfield T, Fullerton SM, Ali-Khan SE et al (2009) Race and ancestry in biomedical research: exploring the challenges. Genome Med 1(1):8
7. Diamond J (2005) Evolutionary biology: geography and skin colour. Nature 435:283–284
8. Rabe JH, Mamelak AJ, McElgunn PJS et al (2006) Photoaging: Mechanisms and Repair. J Am Acad Dermatol 55:1–19
9. Gilchrest BA, Yaar M (1992) Ageing and photoageing of the skin: observations at the cellular and molecular level. Br J Dermatol 127:25–30
10. Glaser DA (2003) Anti-aging products and cosmeceuticals. Facial Plast Surg Clin North Am 11:219–227
11. Jablonski NG, Chaplin G (2000) The evolution of human skin coloration. J Hum Evol 39: 57–106
12. Johnson BL Jr (1998) Differences in skin type. In: Johnson BL Jr, Moy RL, White GM (eds) Ethnic skin: medical and surgical. Mosby, St. Louis, pp 3–5
13. Lavker RM (1995) Cutaneous aging: chronologic versus photoaging. In: Gilchrest BA (ed) Photodamage. Blackwell Science pp, Cambridge, pp 123–135
14. Leenutaphong V (1995) Relationship between skin color and cutaneous response to ultraviolet radiation in Thai. Photodermatol Photoimmunol Photomed 11:198–203
15. Lewis KG, Bercovitch L, Dill SW, Robinson-Bostom L (2004) Acquired disorders of elastic tissue: part I. Increased elastic tissue and solar elastotic syndromes. J Am Acad Dermatol 51:1–21
16. Leyden JJ (1990) Clinical features of aging skin. Br J Dermatol 122:1–3
17. Matzen RN (2004) Preventive medicine: definition and application. In: Lang RS, Hensrud DD (eds) Clinical preventive medicine. AMA Press, Chicago, pp 3–9
18. Mc Curdy JA (1998) Facial surgery in the Asian patient. In: Matory WE (ed) Ethnic considerations in facial aesthetic surgery. Lipppincott Raven, Philadelphia, pp 263–284
19. Montagna W, Carlisle K, Beaverton MS (1991) The architecture of black and white facial skin. J Am Acad Dermatol 24:929–937
20. Ossario P, Duster T (2005) Race and genetics: controversies in biomedical, behavioral, and forensic sciences. Am Psychol 60(1):115–128
21. Quevedo WC, Holstein TJ (2006) General biology of mammalian pigmentation. In: Nordlund JJ, Boissy RE, Hearing VJ, King RA, Oetting WS, Ortonne J-P (eds) The pigmentary system. Blackwell Publishing, Oxford, pp 63–90
22. Rabe JH, Mamelak AJ, Mc Elgunn PJ et al (2006) Photoaging: mechanisms and repair. J Am Acad Dermatol 55:1–19
23. Richards GM, Oresajo CO, Halder RM (2003) Structure and function of ethnic skin and hair. Dermatol Clin 21:595–600
24. Rohde DL, Olson S, Chang JT (2004) Modelling the recent common ancestry of all living humans. Nature 431:562–566
25. Soo-Jin Lee S, Mountain J, Koenig BA (2001) The meanings of race in the new genomics: implications for health disparities research. Yale J Health Policy Law Ethics 17:44

26. Taylor SC (2002) Skin of color: biology, structure, function, and implications for dermatologic disease. J Am Acad Dermatol 46:S41–S62
27. Toda K, Patnak MA, Parrish A, Fitzpatrick TB (1972) Alteration of racial differences in melanosome distribution in human epidermis after exposure to ultraviolet light. Nat New Biol 236:143–144
28. Weinstein GD, Nigra TP, Pochi PE, Savin RC, Allan A, Benik K et al (1991) Topical tretinoin for treatment of photodamaged skin. A multicenter study. Arch Dermatol 127:659–665
29. Weiss JS, Ellis CN, Headington JT, Tincoff T, Hamilton TA, Voorhees JJ (1988) Topical tretinoin improves photodamaged skin: a double-blind, vehicle-controlled study. JAMA 259:527–532
30. Wlaschek M, Tantcheva-Poor I, Naderi L, Ma W, Schneider LA, Razi-Wolf Z et al (2001) Solar UV irradiation and dermal photoaging. J Photochem Photobiol B 63:41–51
31. Carruthers JD, Carruthers JA (1992) Treatment of Glabellar Frown Lines with C. Botulinum-A Exotoxin. J Dermatol Surg Oncol 18(1):17–21
32. Yeatman JM, Kilkenny M, Marks R (1997) The prevalence of seborrhoeic keratoses in an Australian population: does exposure to sunlight play a part in their frequency? Br J Dermatol 137:411–414
33. Yoshida Y, Hachiya A, Sriwiriyanont P, Ohuchi A, Kitahara T, Takema Y, Visscher MO, Boissy RE (2007) Functional analysis of keratinocytes in skin color using a human skin substitute model composed of cells derived from different skin pigmentation types. FASEB J 21:2829–2839
34. Youn JI, Oh JK, Kim BK et al (1997) Relation between skin phototype and MED in Korean brown skin. Photodermatol Photoimmunol Photomed 13:208–211

Index

A
Ablative fractional photothermolysis, 81
Acne
  classification
    acne conglobata, 37
    acne cosmetica, 38–39
    acne excoriée, 39
    acne fulminans, 38
    acne inversa, 37
    acne neonatorum, 34–35
    acne vulgaris, 35
    adult acne, 35–37
    iatrogenic acne, 38–39
    infantile acne, 35
  cosmetological approach
    cleansing agents, 43
    keratolytics, 44
    moisturizing agents, 44
    photoprotection, 45
    sebum regulators, 44
  description, 34
  diagnosis, 41
  etiology
    classical aspects, 39
    diet and weight loss, 39
    sunlight and cosmetics, 39–40
  histology, 41–42
  incidence, 34
  pathophysiology, 40–41
  photodynamic therapy, 118–119
  prognosis, 42
  systemic medical treatment
    hormonal therapy, 48
    oral antibiotics, 47
    oral isotretinoin, 48
  topical medical treatment
    AHAs, 46
    antibiotics, 45
    camouflage, 47
    chemical peels, 46–47
    retinoids, 45
Acne cyst/inflammatory acne, 153, 157
Acne scarring, 206
Actinic keratosis, 117–118, 125, 153, 159–160
Adipolytic therapy, 182, 197–202
Adrenal steroid 21-hydroxylase deficiency (CYP21), 70
Adult acne, 35–37
Alpha hydroxy acids (AHAs)
  acne, 46
  cosmeceuticals, 103
Androgen-secreting tumors, 67
Antiandrogens, 69–70
Antibiotics
  acne, 45
  oral, 47
ATX-101, 196–197

B
Baumann skin type indicator, 6, 7
Biological aging, 208
Biometrical image tools
  confocal Raman spectroscopy, 15
  Dermascan®, 12–13, 15
  reflectance confocal microscopy, 13–14
  Skin Evidence™, 12, 14
  Visioscope® BW 30, 12
Blackheads, 42
Blepharoptosis, 136
Botulinum toxin
  injections, 211
  skin evaluation systems, 9
Botulinum toxin type A (BT-A)
  commercial preparation, 133
  cosmetic usage (*see* Cosmetic use, BT-A)
  dilution, 133
  handling, 134
  immunology, 132–133
  injection technique, 134
  physiology and pharmacology, 132–133
  reconstitution, 133

A. Tosti, D. Hexsel (eds.), *Update in Cosmetic Dermatology*,
DOI 10.1007/978-3-642-34029-1, © Springer-Verlag Berlin Heidelberg 2013

Bowen's disease, 125
Bunny lines, 138–139

C
CAH. *See* Congenital adrenal hyperplasia (CAH)
Camouflage, 47
Carbon dioxide laser, 81
Carboxytherapy, cellulite, 30
Cardiac pacemaker, 176
Cellulite
  anatomical considerations, 23–24
  characterization, 22
  classification, 25
  diagnosis, 25–26
  etiology, 23
  lesions on buttocks, 22
  pathophysiology, 23
  prevalence, 22–23
  prognosis, 30
  semiquantitative skin evaluation, 9
  Subcision® technique
    cellulite classification, 52–54
    complications, 59–60
    contraindications, 54, 55
    indications, 54, 55
    mechanism of action, 55
    patient selection, 54
    postoperative recommendations, 58–59
    preoperative recommendations, 56
    procedure technique, 57–58
  treatments
    carboxytherapy, 30
    Endermologie®, 28
    lasers, 28–29
    liposuction, 29
    manual lymphatic drainage, 26–27
    mesotherapy, 29
    oral treatment, 27–28
    radiofrequency, 28
    Subcision®, 29
    topical treatment, 27
Cellulite severity scale (CSS), 9, 25
Chemical peels, 46–47
Chest/décolleté wrinkles, 141
Clindamycin, 47
Clostridium botulinum, 132
Cone-spray technique, 151, 156
Confocal Raman spectroscopy, 15
Congenital adrenal hyperplasia (CAH), 67
Corneometer-pH-Meter-Sebumeter®, 17
Cosmetic procedures, in Asian skin
  clinical features, 205–208
  methods/products, 210–212
  pathophysiology, 208–210
Cosmetic use, BT-A
  extra facial areas, 141
  lower face
    dimpled chin, 140
    drooping mouth corner, 139
    face lift, 140
    GS, 140–141
    perioral rhytides, 140
  middle face
    bunny lines, 138–139
    cheeks, 139
    infraorbital rhytides, 138
    nasal tip/repeated nasal flare, 139
  upper face
    forehead lines, 137
    glabellar lines, 136
    lateral canthal lines, 137–138
    lateral eyebrow lift, 138
Cosmetological approach, acne
  cleansing agents, 43
  keratolytics, 44
  moisturizing agents, 44
  photoprotection, 45
  sebum regulators, 44
Crow's feet, 137
Cryopeeling, 159–160
Cryosurgery
  advantages, 160
  contraindications, 151
  disadvantages, 160
  history of use, 146–147
  indications, 147–148
  mechanism of action, 146
  patient education, 152
  patient selection, 151
  postprocedure course, 160–161
  procedure technique
    acne cyst/inflammatory acne, 157
    actinic keratoses, 159–160
    hemangioma/hemolymphangioma, 157
    IGH, 152–155
    keloids, 158–159
    oral lesions, 155–157
    seborrheic keratoses, 157–158
    solar lentigines, 155
    sun-damaged skin, 159–160
  products, 148–149
  relevant anatomy, 148
  side effects, 161–162

techniques for, 149–151
uses, 145
Cutometer®, 18

D
Depilation, 70
Dermascan®, 12–13, 15
Dermatoheliosis, 209
Dermatoscope, 2, 3
Dimpled chin (Peau d' Orange), 140
Dipstick technique, 149–150
Direct-current surgical galvanism, 173
Drooping mouth corner, 139

E
Edematous fibrosclerotic panniculopathy. *See* Cellulite
Eflornithine, 71
Elastomer® EM 25, 18
Electrocautery, 173–174
Electrocoagulation, 169–171
Electrodesiccation, 167–169
Electrofulguration, 171
Electrolysis, 70–71
Electrosection, 171–173
Electrosurgery
advantages, 165, 177
adverse effects, 179
burn injury
cardiac pacemaker, 176
channeling, 175
fire hazards, 175
human papillomavirus, 176
clinical applications
direct-current surgical galvanism, 173
electrocautery, 173–174
electrocoagulation, 169–171
electrodesiccation, 167–169
electrofulguration, 171
electrosection, 171–173
complications, 179
disadvantages, 177
history of use, 166–167
mechanism of action, 166
modalities, 167
post-procedure course, 177–178
procedural technique, 174–175
risks, 175
sterilization, 177
Endermologie®, 28
Environmental aging, 208–209
Epilation method, 70
Extrinsic aging, 208–209

F
Face lift, 140
Fat-melting injections, 182
Fitzpatrick skin classification, 5, 6
FotoFinder™, 5

G
18-gauge BD Nokor® needle, 57
Gingival smile/Gummy smile (GS), 140–141
Glabellar lines, 136
Glogau classification, aging skin, 6, 7
Glucocorticoids, 70
GnRH agonists, 70
Griffith's range, skin aging, 8
Gynoid lipodystrophy. *See* Cellulite

H
Hair removal methods
depilation, 70
electrolysis, 70–71
epilation method, 70
photoepilation, 71
Handheld liquid nitrogen device, cryosurgery, 148, 149
Hemangioma/hemolymphangioma, 153, 157
Hematomas, 59
Hemosiderosis, 59
Hexsel and Dal'Forno cellulite severity scale, 53
Hidradenitis suppurativa, 37
Hirsutism
description, 65
diagnostic tests, 68
etiology
androgen-secreting tumors, 67
idiopathic, 66
medications, 67
nonclassical 21-hydroxylase deficiency, 67
PCOS, 66
treatment
antiandrogens, 69–70
glucocorticoid monotherapy, 70
GnRH agonists, 70
insulin-lowering drugs, 69
long term hair removal, 70–71
oral contraceptives, 68–69
temporary hair removal, 70
topical treatment, 71

Horizontal necklace lines and platysmal bands. *See* Platysmal muscle
Hormonal therapy, 48
Hyperinsulinemia, 39

I
Iatrogenic acne, 38–39
Idiopathic guttate hypomelanosis (IGH), 152–155
Idiopathic hirsutism, 66
Infantile acne, 35
Infraorbital rhytides, 138
Injectable treatments, for fat
  deoxycholic acid, 185–191
  detergents and tissue interactions, 192–196
  injection lipolysis, 183
  Lipodissolve®, 184
  lipolysis, 182–183
  Lipostabil®, 184
  mesotherapy, 183–184
  pharmaceutical lipoplasty, 183
  phosphatidylcholine hypothesis, 185
Insulin-lowering drugs, 69
Intense pulsed light (IPL), 80
Intrinsic aging, 208

K
Keloids, 153, 158–159
Keratolytics, 44

L
Labial lentiginous macules (LLM), 156
Laser doppler flowmetry (LDF), 26
Laser resurfacing, 211
Lateral eyebrow lift, 138
Levulan®, 117
LIPO-102 agents, 183, 197–199
Liposuction, 29
Local lipodystrophy. *See* Cellulite
Lupus miliaris disseminatus, 41

M
Macrolides, 47
Magnetic resonance imaging (MRI)
  quantitative skin evaluation, 15
  subcutaneous septa, in cellulite depressed lesion, 24
Manual lymphatic drainage, 26–27
Melasma area and severity index (MASI), 8
Mesotherapy
  cellulite, 29
  injectable fat treatments, 183–184
Mexameter®, 16
Microdermabrasion, 82–83
Minor's test, 9
Mirror™ imaging software, 11
Modified Fitzpatrick Wrinkle Scale, 8
Moisturizers
  acne, 44
  striae distensae, 79
Moschella, 208

N
Nasal tip/repeated nasal flare, 139
Nd:YAG laser, 81
Neck wrinkles, 141
Neonatal acne, 34–35
Nodular BCC, 126
Noninflammatory acne, 35
Nonmelanoma skin cancer (NMSC), 117, 126

O
OMNIA imaging system, 4–5
Open-spray technique, 150–151, 154, 159
Oral antibiotics, 47
Oral contraceptives, 68–69
Oral isotretinoin, 48
Oral lesions, 153, 155–157

P
Papillae adipose, 24
PCOS. *See* Polycystic ovary syndrome (PCOS)
Perioral dermatitis, 41
Perioral rhytides, 140
Photoaging, 206, 209
Photodynamic therapy (PDT)
  actinic keratosis, 125
  advantages, 124
  Bowen's disease, 125
  contraindications, 121
  history of use, 116
  indications
    acne lesions, 118–119
    AK, 117–118
    infective diseases, 120
    NMSC, 117
    photodamage, 119

mechanism of action, 116–117
nodular BCC, 126
patient selection, 120–121
post-procedure course, 124
procedure technique
5-aminolevulinic acid (ALA), 122–123
methyl aminolevulinate (MAL), 123–124
side effects, 124–125
superficial BCC, 126
Photoepilation, 71
Photographic assessment, 2–5
Photosensitizer agents, PDT, 120
Platysmal muscle, 141
Poikiloderma, 210
Polycystic ovary syndrome (PCOS), 66
Primos™ measurement, 10
Protoporphyrin IX (PpIX), 116
Pseudofolliculitis, of beard, 41

Q

Q-switched ND-YAG laser, 210
Qualitative skin evaluation
clinical examination
FotoFinder™, 5
photographic assessment, 2–5
wood's lamp, 2, 4
skin scales, 5–7
Quantitative reproducible facial image analysis, 10–12
Quantitative skin evaluation
imaging measurement tools
biometrical image tools, 12–15
quantitative reproducible facial image analysis, 10–12
three-dimensional skin microphotography, 10
skin feature measure tools
skin barrier and skin surface parameters, 17–18
skin elasticity, 18
skin reflectance instruments, 15–17
Visioscope®, 10

R

Radiofrequency (RF)
cellulite, 28
striae distensae, 81
Reflectance confocal microscopy, 13
Retinoids, 45
Rosacea, 41

S

Seborrheic keratoses, 153, 157–158, 207
Sebum regulators, 44
Semiquantitative skin evaluation
botulinum toxin, 9
cellulite, 9
Likert scale, 7
pigmentary disorders, 8–9
quality of life, 10
skin aging, 8
Seromas, 59
Skin evaluation systems
qualitative
clinical examination, 2–5
skin scales, 5–7
quantitative
imaging measurement tools, 10–15
skin feature measure tools, 15–18
semiquantitative (*see* Semiquantitative skin evaluation)
Skin Evidence™, 12, 14
Skin laxity, 30
Skin phototype (SPT), 204
Skin remodeling, 210
Skin tightening procedures, 212
Skin-Visiometer®, 10
Smokers lines, 140
SmoothShapes™, 29
Solar lentigines, 153, 155
Spironolactone, 69
Striae distensae (SD)
in adolescence, 76
description, 75
differential diagnosis, 76–79
in pregnant women, 76
surgical treatments
lasers, light devices and radio frequency, 80–82
microdermabrasion, 82
sand abrasion, 83
serial superficial dermabrasion, 83
Subcision®, 82
topical treatments
moisturizers, 79
onion extract cream, 80
tretinoin, 79–80
Striae rubra, 76, 77
Subcision®, 29
in cellulite
anatomy, 52
classification, 52–54
complications, 59–60
contraindications, 54, 55

Subcision® (*cont.*)
indications, 54, 55
mechanism of action, 55
patient selection, 54
postoperative recommendations, 58–59
preoperative recommendations, 56
procedure technique, 57–58
striae distensae, 82
Sun-damaged skin, 153, 159–160
Superficial BCC, 126
Superficial dermabrasion, 83

T
Telangiectasias, 210
Tensioactives, 43
Tetracycline, 47
Thermography, 26
Three-dimensional skin microphotography, 10
Topical agents, cellulite, 27
Topical PDT. *See* Photodynamic therapy (PDT)
Tretinoin, 79–80
TriActive™, 28
Tristimulus colorimeters, 16

V
VelaShape™, 28–29
Venous lake, 156–157
Visia™ imaging booth, 10–11
Visioscan® VC 98, 11
Visioscope® BW 30, 12

W
Wood's lamp, 2, 4

GPSR Compliance

The European Union's (EU) General Product Safety Regulation (GPSR) is a set of rules that requires consumer products to be safe and our obligations to ensure this.

If you have any concerns about our products, you can contact us on ProductSafety@springernature.com

In case Publisher is established outside the EU, the EU authorized representative is:

Springer Nature Customer Service Center GmbH
Europaplatz 3
69115 Heidelberg, Germany

Batch number: 09225037

Printed by Printforce, the Netherlands